COLD WAR RESISTANCE

Cold War Resistance

THE INTERNATIONAL STRUGGLE OVER ANTIBIOTICS

Marc Landas

Potomac Books
AN IMPRINT OF THE UNIVERSITY OF NEBRASKA PRESS

Manufactured in the United States of America.

♾

Library of Congress Cataloging-in-Publication Data
Names: Landas, Marc, 1972– author.
Title: Cold war resistance: the international struggle over antibiotics / Marc Landas.
Description: Lincoln: Potomac Books, an imprint of the University of Nebraska Press, [2020] |
Includes bibliographical references and index.
Identifiers: LCCN 2019046695
ISBN 9781640121058 (hardback)
ISBN 9781640123663 (epub)
ISBN 9781640123670 (mobi)
ISBN 9781640123687 (pdf)
Subjects: LCSH: Antibiotics—History. | Antibiotics industry—History. | Drug resistance in microorganisms. | Cold War—Biological warfare.
Classification: LCC RM267 .L35 2020 | DDC 615.7/922—dc23
LC record available at https://lccn.loc.gov/2019046695

Set in Minion Pro by Mikala R. Kolander.

For Nora, Heily, and Angelica

COLD WAR RESISTANCE

INTRODUCTION

The demon was out there. Lurking. Shifting. For months, reports from across the globe circulated warnings. What started as a trickle grew into a stream. A new variation of an old enemy emerged from the prokaryotic kingdom, bearing its microbial teeth and rabid stare, only to recede into the shadows. It was *Escherichia coli* (*E. coli*) like the world had never seen. Once it surfaced, scientists the world over hoped to never see it again. They remained on alert now, monitoring the global flow of microbes. China was ground zero with its live animal wet markets, spotty regulation, and insatiable carnivory. It was also half the world away.

Then a woman walked into a Pennsylvania hospital, and everything changed. An innocuous visit. Only it wasn't. Her appearance at an unidentified facility—let's call it St. Elsewhere—in April 2016 kicked off a chain of events that would culminate in a rapid stream of doomsday news articles. This woman—let's call her Jane—caught a bug, something she could not quite shake. Her stomach may have felt as if it was cramping. Maybe she suffered from frequent or uncomfortable urination or a combination of both. A cloudy discharge would not have been out of the ordinary. Maybe she even had a low-grade fever. While general enough, her symptoms would have tipped doctors off to a few possible diagnoses. Chances are Jane had a urinary tract infection (UTI).

A condition common enough to be almost routine, UTIs occur when *E. coli* finds its way into the reproductive tracts of women. It is the second most common infection in adults, accounting for an average 8.1 million visits to the doctor each year. For various reasons, men are less susceptible to infection, though not immune by any means.

Jane's health care providers probably prescribed Z-PAK (six tablets of azithromycin) on the spot and sent her on her way. At this point, only a select few people knew the truth. The public record does not disclose who the woman was or even in what part of Pennsylvania the incident occurred. It's the clearest indication of the public health officials' alarm at the germ's appearance.

The doctors at St. Elsewhere took the urine sample and sent it to the Walter Reed Army Institute of Research in Silver Spring, Maryland. They did so not on a hunch but rather by design. Jane had tested positive for bacteria producing extended-spectrum beta-lactamase (ESBL), a form of antibiotic resistance that destroys certain types of antibiotics—in particular, penicillins, cephalosporins, and monobactams.

Spotting the case involved a degree of luck. The facility happened to be a military outpatient center. A normal hospital would not have forwarded the sample. It would have stayed put for the world to miss.

On May 12 Dr. Kurt Schaecher sat in his laboratory at Walter Reed, carrying out routine tests on urine samples collected from military hospitals around the country such as the one Jane had visited. Earlier that month, researchers at the institute began testing ESBL-positive samples for colistin resistance. It was part of a deliberate program to monitor whether bacteria with the gene that made them immune to the antibiotic had reached the United States. Since it first emerged in China in November 2015, the specific strain of *E. coli* had not appeared, but scientists tend to be realists and not idealists. It was only a matter of time. For months Schaecher had been concerned about the slow but steady stream of global reports mapping the microbe's march.

Concern about bacteria unaffected by colistin stems from the antibiotic's critical role as the last line of defense against infection. If a microbial target displays resistance to many different antibiotics, or multidrug resistance, colistin is brought out and, in most cases, does the trick. But there are drawbacks. One of the reasons colistin still works, even though it is almost fifty years old, is because doctors seldom used it. The drug's toxicity made it hard to justify prescribing it, especially when other less harmful options existed. In fact, for years, health care professionals relied on carbapenems as their final option antibiotic—that is, until carbapenem-resistant *Enterobacteriaceae* (CRE) began spreading around the world at a furious clip. Making matters worse, CRE tended to carry multidrug resistance to various antibiotics with it. Their genes were somehow linked. Thus came colistin's rise and the concern about its fall. Just like that, a doomsday scenario was on the table. What would happen if the new colistin-resistant bacteria swapped genetic material with CRE?

Schaecher called Patrick McGann, a microbiologist and the chief of molecular research and diagnosis at the Multidrug-resistant Organism Repository and Surveillance Network (MRSN). He informed McGann of his discovery. It would need to be double-checked, even triple-checked. More intensive tests needed to be performed to ascertain the nature of the invasion. If the colistin-resistant bacteria had, in fact, made its way onto American shores, a whole battery of emergency procedures would fall into place.

Making a spot judgment about the significance of Schaecher's discovery was unwarranted. Bacteria could often develop isolated instances of resistance that appeared due to spontaneous mutations. Those were okay. They fizzled, then faded like sparklers on the Fourth of July. It was the resistance encoded into bacteria's deoxyribonucleic acid (DNA), its traits passed down between generations, that posed the true danger.

McGann did not take any chances. He drove to Schaecher's lab and picked up the samples himself. When he returned to his lab, he labeled the bacteria "*E. coli* MRSN 388634." Next, he performed a basic test to determine whether colistin had any effect on the bacteria. Called microbroth susceptibility testing, the technique consisted of placing bacteria into a series of tiny wells, then adding mixtures of reagent and varying amounts of antibiotic. The degree to which the bacteria is cleared from a sample is indicated by a change in color. It is a quick means of determining whether a drug affects a bacteria and the minimal quantity of antibiotic necessary to elicit a response.

The results matched: the bacteria exhibited the phenotype for colistin resistance. The possibility must have been equal parts exhilarating and terrifying. Still, he refrained from reading too much into it. He did not rush to sound any media alarms. He let it sink in. This was the exhilarating part. A significant finding. A moment in U.S. scientific history (infamous, no doubt). The beginning of the end? Hopefully not. Anyway, an initial identification was just the first step in a well-defined series of tests his lab would need to perform. The terrifying step was yet to come.

Science tends to work in increments. Eureka moments are far and few between. There is no blaze to discovery. After an initial discovery, a meticulous collection of facts ensues. The scientific method ad nauseum. Rushing the process often leads to disastrous results. Mistakes could ruin a career. This case would go by the books, no matter the implications. A clearer picture would develop in its own time.

The research team needed to establish the presence of the mobilized colistin resistance (mcr)-1 gene that is known to result in a colistin resistance. Confirming its presence with a more precise test than the quick-and-dirty microbroth susceptibility method was the team's first priority. Rather than looking for the smoke to deduce the fire, the most reliable indicators pointed to the fire itself. Once mcr-1 was confirmed, establishing the gene's exact location on *E. coli* MRSN 388634's genetic material became critical. This was the step everyone feared in the back of their minds. Soon they'd know whether the resistance gene sat on a section of the bacteria's genome that was readily transferred to other prokaryotes.

While McGann attended a meeting, his team at Walter Reed began the painstaking process of painting the enemy's portrait. Things hadn't hit the "urgent" point yet, but the potential and inertia were there. All of the evidence so far seemed to be moving them in that direction. The simple fact that the sample had tested positive made further testing that much more imperative.

The first significant step in understanding the nature of the bacteria was subjecting it to a process called real-time polymerase chain reaction (real-time PCR). PCR works by using an enzyme that crawls along a single strand of DNA, replicating it one base pair (bp) at a time and detaching itself at a predetermined point. Each time the polymerase makes a pass on the DNA, another perfect replica is produced. The process repeats itself until a detectable segment of the genetic material is present. That end product can then be analyzed using PCR analysis software and compared in a database of genetic cartridges. Since it was discovered in the 1980s, the process has revolutionized laboratory work, particularly in detecting the presence of specific genes.

Kathy "Ana" Ong, one of McGann's team members, performed the test. In one half-inch well at a time, she used a micropipette to mix reagent, assay, and *E. coli* MRSN 388634's genetic material. After working feverishly, the PCR machine quieted, and McGann's team had their result: the mcr-1 gene was present. No room for doubt now. It was important but not altogether unexpected. It just made their findings official enough to go public with them. It ticked the first box.

Ong texted McGann about the positive result. He replied, "You're shitting me."

"We had to drop everything else to get this done," he would later recall in a *Washington Post* article. "When the test came back positive, all hell broke loose."

He indicated that the lab's team should move immediately to the next step—whole genome sequencing. Once that was completed, they would be able to determine whether this particular strain of *E. coli* had ever been seen before or whether it represented an entirely novel type of bacteria. Most important, they would be able to determine exactly where on the microbe's genetic material the mcr-1 sequence was located. They needed to determine whether it resided on a chromosome or a plasmid. The difference between the two was immense.

The identification process moved to a pair of much larger, more imposing, and more complex machines. The PacBio RS II and MiSeq benchtop sequencer have become staples in laboratories across the globe. They allow scientists to take an organism's DNA—in this case, *E. coli* MRSN 388634—and determine the exact code. It's a painstaking process only made possible by modern robotics and increased computer processing power. Both machines performed the same task, only at different speeds, with the former taking seventy-two hours and the latter in eight days. The results of each sequencer would be used to confirm the other's.

Everyone held their collective breath.

Three days later, the results were waiting. Almost a week after that, confirmation arrived from MiSeq. It was definitive and terrifying. *E. coli* MRSN 388634 not only carried the mcr-1 gene but also bore the genetic sequences for fifteen additional types of antibiotic resistance. And while resistant bacteria are well known for carrying multiple resistance, the sheer quantity contained within the single organism was breathtaking.

Now that *E. coli* MRSN 388634 had been identified, the researchers had a story. It had been seen before. It belonged to a strain first identified in 2008 in a urine sample taken in the United Kingdom. The strain appeared again in Italy that same year. The Italian culture differed from the British one in a very important way: in addition to being resistant to colistin, it also carried the genes blaKPC-3 and blaCTX-M-55, which code for carbapenem resistance. If the genes for carbapenem and colistin resistance were teamed together in more bacteria, the two most effective antibiotics remaining in doctors' arsenal no longer mattered. The way some bacteria swapped genes, the idea that it was only a matter of time until these genes paired with the more common forms of resistance was far from remote. Public health officials labeled it a doomsday scenario. A return to the Dark Ages before penicillin and sulfa drugs just took a big step closer to existence. Infections would be untreatable; simple surgery, impossible; an inadvertent paper cut, a possible death sentence.

The next secret *E. coli* MRSN 388634's sequenced genome revealed suggested it truly was only a matter of time. What started off badly just got worse.

Bacteria possess a unique genetic quirk that, from an evolutionary point of view, stacks the deck in their favor against just about every other organism on the planet. DNA tends to be wrapped around proteins for the vast majority of the earth's creatures. Taken together, they are called chromosomes, and as far as individual genes are concerned, they are pretty massive. The primary means organisms have of passing their chromosomal DNA to subsequent generations is by sexual reproduction. While effective, it is limiting. It prevents dogs from mating with sea lions. It's a bit of a process, even for unicellular microbes, and ensures that genes cannot be passed between different types of bacteria, or horizontally, so to speak. They can only be inherited by subsequent generations—that is, vertically. An *E. coli* cannot pass its chromosomal DNA on to *Staphylococcus aureus*.

However, bacteria have an extra piece of DNA called a plasmid floating around its cell independently of the chromosome, which is almost anchored in place. This tiny snippet of DNA, often referred to as a replicon, is not technically alive, but it is able to reproduce on its own, much like a virus. Unlike chromosomal DNA, plasmids can be passed horizontally between different types of bacteria by a process known as conjugation. It allows them to share genes that are useful for survival.

Antibiotic resistance is often promulgated in this way.

According to the research paper published by McGann and his team, *E. coli* MRSN 388634 possessed two plasmids. The larger of the pair, pMR0516mcr, registered at 225,707 base pairs, and it dwarfed its 47,000-bp partner. The mcr-1 gene was located on the larger of the two, enabling it to be transferred horizontally with any bacteria it encountered. It was almost as if *E. coli* MRSN 388634 could sneeze and pass on its resistance. For some perspective, think of it this way: The average human body, inside and out, carries roughly 39 trillion bacteria. Multiply that by the number of human beings on the earth now—7.5 billion—and you get 2.925×10^{23} bacteria on people alone. That number does not include the bacteria in the environment. A quick glance at the number should tip even the most unscientific-minded person off to the likelihood of just a few of those germs being engaged in beneficial transactions.

And that realization is what must have scared the experts.

Once the genome was pinned down, McGann notified his colleagues at the Department of Defense (DOD), the Centers for Disease Control and Prevention (CDC), the Department of Health and Human Services, and the Department of Agriculture. He set in motion a chain of events that had been mapped out and mandated months before in the Barack Obama administration's National Action Plan for Combating Antibiotic Resistant Bacteria. It had been designed for events just like this one.

The DOD began informing its stakeholders about the appearance of colistin-resistant bacteria on American shores, and the other agencies began issuing alerts. Press conferences came soon afterward, followed by a tidal wave of apocalyptic news articles.

The demon had, in fact, arrived. And it was worse than anyone thought.

COLISTIN-RESISTANT BACTERIA RANK RATHER low on my list of daily concerns. Every day, when I open my eyes, I pine for a shot of caffeine. It consumes my thoughts, so I wobble my way into the kitchen. In a daily testament that miracles do happen, the pot of coffee gets made without scalding my palms or scorching my pajamas. Drip coffee. Pressed coffee. Percolator coffee. Cafetière. Instant. I've done it all, and at 6:30 a.m., I'm always splashing a bit of milk into my brew. While I may have pondered the utter genius of passing boiling water through roasted coffee grounds, I can guarantee you that I did not think about *Escherichia coli* once during the process.

I read and listen and watch the news while sipping away. My smartphone commands my attention. My thumbs swipe the screen on autopilot, flipping through my various email accounts, news aggregators, and Twitter feeds. Facebook Messenger, WhatsApp, LINE, WeChat, Snapchat, Signal, Viber, and my normal text messages connect me with friends. Unless there's some coverage of an outbreak of food poisoning—hello, Chipotle—I still haven't given the prokaryotic kingdom a morsel of my thought. At 7 a.m., I doubt I'm alone in my neglect.

If it's a weekday—or even weekends—I'm rushing out of the door sans breakfast. I'll catch another coffee on my way to my destination. If I'm feeling rich, I'll splurge on a bagel with the works. That would be an ideal time for the notion of bacteria to enter my mind, but who in the world thinks "bacteria" before digging into some cream cheese and lox? The moment passes without microbial incident.

While I'm at my job, my mind is occupied with other things. Did my sports teams win? Should I buy that ugly new phone or watch? How long till lunch? Does my girlfriend still love me?

Sometimes, I even think about the work I should be doing. *Klebsiella pneumoniae*? Not so much.

If it's a weekend, I might take the time to make breakfast. Eggs, home fries, baked beans, toast. Awesome. Reaching for the half-filled carton of brown, free-range, organic beauties, I should give salmonella a token thought. It loves eggs so much it lives in them. (Even my adoration has its limits.) Of course, what I'm really thinking about is whether an omelet or sunny-side up or poached eggs suit my fancy. After all, the eggs are in the fridge—as we Americans do—so they should be contamination free by default.

That's not to say that nobody thinks about bacteria daily. Bacteriologists obviously do. It's their job. Doctors and nurses, the same. Par for the course. People in the food industry think about them too. It's a part of their job, one that I sometimes wish they'd pay more attention to. These people are exceptions to the rule, though.

Of course, at times humanity's uneasy coexistence with microbes gets thrust into the limelight. Food-borne illnesses dominate the discourse. Salmonella, *E. coli*, and listeria feature prominently in the gastronomy-gone-rogue narratives, and thankfully, fatalities seem to be the exception of late.

Not far behind, methicillin-resistant *Staphylococcus aureus* (MRSA) casts a black pall over health care facilities worldwide. It's the famous rascal among a family of rakes. Since the late 1950s, the medical and scientific communities have met this most opportunistic of microbes head-on. At first, they limited its reach to hospitals, where it colonized everything from plastic medical tubes to the air circulating through vents. It latched onto open wounds and slipped into patients' bloodstreams. Infection led to tragedy.

In recent years, MRSA shot to the public's attention thanks to the popular media's sensational branding of "flesh-eating bacteria," which represents an unhelpful and inaccurate representation of the condition. (Even when bacteria manage to infiltrate our collective consciousness, we defer to Hollywood tropes rather than attempt to understand the bleak reality at hand.) Ask someone about necrotizing fasciitis, and you'll get a blank stare. Mention flesh-eating bacteria, and I guarantee a glimmer of awareness.

Truth is, antibiotic resistance proves less compelling for a general population accustomed to the immediacy of the human immunodeficiency virus and acquired immune deficiency syndrome (HIV/AIDS) and the hysteria of avian influenza. Even the story leading this introduction falls short. Never mind that it essentially points to the paved road from here to hell; it still lacks that final punch to make it memorable. The story is difficult to connect with. Blood wasn't pouring out of any orifices. Virus-filled vomit wasn't being projected halfway across the room. Even less forgivable to a modern, popular science narrative, nobody died. The patient had a UTI.

Why is this a big deal? Because your average citizen who reaps the advantages of living in an antibacterial world—that is to say, being alive—is clueless about the disaster looming down the road.

Daily existence would be different had penicillin and its descendants never been discovered and developed. I was born and raised during the antibiotic era. I reap its benefits every time I cut my finger while cooking and don't even bat an eyelash. I have bacitracin, so it's all good. When I travel to a country where everything from freshly washed salad to ice cubes represent opportunities for bacterial ambush, I take solace in knowing that when push comes to shove, I have my bottle of amoxicillin. Should I need surgery to fix my bum back, I'm more concerned about the duration of my convalescence than the fact that my body would be cut open and exposed to legions of foreign bacteria. At any other time in history, I'd be taking stock of my life instead and wondering whether the world would really continue to turn once I passed. To say that we take antibiotics for granted is an understatement.

And yet, it's out there. Resistance. The darkness hugging the horizon. The secondary hospital—or nosocomial, in medical parlance—infections that greet immunocompromised patients at hospital entrances and never leave their sides for the length of their stay. The slimy biofilms that form inside medical equipment, impervious to sterilization and imperious in their unity. The potent bacteria incubating in factory farms, given free rein to live long and prosper. The flora we carry on our skin, in our mouths, and in our guts that are benign until they are not. Bacteria are constant threats.

According to the CDC, eighteen specific forms of resistance pose a significant danger to the well-being of Americans. Seventeen are bacterial and one is fungal. Employing a three-tier grading system of urgent, serious, and concerning, the CDC system consists of germs that cause familiar and not-so-familiar diseases. The common infections that would become untreatable in a resistant world—

pharyngitis, pneumonia, tuberculosis, typhoid fever, meningitis, gonorrhea—are truly terrifying because treating them is so routine today. Then there are all sorts of infections we tend to shrug off as "stomach bugs." They would all become life-threatening conditions, as would common everyday surgery.

For scientists and health professionals, however, the most horrific bacteria are the ones displaying resistance to a range of drugs. Those bacteria include extended-spectrum beta-lactamase *Enterobacteriaceae*, multidrug-resistant *Acinetobacter*, vancomycin-resistant *Staphylococcus aureus*, and carbapenem-resistant *Enterobacteriaceae*. The latter occupies a particularly troubling place because of carbapenem's role as one of the last-line-of-defense weapons doctors have to combat other untreatable infections. In addition, the genes that code for its activity tend to be associated with other types of resistance, making it impervious to treatment. Yet, as with colistin-resistant bacteria, the most troubling aspect of CRE is not the microbe itself but with its potential as a pan-drug-resistant gene vector swapping plasmids with other bacteria. It carries the power to avoid antibiotics in its pocket and is ready to hand out its talents like personal calling cards.

We live in a bacterial world. They rule everything, sight unseen. Long after we've become extinct and only brittle hints of our existence litter the earth, they will be here. Bacteria are active and vibrant and consistent in their march. Meanwhile, human beings are as fickle as their attention spans are short. People are not personally invested in antibiotic development though they benefit from it regularly. As a result, available and effective treatments lag their bacterial opponents. If people do not press governments and corporations, the inaction to develop new, effective treatments will continue.

ON JUNE 2016, OVER the course of an afternoon, twenty-four members of Congress peered from their perches on Capitol Hill. Four scientists faced them, a moat of empty swivel chairs separating the two parties, perhaps for safety but most likely for symbolism. The optics of power politics were on full display. A new form of antibiotic resistant bacteria had invaded America, and these politicians on the House Subcommittee on Oversight and Investigations wanted answers. The meeting revolved more around rehashing oft-repeated notions of antibiotic resistance, however, than about fighting the onrushing scourge. Considering its affirmative title, "Combating Superbugs: U.S. Public Health Responses to Antibiotic Resistance," the session proved disheartening. The image of hamsters sprinting on wheels comes to mind.[1]

The positive result for colistin-resistant *E. coli* represented a breathtaking paradigm shift in American epidemiology. But it was the earthquake that no one but the scientists felt.

Long before the hearings, CDC director Thomas Frieden offered the most succinct analysis of the situation. "The medicine cabinet is empty," he declared.

What he left out in his full statement was an explanation as to why. Had he elaborated, he would have had to point out the inaction of pharmaceutical companies and government politicians such as the people in the room. What would be implied throughout the hearing but nobody dared utter was that it did not have to be this way. Yet, there they were, proof that it was.

Representatives from the Centers for Disease Control and Prevention, the National Institute of Allergy and Infectious Diseases (NIAID) of the National Institutes of Health, the Biomedical Advanced Research and Development Authority (BARDA), and the Food and Drug Administration (FDA) took turns explaining their respective agencies' roles in the war against antibiotic resistant bacteria. They shuffled papers, tweaked their notes, and waited patiently while their colleagues read from prepared statements. Congress granted them five minutes each. Their words were entered into the record for legislative posterity.

Dr. Beth Bell, director of the National Center for Emerging and Zoonotic Infectious Diseases at the CDC: "The identification of mcr-1 vividly illustrates our domestic and global challenges of antibiotic resistance. Mcr-1 was first identified in China in November of last year, and in less than six months, had been identified in a human and two animals in the United States. Antibiotic use anywhere can potentially affect any one of us."

Dr. Dennis Dixon from the Division of Microbiology and Infectious Diseases at NIAID: "NIAID recently awarded funding for research projects to develop non-traditional therapeutics for bacterial infections and funds clinical studies, testing new formulations, dosing regimens or combination therapies of currently licensed drugs such as colistin."

Dr. Richard Hatchett, acting director at BARDA: "We have achieved notable success. Our portfolio is quite mature at this point. Five BARDA products are in Phase 3 clinical development, and two have completed the pivotal studies required for FDA approval. . . . Several products showed promise for the treatment of infections due to carbapenem-resistant Enterobacteriaceae."

Dr. Janet Woodcock, director of the Center for Drug Evaluation and Research at the FDA: "Drug development in this area remains fragile and weak. The incentives that have been put in place apparently are not enough to overcome the scientific challenges that the industry faces in finding new targets and developing these, and then actually making money on them."

The hearing touched on the issues that tend to arise in any discussion of antibiotic resistance. At this point in the game, it's almost by rote. Improved stewardship of antibiotic use with quicker testing and diagnosis decreases inappropriate prescriptions. The days without antibiotics is near. While the participants' intentions might have been noble, the most striking thing about the session was the general lack of ideas and creative approaches to a nearly sixty-year-old problem. The role of politicians as investigative critics did little to facilitate the process. Their questions lacked insight and sometimes even preparation.

There was nothing contentious about the ensuing session. On the contrary, the exchanges between the subcommittee members and their expert witnesses maintained an even, congenial keel. As Rep. Tim Murphy (R-PA) said, "We're on the same team. We're just trying to help." Yet for all the cooperative back-patting, there was a striking lack of urgency.

The BARDA Combating Antibiotic Resistant Bacteria Accelerator (CARB-X) program appeared to be the afternoon's exception. Touted by BARDA's acting director, Dr. Richard Hatchett, as an incubator for novel approaches to the antibiotic program that fast-tracked promising drugs through time-consuming test phases, the program offered the most promise.

"Innovation frequently occurs in small biotechnology companies and in academic laboratories with limited resources and expertise to move product candidates forward," Hatchett said, reading from a prepared statement. "In such circumstances, promising early stage candidates often fail to advance. The accelerator will serve as an incubator for new products and explicitly seeks to improve success rates in the early stage antibiotic pipeline."

Yet, when the commission returned to the program during the question-and-answer session, the initial promise fell flat upon closer inspection. The exchange with Rep. Marsha Blackburn (R-TN) is telling.

"Going back into February," she said, "BARDA established the accelerator to support in research and development. . . . We've been so interested in that. . . . I would like it if you could take just a minute and talk a little about the specific candidates that you all have put in, about some of the vaccines or the microbials, some of the alternative therapies that you are reviewing in that program."

"Just to be clear, the accelerator has not been established yet," Hatchett replied. "We put out this solicitation earlier this year, and we've received the proposals, we had a good response. And we actually are in the process of negotiating with the lead candidates right now. So, we have . . ."

"Okay, when you say a good response, quantify that for me a little bit."

"I believe we had five proposals," he replied.

Five proposals.

Blackburn continued to press Hatchett for a timetable for how quickly BARDA's not-quite-existent accelerator could have something to show for its efforts (and Congress's money, presumably). "And what is your expectation once you are able to populate the accelerator basically? How long do you think it will be before we begin to see next generation products that are ready to go to the marketplace?"

Hatchett explained the difference between allowing the drugs to develop without aid from BARDA. It's a question of decades versus a few years. "The things that are in the accelerator are not going to pop out of the accelerator right into the marketplace. They're going to be brought to the stage of clinical—"

"Fine," Blackburn said, cutting him off.

"It would take several years," Hatchett continued.

Blackburn was not content. She persisted, "We understand that but we—when we look at some of these drugs that are taking 10 years, 12 years to get through the process and you look at the entire compendium and you looked at what goes on with them, the innovators working with the FDA. Our hope is, is that we're going to see your process work and help to push this to the marketplace sooner . . . that there will be some efficiencies. We know you've got some challenges, but we are hopeful there will be some efficiencies in moving it forward."

Finally understanding what was expected of him, Hatchett drew a parallel between the *Zaire ebolavirus* outbreak in 2014 and the subsequent development of a potential vaccine. Stating that it had taken only a couple of years, he received a reprieve.

Satisfied that she had altered the laws of nature during a congressional hearing, Blackburn concluded, "That's helpful. That's what we want to hear."

Colistin-resistant bacteria aren't the only problem. Daily life conditions us to think locally. It's understandable. Except on rare occasions, distant events bear little impact on our daily frustrations. War in the Middle East cannot compete with the frustration that shoots through your body when traffic bottlenecks at the same point on your way to work. The latest nuclear bomb test by the North Koreans—distressing as it may be—cannot compete with the irritation at discovering thousands of dollars' worth of unexplained charges on your credit card statement. And tyranny abroad cannot compete with the undeterred tyranny at home posed each month when bills begin rolling in. We focus on what's in front of us and deal with the wider world as an afterthought.

It's easy to analyze antibiotic resistance along similar terms. An estimated 2 million resistant infections occur annually in the United States. This results in a projected $25 billion–$30 billion additional health care costs on top of twenty-three thousand deaths. They are daunting figures, yet they represent a very limited statistical slice of the pie. The European Union reports similar figures, estimating roughly twenty-five thousand deaths and economic losses around 1.5 billion euros. Studies project the trend to worsen.

Around the world, new strains of resistance emerge like buds in a spring meadow. Colistin-resistant *E. coli* prove that no amount of walls or restrictions can control its spread. It originated in China, moved to Europe, and then breached American shores. That's the way it works these days.

Different regions possess very distinct profiles of antibiotic resistance. While resistant bacteria travel between continents with ease, a country's resistance spectrum nonetheless often reflects conditions particular to that place—for example, the specific drugs prescribed in the country.

Like most countries, Japan's antibiotic resistance problem threatens its population every day. Recent years have seen the increasing prevalence of multidrug-resistant bacteria while options for treatment shrink in inverse proportion. While the same bacteria that circulate around the world are present in Japan, local antibiotic resistance exhibits subtle differences compared with the rest of the world.

In the early 1990s, Japan experienced a significant rise in methicillin-resistant *Staphylococcus aureus* infections in hospital settings, mirroring the worldwide trend. Genetic lineage analysis of nosocomial MRSA strains reveals the existence of seven primary types (as opposed to community-associated MRSA, which differs from nosocomial strains); however, MRSA in Japan is still relatively treatable with glycopeptide antibiotics such as vancomycin. The same is not the case in the United States, where vancomycin-resistant strains of *Staphylococcus aureus* (VRSA) are prevalent. This discrepancy is thought to be attributable to the horizontal transmission of resistance from vancomycin-resistant enterococci (VRE) to VRSA. Historically Japan has exhibited low detection rates of VRE, possibly explaining VRSA's absence.

Another example of resistance differing due to local conditions is *Haemophilus influenzae*. Initially treatable with ampicillin, it began to exhibit resistance to penicillin-derived antibiotics in the 1980s through the production of beta-lactamase. For whatever reason, that same strain decreased in Japan a decade later, only to be replaced by a genetically different strain called beta-lactamase-negative, ampicillin-resistant *Haemophilus influenzae*. The rise of this strain is thought to be the result of an increased use of cephem antibiotics, such as cephamycin, in Japan versus the rest of the world.

Of all the countries actively reporting antibiotic resistance, India offers the starkest illustration of the effects local conditions play in the development of antibiotic resistance. A quick glance at the statistics gives the impression of an antibiotic wasteland. Some bacteria such as *Klebsiella pneumoniae*, *Escherichia coli*, *Enterobacter aerogenes* and *E. cloacae*, and *Acinetobacter baumannii* show nearly 100 percent resistance to multiple antibiotics. A host of others exhibit upward of 50 percent resistance. Considering the ease at which resistant strains circumnavigate the globe, the situation in India is truly frightening.

The reasons behind the deteriorating situation in India are complex. Unlike most Western nations, where agricultural uses have greatly contributed to antibiotic resistance, its development in India stems from human health. With a population of nearly 1.252 billion people, India boasts one of the highest infectious disease burdens in the world. Coupled with a poor public health infrastructure, doctors and patients rely on medicine to treat a wide spectrum of diseases and often inappropriately. India was the world's largest consumer of antibiotics for human health in 2010. Because of India's increasing affluence, antibiotics are more readily available there now than in the past. Overall, this is good as a large portion of India's population has access to life-saving drugs; however, regulation has not kept pace. Over-the-counter sales are common. It has gotten to the point where India's nonprescription sales of carbapenems are among the highest in the world and are a major contributor to the wave of CRE and other gram-negative microbes around the world.

However frightening an outlier India may seem, it may soon be the worldwide norm should we fail to develop new classes of antibiotics. If the head-spinning rapidity of colistin resistance's spread from China proves anything, it is that little can prevent a super germ from hitching a ride on a boat or a plane or even a spacecraft. Antibiotic resistance is a global problem exacerbated by the mesh of disease that modern travel's crisscrossing routes have created. Man's impotence in the face of the prokaryotic kingdom's relentless march forward has never been more evident.

A simple analysis? The situation is desperate.

CAPITALISM GIVETH, CAPITALISM TAKETH. During the post–World War II years, the urgency with which pharmaceutical companies pursued antibiotic research and development gave credit to the title of "miracle drugs." From the soil—where most of the discoveries were derived—an amazing cornucopia of bacteria-bashing chemicals sprouted. Tilling the soil. Harvesting of medicine. Images of scientists, cloaked in white and wielding their tools, adorned the covers of magazines, and some, such as Selman Waksman at Rutgers (then primarily an agricultural institute) and with Merck and Company, passed into scientific lore like an antimicrobial Johnny Appleseed in reverse. Profit motive compelled them to achieve incredible discoveries, yet they made bold choices nonetheless. They stood to lose piles of money, especially during those early uncertain years; they persevered and, to their credit, literally hit pay dirt.

Then complacency set in.

If credit is granted for their achievements, criticism must be doled out as well. The turnaround from sprinting between discoveries to pure neglect is nothing short of a crime. In the face of the world's dwindling antibiotic arsenal, the lack of urgency between governments and pharmaceutical companies is startling. It's hard to imagine that both parties understand what is at stake because when the impetus is there, the public and private sectors take decisive strides toward whatever goal they set. It happened during World War II with the development of penicillin. As a more recent example, the 2016 outbreak of Ebola resulted in potential vaccines being developed within a few years.

The antibiotic industry died in the early 1980s. Today, research and development languishes in a state of perpetual limbo. Most companies have stopped looking altogether. In fact, out of roughly thirty-four companies with antibiotics in clinical development, only five rank in the top fifty pharmaceutical companies by sales. Smaller and nimbler biotechnology start-ups assumed the responsibility, but they lack the robust funds and network of connections the giants of Big Pharma can muster. In fact, they are considered "pre-revenue," meaning they have no products that have made it to market yet. The new paradigm impels them to make their discovery in the hopes of being acquired by a large company such as Pfizer or GlaxoSmithKlein. Even then, nothing is guaranteed since the industry has labeled antibiotics as unprofitable. Unlike diseases that treat chronic, incurable conditions that require a lifetime of medicinal purchases, antibiotics function as efficient and effective cures. A few doses and you're done. It's not an appealing proposition for stockholders and analysts.

In the meantime, a search for solutions continues. In an attempt at incentivizing the pharmaceutical industry—essentially dangling a cash "carrot"—the government has extended patent exclusivity so that companies can delay being undercut by generic versions of their drugs. In addition, it has fast-tracked certain drugs the FDA has deemed to address urgent issues. While helpful it does not go far enough. The pharmaceutical industry has refused to bite, exposing a lack of ideas at a governmental level.

Making due with what they have, scientists are scrambling to discover new drugs and novel classes of antibiotics that rely on different strategies than past drugs. According to a study conducted by the Pew Charitable Trusts, as of September 2016, forty new drugs were in development with fourteen in phase 1 clinical trials, thirteen in phase 2, eleven in phase 3, and two drugs under review by the FDA. As the study notes, "However, given the inevitability that some of these antibiotics will fail to win approval, it is clear that there are too few drugs in development to meet current and anticipated patient needs."

Researchers have also turned to an old-but-new approach to antibiotic research and development. Long ignored by Western scientists, bacteriophages and botanicals—essentially herbal medicines—formed the backbone of Russian and former Soviet bloc pharmaceutical companies since the Cold War. A long tradition in those areas allowed them to be employed as stop-gap measures since years of U.S.-led embargoes and questionable economic approaches resulted in chronic shortages of drugs and production supplies that never completely abated until after the Berlin Wall fell. Now biotechnology companies are taking a second look at them—no longer tainted by politics—as possible solutions to the current antibiotic crisis. Bacteriophages, in particular, offer drug designers a more targeted approach compared with the nuclear-option, broad-spectrum antibiotics that exacerbated the resistance problem. One can only ponder what our current situation would be had we been less reliant on drugs that obliterated bacteria en masse, thereby increasing the selective pressure for resistance.

The fact remains that after a promising start, the antibiotic development paradigm no longer works. Misplaced priorities—corporate, governmental, and public—have exacerbated the problem. To be clear, they and their policies are not the cause of antibiotic resistance, which is a natural phenomenon probably as old as bacteria themselves. Still, by placing profits ahead of progress, pharmaceutical companies have endangered the public, and by placing politics ahead of the greater good, governments have squandered the closest thing science has come to a medical magic bullet.

EVEN BEFORE PENICILLIN BECAME available to the public, five years to be exact, the first studies describing penicillin-resistant strains of bacteria had been published in scientific literature. Since then, data has been accumulating so that by 2019, over seventy-five years' worth of findings are available for study. Despite the field's shortcomings, consensus among researchers and public health officials have produced a number of points designed to slow the creep of resistant bacteria. To achieve this goal, the World Health Organization devised a global action plan with five strategic objectives that are based on factors believed to foster antibiotic resistance:

to improve *awareness* and understanding of antimicrobial resistance,

to strengthen knowledge through *surveillance* and research,

to *reduce the incidence of infection*,

to *optimize the use* of antimicrobial agents, and

to develop the economic case for sustainable investment that takes account of the needs of all countries and increases investment in new medicines, diagnostic tools, vaccines, and other interventions.

Each of the points addresses an aspect of how antibiotic resistance is believed to arise. The first ensures that the correct drug is only used against bacteria susceptible to it. Incorrect usage fails to kill the disease-causing bacteria while allowing resistant forms to arise. The second point deals with basic research and the fact that only by properly studying bacteria and antibiotic resistance can they be addressed. The third point states the obvious: avoiding infection reduces the chances of resistance. This also entails preventing circumstances ripe for acquiring infections, such as war and its aftermath where critical urban infrastructure is often destroyed. The fourth point means not only using the right antibiotic but also administering it in adequate doses that are known to kill targeted bacteria. Inadequate dosage (as seen in counterfeit drugs), incomplete treatments (disrupted by conflict zone conditions), and subtherapeutic doses (as seen in agriculture settings)—all play roles in fostering antibiotic resistance.

It cannot be stressed enough: the book does not suggest that the Cold War caused antibiotic resistance in any form. The ability of bacteria to circumvent man-made chemotherapeutic drugs, beginning with sulfonamides, existed way before they were discovered. The aim of this work is to demonstrate how the tug-of-war between the East and the West created conditions that common scientific consensus believes foster antibiotic resistance.

1

German bombs fell on Britain from Bristol to Edinburgh. Like the Royal Air Force, the Luftwaffe blurred the line between military and civilian targets until the two merged into one. Nothing was off-limits, not even centuries-old landmarks. Once considered safe, they became prime targets for their symbolic value. Months earlier, in October, thousands of tons of incendiary bombs showered the city of London in a concerted effort at taking down Christopher Wren's magnificent dome. The Germans wanted St. Paul's Cathedral reduced to ashes. That night, they failed. That would not always be the case. All of England's famous landmarks stood on alert, ready for the fateful moment when sirens would warn them of an imminent attack. At the behest of Prime Minister Winston Churchill, the country kept moving as if the incendiaries and the Heinkel He 111s amounted to minor inconveniences. Life in Great Britain would go on as normally as possible.[1]

Oxford University, Europe's second-oldest institution of higher learning behind Bologna, could have been hit any time. Unlike St. Paul's, it could have been considered a military target, though rumors suggested an early agreement existed between the Nazis and the British not to target each other's universities. Each day without a bombing increased the likelihood of one happening. It was a question of not if but when. Undeterred, the university's staff continued working. Classrooms remained open. Countless labs continued churning out papers for publication and reporting the discoveries being made in spite of the circumstances.

In 1941 nothing at the university would prove as significant as the research being conducted on the mold *Penicillium notatum* in Howard Florey's laboratory at the Sir William Dunn School of Pathology.

Despite the knowledge only they possessed, Florey and his primary research partners, Ernst Chain and Norman Heatley, found themselves a few steps short of the miracle they sought.[2]

For three years, Florey, Chain, and Heatley labored in the hopes of isolating and identifying the active antimicrobial element in the mold. The trio had been working together since 1937. A taciturn Australian, Florey kept people at a distance for the most part, but when it came to scientific collaboration, he understood the necessities of sharing thoughts and information. To his credit, he valued a keen mind over an amicable personality. Hiring the mercurial biochemist Ernst Chain to join his laboratory proved it. Their personalities and temperaments were opposites, yet a common scientific curiosity overrode any differences. They worked on problems ranging from the nature of cancerous cells to the mechanisms of lysozyme activity.

Along with many other Jews during the 1930s, Chain fled Germany during Adolf Hitler's rise to power. He found acceptance in Oxford, at least scientifically. He would be tasked with isolating and purifying penicillin's active antibacterial element.

Norman Heatley's disposition was more in line with Florey's. Being a stickler for methodology made him the ideal researcher to be tasked with deciphering the conditions for growing *P. notatum*, a notoriously unstable chemical. It was a thankless job that had bested many researchers before him, smothering their hope for glory like a rag on a match. In the end, it would prove the hardest of penicillin's mysteries for the Oxford team to unravel.

Henry Harris, the famed Australian cell biologist who studied under Florey, summed up the men's roles when he quipped, "Without Fleming, no Chain or Florey; without Chain, no Florey; without Florey, no Heatley; without Heatley, no penicillin."[3]

Over a decade earlier, Alexander Fleming discovered by chance that something in *Penicillium notatum* exercised an inhibitory effect on bacteria growing in discarded petri dishes in his lab. It was normally considered a pervasive contaminant, but Fleming had the wherewithal to investigate further. His hunch proved well-founded. The mold did, in fact, appear to kill bacteria. Exactly what caused the effect remained a mystery, one that he would never solve. He did, however, publish his findings in a *British Journal of Experimental Pathology* article that launched a medical revolution.[4]

For the most part, the scientific community ignored penicillin or at least failed to take notice of Fleming's article amid the flood of research published annually. Scientists who did take an interest—Roger Reid in the early 1930s and Harold Raistrick in 1932—found frustration by the flaskful, thanks to penicillin's unstable nature. No sooner had they isolated it—whatever "it" was, since at that point they hadn't a clue—they watched their hard work dissolve into oblivion. Catching water with a net appeared more likely than isolating *P. notatum*'s active element. As far as chemicals went, whatever made the mold lethal to bacteria also made it a headache to pin down. Yet where other scientists saw an insurmountable obstacle, Florey, Chain, and Heatley realized an opportunity.

They set out to isolate and then identify the active ingredient in whatever Fleming had discovered. It could have been anything, from a small molecule to an enzyme. Early bets were on the latter. Once the active substance was isolated and identified, its mechanism of action would be easier to define. Florey's team had a hunch that the blue mold might prove to be special if given the chance.

By late 1940 the team members had accomplished much of what they had set out to do at the start of their investigation, despite the constant *Penicillium* production challenges. Thanks to Chain's early efforts, the researchers established that the antibacterial activity originated in an active substance—a molecule—and not an enzyme as initially suspected. Penicillin extraction had been a major challenge for previous researchers such as Raistrick, Reid, and Fleming due to its unstable nature. The Oxford team had accomplished this by 1939.

Not only that, they had managed to achieve upward of 80 percent purity, clearing the way for the eventual X-ray crystallographic analysis of the substance's structure. Once penicillin's configuration was established, deciphering its antibacterial mechanism would be possible. Moreover, it was the first step in producing the molecule synthetically, something most chemists considered a distinct possibility.

Animal testing proved that penicillin posed little threat of toxicity, and by the beginning of 1941, limited trials were being conducted on human patients under controlled conditions. By doing so, scientists hoped to establish its safety and efficacy in humans and determine against which bacteria penicillin was most effective. The initial catalog was impressive: gonorrhea, meningitis, *Staphylococcus*, *Streptococcus*, anthrax, and gas gangrene, to name a few.

Heatley made considerable strides in mold production, greatly increasing the meager amounts Chain initially grew in pie trays. He experimented with various dilution and diffusion assaying methods until he found the optimal technique—diffusion—which he then set out to improve. He also designed and constructed an automated extraction apparatus called a countercurrent machine that simplified the laborious task of separating penicillin from its reagent. Still, despite the numerous improvements, inefficiencies plagued the production process, particularly when scaling up from growing mold in a few tiny flasks to hundreds, if not thousands, of larger ones.[5]

The Oxford group still relied on the same technique Fleming had used. It entailed growing the mold culture on the surface of a medium consisting of sugar and inorganic salts. After five to ten days, the liquid under the mat of *Penicillium notatum* was used as the source of penicillin. The active ingredient was then extracted from the liquor and dried. The process was known as the surface culture fermentation method of growing mold. On a small scale, it worked fine enough. Even a modest scale-up was problematic, though. Contamination was an immediate concern, and the idea of washing thousands of flasks and removing all harmful residue seemed impossible. Distributing a medium into the vessels and ensuring uniform growth proved another challenge. Ensuring each flask received the same amount of inoculum and dispensing spores under aseptic conditions were yet other problems. In fact, maintaining aseptic conditions during the entire process was a daunting task.

And there was another slight problem. After the *Lancet* published the first paper regarding the isolation of penicillin, researchers around the world grasped the same potential the Oxford men did years earlier. Some even wrote to them and requested samples. When a group of researchers at Columbia University—Martin Henry Dawson, Karl Meyer, and Gladys Hobby—queried Chain for the Oxford *P. notatum*, he obliged.[6] However, when Nazi scientists sent a formal request to Heatley through the Swiss Embassy, the lab declined.[7] One thing both requests had made clear: the race to produce penicillin had started.

At the most inopportune moment, Florey's lab had arrived at an impasse. To take the penicillin research further, the team needed yields much greater than what an Oxford laboratory could supply. Florey believed the pharmaceutical industry held the key. Unfortunately, when he canvassed the English pharmaceutical landscape, he met with collective skepticism and indifference. The experience was instructive. It disappointed but did not devastate. He had one proverbial ace up his sleeve.[8]

During the early stages of research into penicillin, Florey had received a grant from the Rockefeller Foundation. He decided to try his luck with it again. The foundation had seen promise in his research once; he believed the group would see it now, especially after the significant amount of work he had already done. If his proposal found receptive ears, he would not only have access to the organization's deep monetary reserves but also to its connections in industry and academia. As luck would have it, Warren Weaver, the head of the foundation's Natural Sciences Division, was convalescing in London.[9]

The American immediately recognized penicillin's potential. He informed Florey the foundation would cover his travel expenses to the United States if the scientist could get permission from Whitehall to leave the United Kingdom. The Rockefeller Foundation would then facilitate meetings with potential partners. The rest was in Florey's hands.[10]

Constraints imposed on Florey by the British government and the Rockefeller Foundation forced him to make a choice. The entire team could not make the voyage. Because the purpose of going to the States was to find a partner to help produce penicillin, Florey chose Heatley since he knew the process better than anyone. Preparations for the trip proceeded in secrecy. Wartime requirements forced them to keep the mission under wraps until their departure date. It was bound to cause friction in the laboratory.[11]

When Chain saw them with their bags packed on the day of their departure, he understandably felt a tinge of betrayal. It reinforced his suspicions that anti-Semitism was rampant at Oxford. After a brief confrontation between the three, the matter was put to rest. Chain was left behind.

The German would later reflect, "I left the room silently but shattered by the experience of this underhanded trick and act of bad faith, the worst so far in my relationship with Florey. It spoiled my initially good relations with this man forever."[12]

The incident caused irreparable damage to their relationship and had implications that would play out in unforeseen ways when the war ended.

A wartime flight through British airspace had its downsides, among them possibly being shot out of the clouds by a hostile plane or an antiaircraft gun. These concerns weighed on the researchers' minds. Yet nothing could deter them from making the Pan American flight from London to Lisbon, then on to New York City. If the actions of the U.S. government were any indication, it shared their enthusiasm because when the airline scoffed at granting Florey and Heatley seats to New York City, the State Department intervened. Within three days, the Oxford men sat on the tarmac, waiting for takeoff. The journey would change history, mostly for the better.

JOSEPH STALIN HAD GONE missing. After the most humbling week of his life, starting with the German invasion of Soviet territories on June 22, 1941, and ending with the fall of Minsk, the *vozhd* (leader) had had enough. He had misjudged Hitler. His military decisions bordered on farcical. His legacy as Vladimir Lenin's successor and as the champion of the Communist cause suffered with every setback. The fascists were winning. Stalin's exasperated declaration—"Lenin left us a great legacy. We, his heirs, have pissed it all away."—represented a rare public display of vulnerability.[13] His subordinates, maybe even the entire country, sensed a change in their leader. Whether permanent or fleeting, his weakness became palpable. For perhaps the first time, the "Man of Steel" grappled with a crisis of confidence.

Hitler's onrushing Wehrmacht crushed the Red Army at every junction. The figures for the first months of the war tell a story of near-complete domination. As Operation Barbarossa unfolded,

Stalin played down the losses. Official Soviet military and civilian reports claimed minor casualties and fantastical exaggerations that the enemy had been repelled and suffered heavy losses. Quite the opposite was the case. Soviet sources underreported figures across the board.[14]

When Operation Barbarossa commenced in the early hours of June 22, Stalin was informed immediately. Against the advice of his advisers—military men, something he was not—Stalin ordered his troops not to react. He refused to believe an actual invasion could happen and that Hitler would double-cross him in such a disrespectful manner. Instead, he sent Vyacheslav Molotov, his second in command, to meet the German ambassador Friedrich von der Schulenburg. Molotov's words voiced the disbelief that trickled down from his leader. Sounding like a jilted lover, he asked, "Why did Germany sign a non-aggression pact only to break it so easily?"[15]

While Stalin soul searched for answers, the many moving parts of the Second World War continued. Winston Churchill. Benito Mussolini. Adolf Hitler. And in the background, silent and pulling strings, Franklin Delano Roosevelt (FDR).

In 1941 Harry Hopkins covered more international miles than did his boss, FDR. Since his time running the New Deal's behemoth Works Projects Administration, Hopkins's responsibilities had expanded into various unrelated diplomatic fields. A social worker by trade, he had essentially become FDR's personal emissary over the past year. He already possessed unrivaled access to the president's ears; now he traveled the world as his eyes. Hopkins did so at great personal risk, in this instance flying with a squadron of bombers from the United States to London and on to Moscow.[16]

Operation Barbarossa began just as Hopkins finished negotiating the Atlantic Conference, which would occur between Roosevelt and Churchill. Upon hearing the news of the battle, he grasped the profound implications of Hitler's decision, as did the president, who observed, "It was Hitler's first big political miscalculation."[17] Hitler's fighting a war on two fronts relieved some pressure from Great Britain, at least for the time being. The Russians needed to withstand the Nazi onslaught, however, and considering the speed at which France had capitulated, nothing could be taken for granted. In fact, the news coming from the Soviet front was far from encouraging. Some American experts predicted Moscow would fall within days. So on June 23, Hopkins sent a telegram to Washington suggesting he visit Moscow to assess the situation. Roosevelt agreed. He was willing to extend the Lend-Lease program—his way of aiding Great Britain without a formal declaration of war—to the Soviet Union but needed to be sure the Soviets would still be able to fight.[18]

The American Embassy arranged a prompt meeting between Stalin and Hopkins. The simple fact that it took place so quickly proves the importance the dictator placed on the visit. Their initial meeting lasted four hours. During that time, Hopkins conveyed a personal message from Roosevelt: the American president "wished to aid the Soviet Union in its fight against Hitler." He informed Stalin that Churchill had authorized him to say that Britain was eager to help as well. When asked for his immediate needs, the vozhd replied, "Give us anti-aircraft guns and aluminum and we can fight for three or four years."[19]

Hopkins asked for an honest analysis of the Soviet Union's potential to continue fighting. Stalin impressed on him that Hitler had underestimated Russia's strength and resolve, as well as the logistical challenges the country's terrain presented. Already the Wehrmacht's supply and communications lines were extended. The fall rains beckoned and would make the dirt roads impassable. After that, the brutal winter winds would descend. His words gave the impression that the worst had passed. Perhaps he believed it.

There was no contradicting him, of course. Therein lay the problem. Stalin's consistent error. In some ways, his fatal flaw. He thought he knew everything. In the initial stage of the war against Germany, he believed he understood necessary tactics better than his generals did. It was not until he began deferring to them that the tide began to turn. Even then, he came face to face with yet another of his self-inflicted crises: most of his experienced and knowledgeable senior military officers had been executed during his Great Purge of 1937–39.[20]

Starting in 1936, Stalin used a perceived threat against the Soviet state as an excuse to embark on a vindictive and bloody campaign against his own citizens. The first victims were Stalin's political rivals.

Following the murder of Sergei Kirov, Stalin orchestrated the arrest of dozens of opposition leaders in Leningrad and oversaw their show trials. Tribunals found them guilty and sentenced them either to death by firing squad or to imprisonment. The wave of incriminations spread throughout the city. Under the direction of Nikolai Yezhov, thousands of Leningraders met the same fate as Stalin's enemies.

After the Kirov affair, the purge shifted to Moscow, where a supposed plot to murder Stalin by Kremlin support staff was uncovered. After a fresh wave of arrests and show trials, guilty sentences were meted out. The hysteria in the capital reached levels heretofore unseen even in Leningrad. With all opposition politicians pacified, Stalin turned his attention to other sectors of society. First, he went after the economic sector, then the industrial sector. Then in June 1937, after being tortured, many senior military officers received death sentences based on trumped-up charges of belonging to an "anti-Soviet Trotskyite military organization." The depletion of these top generals exacerbated the Red Army's dire initial months of Operation Barbarossa.[21]

During the course of three years, terror reigned in the Soviet Union; all facets of society were deprived of their brightest talents. Mediocrity was exalted in the name of party politics and Communist dialectics. Basic tenets of economics, linguistics, engineering, physics, and chemistry were redefined according to Stalin's diktat. For the first time in history, the idea of science was denigrated as being bourgeois and worthy of destruction. It heralded a Communist revolution of knowledge. In the life sciences, the upheavals went through the person of Trofim Lysenko. A giant in Soviet science, his name would become anathema to genuine research around the world.

EVER SINCE HITLER'S TANKS rolled into Poland in 1939, domestic politics forced Roosevelt to toe the line between aiding Britain and France and declaring war outright, something the isolationist element in the country refused to consider. Day after day, the Roosevelt administration pricked the Nazis with provocations in the Atlantic Ocean and with the occupation of Iceland. Some historians suggest his actions were designed to force Hitler to retaliate. (He never fell for it.) Yet despite the country's stated neutrality, anyone with eyes could see its factories were cranking out ships, trucks, aircraft, and munitions. Like Lend-Lease, America's factories were engaged in the war indirectly. Everyone recognized it for what it was—a prelude to war. Quite simply, Roosevelt was using his Republican-imposed time in isolation to prepare for an inevitable conflict.

Apart from industrial preparations, Roosevelt was eager to exploit the strides American scientists had achieved in the years between the First and Second World Wars. They had catapulted the United States from a scientific backwater to a world leader, thanks to liberal spending on university-based research. He grasped how technology, especially mustard gas and tanks, had shaped the previous war and refused to allow the United States to be caught on the wrong side of the trend. Ever attentive to his boss's needs, Hopkins was well aware of this; so in 1939, when FDR's uncle suggested meeting an ambitious scientist with a genius for administration, he relented. The meeting with Vannevar Bush, the vice chairman of the National Advisory Committee for Aeronautics (NACA) and the chairman of the Carnegie Institution of Washington (CIW), took place in early June 1940. After reading a brief memo describing the proposed National Defense Research Committee (NDRC), Hopkins wasted no time setting up a meeting with the president.[22]

In the late afternoon of June 12, Hopkins accompanied Bush to the meeting with Roosevelt.[23] If everything went well, everyone would get what they wanted. The scientist would get his funding, and the politician would get his advanced weaponry.

After greetings and a few pleasantries, Bush got straight to the point. He handed the president a single sheet of paper with a concise description of how he would bring science into the service of the military and the country. It listed six items:

> 1. The NDRC would be attached to the National Defense Commission.
>
> 2. Composed of Chairman, members from War, Navy, Commerce, National Academy of Sciences, plus several distinguished scientists or engineers, all to serve without remuneration.

3. Function, to correlate and support scientific research on mechanisms and devices of warfare (except in field covered by NACA).

4. Concerned with research rather than industrial development or manufacture.

5. Supplied with funds for office staff, and for financing research in laboratories of educational and scientific institutions or industry.

6. To aid and supplement, and not to replace, activities of War and Navy departments. An Army and Navy officer detailed to work with chairman.[24]

After voicing a few observations, Roosevelt wrote "OK—FDR" on the paper, and that was it.[25] Bush and the president were satisfied, and Hopkins made it all happen.

DEMONSTRATING THE ANTIBIOTIC'S CURATIVE powers could never be put on display until someone solved the production shortage problem. Frustrations the Oxford team experienced during the first clinical trials of penicillin provided the impetus to seek help producing penicillin at home and then abroad. Despite achieving promising results with patients, Dr. Charles Fletcher, a clinician tasked with administering the drug, faced dwindling supplies every day. Still unable to produce significant amounts of penicillin in an adequate time, the Oxford team recycled whatever the patient excreted in their urine. While this approached worked to a limited degree, the yields decreased each round.[26] If patients failed to recover after the first or second dosage, the likelihood of a fatal relapse ballooned.

That proved the case with Albert Alexander, an Oxford policeman who had scratched his face while working in his rose garden. The scrape became infected with staphylococci and streptococci, which then spread to his eyes and scalp. He received sulfa drugs, but they proved ineffective. An experimental dosage of penicillin was the next option. After receiving a loading dose of 200 milligrams, followed by three injections of 100 milligrams every three hours, his health improved. Heatley wrote in his journal that there was "dramatic improvement," so they decided to increase the amount. Considering Alexander's desperate condition prior to treatment, there was much celebration.[27]

Fletcher later recalled: "Chain dancing with excitement at the possibility of a real triumph in medicine, and Florey reserved and quiet but nonetheless intensely thrilled by this remarkable clinical story that I had to tell. . . . I remember him [Florey] saying to me, 'This is the sort of thing that only happens to you once in a life'—and I remember thinking, 'Well, I wish it would happen to me,' and how privileged I was to be taking part in this work."[28]

Their elation was short lived. The supply of penicillin had been spent, and the last remaining doses were administered to a new patient. Alexander's health then deteriorated quicker than it had improved. On March 15 he died of septicemia.[29]

Incidents such as Albert Alexander's must have been on Florey's and Heatley's minds as they disembarked from their Pan American flight at LaGuardia Airfield on July 2. After almost a week in transit, they arrived to a schedule packed with meetings. The Rockefeller Foundation delivered as promised. For Florey, in particular, the term of their three-month visas would be spent shuttling from one potential partner to the next, pitching penicillin as "Erlich's magic bullet." After stopping at their hotel to drop their bags, they headed for an update with Warren Weaver at the foundation's headquarters.

Their first official meeting the following day involved a visit with the head of the Rockefeller Foundation's Medical Sciences Division, Dr. Alan Gregg. Getting him on board as a vocal supporter would make their time in the States easier. He was one of the top officials at the organization, and it was important to demonstrate that its money was not being wasted.[30]

Florey battled exhaustion to summon up a moving and convincing account of their research thus far, including the many highs and multitude of lows. In a measured tone, he correlated the initial grant bestowed by the foundation with the strides the team had made. His lab's achievements were also theirs. This acknowledgment implied that they also shared the disappointments. He recollected Albert Alexander's startling recovery and death. If only more penicillin had been available . . . Without it being voiced outright, everyone knew his death was preventable.[31]

Heatley would later recall the afternoon. "The Professor spun the penicillin tale in a real expert way. I remember him best for that performance—and he was so tired after that long journey. . . . It was unemotional, but still very telling. And in a startling sort of way, it revealed the wide grasp of his scientific mind. Even though I knew the subject well, he showed me new facets, and I realized suddenly how great a man he was. . . . I count that hour in Gregg's office as one of the great experiences in my life."

To close the presentation, Florey handed Gregg an advance copy of an article due to be published in the *Lancet*. It might have been early days, but they could not have asked for a better start.[32]

Florey and Heatley next met with members of the National Research Council, formed by the National Academy of Sciences in 1916 at Woodrow Wilson's request. After hearing about penicillin's promise, Dr. Lewis Wood provided them with an introduction to someone he thought could further their investigations. If anyone would understand what penicillin offered and what its production might entail, it was Dr. Charles Thom, a mycologist in the Bureau of Plant Industry at the U.S. Department of Agriculture (USDA).[33] Over a decade earlier, he had been responsible for identifying Alexander Fleming's mystery mold as *Penicillium notatum*.[34]

Florey's argument evolved each time he spoke. In a shrewd move that suggests Florey was beginning to grasp the immense implications of his research and what it would mean for a country inches away from a war footing, he presented his findings to Dr. Thom in terms of how it would benefit American soldiers when they entered combat.[35] Undoubtedly, he detailed how penicillin effectively treated the onset of gas gangrene. Whether the strategy of linking penicillin to America's march toward war was prudent is impossible to know. It probably represented the first time the development of penicillin was overtly politicized. Considering the climate, chances are that it would have happened anyway. However, the fact remains, whenever science and politics mix, positive developments seldom result.

On top of tying the development of penicillin to a pending crisis, Florey's presentations carried the implicit acknowledgment that he had discovered Ehrlich's magic bullet. More than anything, this news would have caused the most excitement for his audience. It would also have prompted a considerable amount of skepticism.

Eventually the penicillin production trail ended up at the Department of Agriculture's Northern Regional Research Laboratory (NRRL) in Peoria, Illinois. While it took a daisy chain of presentations and referrals, Florey and Heatley were in the right place, sitting across from Dr. Orville E. May, director of the NRRL, and Dr. Robert Coghill, head of the Fermentation Division. They discussed the mold, its attributes, and its fickleness.[36] This meeting seemed less like an audition and more like a conference, because this time the audience possessed a deep understanding about the complexities that producing penicillin presented. And unlike previous encounters, these men had more in common with Heatley, the brewmaster, than with his boss. In fact, the entire organization, recently exiled in Peoria after being kicked out of their longtime headquarters in California, consisted of experienced microbiologists, chemists, and mycologists dedicated to tackling problems like penicillin. If any place was tailor made for developing more efficient production methods, this was it.[37]

The parties reached an agreement in no time. The NRRL would employ all its considerable know-how to the problem of increasing the yield and purity of penicillin. The researchers also asked that Norman Heatley remain with them. He possessed the deep knowledge of the mold only firsthand experience could provide. That alone made him invaluable. His salary and incidentals would be covered by the Rockefeller Foundation.[38]

May voiced his feelings about helping Florey and Heatley a few weeks later in a memo to Henry Knight, the chief of the USDA's Bureau of Agricultural Chemistry and Engineering. "I feel that this whole problem is of significant importance and may well eventuate into a very far reaching contribution. In my opinion, this laboratory can contribute extremely valuable assistance in the solution of the various problems surrounding the production of penicillin because of the quite varied experience which members of the staff have accumulated in the fermentation field."[39]

Florey left Peoria to continue pitching penicillin with varying levels of success. He met with less enthusiasm—much less—during his meetings with U.S. pharmaceutical companies. Each reluctant or disbelieving expression must have sapped his energy by a notch. Undeterred, he crisscrossed the country like an old-time salesman peddling his miraculous elixir. The best responses he received were tepid assurances from a handful of companies, including E. R. Squibb & Sons and Lederle Laboratories, that they would consider it.[40] No contracts. No pledges of support. Definitely no monetary offerings. Only noncommittal expressions of interest. Their priority lay in making a profit, and their conservative approaches reflected more than a little skepticism. In their expert opinions, penicillin would never be a moneymaker, regardless of its potential benefits.

As disappointing as Howard Florey's pharmaceutical endeavors proved, he felt confident he'd find a receptive ear at Connaught Laboratories in Canada. A massive institution with coffers to bear, it nominally figured as part of the University of Toronto. In reality, it was a semiautonomous fiefdom with a considerable international reputation.

On August 28 Florey walked into a meeting with Robert Defries, the institution's director. Also present at the meeting, at the director's request, was Ronald Hare. An alumnus of Almroth Wright's laboratory, he had worked with Fleming and played an instrumental role in the discovery of penicillin. It was his intuition of checking the local weather reports that had led to deciphering how Fleming's mold took root in the famous petri dish by the window. Hare's presence, almost providential in occurrence, must have encouraged Florey to the point of certainty.[41]

Beyond Hare's influence, everything about Connaught Labs seemed tailor made for penicillin research and production. The company boasted some of the top scientific minds in the world, the funding to support them, and the practical knowledge that results from melding the two together. On top of that, it belonged to the British Empire. The staff and Florey were practically compatriots and everything that went along with that. A common vantage point. Similar roots. A regent's sideward-turned profile gracing their currencies. Most important, they shared a common Nazi enemy since the Canadians were already at war. If penicillin's curative aspects could be realized, their men would be among the first to reap the benefits. It must have seemed a reasonable assumption to believe the pieces were in place for a significant commitment.

He couldn't have been more wrong.

The level of disbelief that greeted Florey shocked him.

Hare described what he heard as an "almost incredible story," a backhanded claim that seemed aimed at discrediting the entire endeavor. As they considered the facts presented to them, Defries and Hare grasped the complexities inherent in the production process and did not fancy their chances. They consulted with the chemists at Connaught Labs. Hare later recalled, "When they asked us how we proposed to produce penicillin, and we told them by growth of the mold in containers of some kind, they laughed at us and predicted that by the time we had spent a great deal of time, money, and effort on something so futile, they, the chemists, would have found a way to synthesize it. We must have been unlucky with our choice of chemists because penicillin cannot, even now [1970], be synthesized in any quantity."[42]

Defries added to the insult by questioning penicillin's usefulness even after reading both of the *Lancet* articles Florey wrote. The lab director insinuated that it only worked against *Staphylococcus*, contrary to the published scientific literature he had just read. According to Eric Lax, in his book *The Mold in Dr. Florey's Coat*, "Defries, for reasons that were never recorded but which a bitterly disappointed Florey rejected as 'fallacious,' declined to be of any help. Hare felt that Florey had never forgiven him, and in the case of Defries, he was probably right."[43]

In fairness, Connaught Labs was not alone in its hesitancy; rather, its reaction was the norm. Even the Americans Florey conferred with had similar reservations, as a later memo by A. Baird Hastings—the biochemist and Committee on Medical Research (CMR) member—demonstrates: "It was the impression of the Committee that the difficulties of manufacture were so great and the probable cost of treating so large that penicillin could hardly be expected to become a drug of practical significance during this war."[44]

IN RETROSPECT, IT WAS a friendly dinner on August 7 between Florey and an old professional acquaintance, Alfred Newton Richards, that would bear fruit. The two had worked together because of Florey's 1929 Rockefeller traveling grant. At the time, Richards was conducting extensive research in kidney function and whether its primary mechanism worked via reuptake/filtration or excretion. He was the more senior of the two and was well known for his work modernizing U.S. medical schools, first at Columbia University and then at University of Pennsylvania. Florey's term at Richards's lab clearly had left a good impression. Their meeting attests to that.[45]

As they sat in Richards's social club, the Oxford man donned his penicillin salesman hat and mustered whatever enthusiasm he could. On some level, Florey must have wondered why people weren't falling over to fund the penicillin project.

In the end, Richards's excitement would trump every tepid nod Florey ever received.

EVEN AS HITLER'S TROOPS marched toward Moscow and Leningrad, Stalin's merciless state apparatus churned on autopilot. Not even the threat of impending doom within the Soviet Union could halt its machinations. With every sector of society, industry, and government paralyzed with terror, uncertainty overwhelmed daily life. Self-preservation took precedence over productivity, initiative, and creativity. Neighbors hurled baseless denunciations at each other as a means of defense. With the mechanisms of persecution in place, people were sent to the gulag or executed with an efficiency that aspired to Nazi levels. Meanwhile, a small but significant segment of the population grasped the opportunity chaos presented. Vacant positions. Questionable relationships. Vulnerable ideals. The time was ripe for a power grab, and it happened publicly in the field of Soviet biology.

In early July 1941, Trofim Lysenko's ascendency to the unofficial head of Soviet biology neared completion while his arch rival in science, Nikolai Vavilov, languished in a Moscow prison. Under normal circumstances the notion of one of Russia's most important scientists being supplanted by someone with questionable knowledge of his field and whose experiments were conducted with flawed methodology would seem absurd. But this was not a normal time, and it happened.[46]

After years of positioning himself as the proletarian champion of a new Soviet biology, Lysenko had just about cleared the path to begin his ascent to the official zenith of his field. He achieved this by way of a novel and native field called agrobiology, which he pioneered in 1932. A creation of his imagination, it melded traditional agricultural techniques with questionable evolutionary science polished with cherry-picked portions of Marxist ideology. Together with I. I. Prezent, a member of the Communist Party and a lawyer by training, Lysenko published a paper—his first—that proposed the existence of two competing strains of biology. It posited the primary and only true form was a socialist biology embodied in the formulation of agrobiology and championed by the two men. The second and illegitimate strain of biology was a capitalist bourgeois version inherited from pre-1917 days. This claim was a logical extension of an idea that took root after Stalin's rise: science, in and of itself, was bourgeois and ripe for destruction.[47]

Central to this argument was the concept of evolution and, more specifically, the notion of the gene as a unit of inheritance. According to Lysenko and his apostles, the chromosome did not exist and was simply a Western counterrevolutionary construct. While acknowledging the basic evolutionary tenet of inheritance, Lysenko took exception to Charles Darwin's notion of competition and the idea that heritable traits were passed along in that manner. In other words, external factors—that is, the environment—held the key to evolution. Lysenkoists insisted that traits were acquired and transmitted by a process more akin to Lamarckian evolution.[48] While by no means entirely original—an odd strain of Marxist Darwinism had been debated in Russia since the Bolshevik Revolution—agrobiology represented an especially crass reading of Darwin and Jean-Baptiste Lamarck that was propelled by misunderstandings rather than hampered by them. Lysenko and Prezent renamed the new synthesis of evolutionary ideas to exalt its Marxist status—Soviet creative Darwinism.

It became the sword wielded by Lysenko and his followers, as he felled his rivals with ease. With each strike, its blade sharpened and steel strengthened. He tied it directly to his approach to agriculture and suggested that any criticism of agrobiological techniques was counterrevolutionary. The critic was accused of displaying a lack of enthusiasm for the goal of Soviet agriculture. It was a classic case of if you are not with us (socialists), you (capitalists) are against us. As with all ideologues, nothing existed between the extremes. Stalin's lack of disapproval signified a tacit approval.

Lysenko proved a capable administrator and natural politician. He trained his sights on the bastions of genetics in the Soviet Union—its agricultural institutes. Lysenko emerged triumphant.

VANNEVAR BUSH WAS A decisive man. The angularity of his features coupled with his steel-rim glasses and silver hair reflected his sober disposition. He had a Warren Buffett–style folksiness in the way he spoke that could be disarming, but as with Buffett, it belied a sharp, unapologetic pragmatism. During his time in charge of the Carnegie Institution of Washington, he demonstrated the trait time and again as he cut, slashed, and burned entire research departments he considered superfluous or, still worse, "marginal" to the hard sciences. CIW's funding and support for programs associated with history, archaeology, sociology, and psychology evaporated at a pace historian I. Bernard Cohen described as "little short of catastrophic." According to a former colleague, "[Bush] had the self-confidence that he could confront and comprehend any problem. . . . And that gave him the confidence to wade into questions that other people might avoid."[49]

Yet, however distressing Bush's views might have been for social scientists, they provided an unquestionable boon to the hard sciences of chemistry, biology, and physics. They no longer had to share the CIW's budget. There was little doubt about his dedication to pure and applied science.

When President Roosevelt approved the establishment of the National Defense Research Council, Bush's long-held vision of creating a grand research system consisting of military, academic, and industrial organizations came a step closer to fruition. Long before the military-industrial complex became codified in the 1950s, Bush understood the inherent commonalities between various types of research institutions and how they could be coordinated to maximize their output. Rather than working in complete isolation, he felt their efforts should be synchronized. Addressing a single problem from as many different angles as possible created solutions. Moreover, for Bush, science in the service of the military was of utmost importance. Invariably, the first question he asked when presented with a proposal for a new project ran along the line, "Will it help win a war; this war?" A year after forming the NDRC, FDR would provide the canvas for Vannevar Bush's vision to become a reality.[50]

In July 1941 Executive Order 8807 created the Office of Scientific Research and Development (OSRD). It replaced the NDRC with a larger, more ambitious organization. Whereas the older body functioned in a consulting capacity with a limited budget, the executive order empowered the OSRD to play a much more proactive role in facilitating research projects by increasing its budget and authority; yet, that did not mean Bush simply threw money at projects and barked orders. He was too savvy an administrator to engage collaborators that way, and he understood how to stretch a budget, regardless how sizable. Instead, one of the major strategies the OSRD adopted with its contractors entailed "encouragement," wherein companies received incentives such as tax breaks and preferential treatment beneficial to accomplishing the goal. Under this scheme, any contractual ties were kept minimal and loose. The OSRD served more of a facilitating role than an organizational one.[51]

At the behest of the president, the OSRD expanded its mandate to include research in military medicine, something Roosevelt knew would eventually filter down to the American public. Central to that effort was the creation of a new research organization within the OSRD, the Committee on Medical Research.[52]

According to Executive Order 8807, "The Committee on Medical Research shall advise and assist the Director in the performance of his medical research duties with special reference to the mobilization of medical and scientific personnel of the nation." Its primary duty consisted of analyzing proposals pertinent to military medicine and then recommending the best ones to Vannevar Bush. It would also monitor approved programs and report progress to the director.[53]

The CMR consisted of four presidential appointees and three other members chosen by the secretary of war, the secretary of the navy, and the administrator of the Federal Security Agency. The first meeting was held on July 31, 1941. Leading the meeting was the head of the committee, A. N. Richards.[54]

Weeks later, the chairman returned from his face-to-face meeting with Howard Florey enthusiastic about the briefing and presented the case for penicillin to his fellow committee members. Unbeknownst to Florey at the time of their meeting, Richards would become penicillin's most influential benefactor and champion. Still, the same old concerns about production cropped up plus another one specific to the CMR's organization.

As part of the OSRD and as defined in Roosevelt's executive order, the CMR's mission was to facilitate research to reach stated national goals. The problem with penicillin—at least in the way Florey had presented it—was not so much a question of inquiry as it was of industry. The Oxford man asked for help in addressing a shortage of the chemical; thus, the task fell outside the purview of the OSRD.

Richards refused to allow semantics to derail a discovery he believed could have real, positive implications for the pending war and for humanity. It would not be the last time he pushed the development of penicillin forward by sheer force of will.[55]

Meanwhile, time was running out in Peoria. Heatley continued working on the penicillin fermentation process with the help of Andrew J. Moyer. Heatley's visa and contract with the Rockefeller Foundation had been extended to give him a fair chance at discovery.[56] However, the NRRL continued to have reservations regarding how much of its resources to invest in the production of penicillin. The longer the investigation dragged on, the less eager the lab was to continue. Other more important subjects demanded its attention. This point was made clear during a September 29 meeting between Dr. Charles Thom and H. T. Herrick, the assistant chief of the USDA's Bureau of Agricultural Chemistry and Engineering.

According to Herrick, "I told Dr. Thom that it was my opinion that the Northern Regional Research Laboratory was not interested in concerning itself with the problem any more than it already is—that is acting in an advisory capacity to Dr. Heatley. . . . It is my recollection that you [Orville May] said you had too much planned for the Fermentation Division to give any further consideration to the production of Penicillin."[57]

On October 2 the CMR convened and resolved to move forward with Dr. Florey's penicillin proposal. Richards was "authorized to suggest to interested persons the desirability of a concerted program of research on penicillin involving the pooling of information and results; and if the responses are favorable, to proceed to arrange for a conference on the subject."[58] The meeting occurred six days later. Present in the room were representatives from the companies Merck, Chas. Pfizer, E. R. Squibb & Sons, and Lederle Laboratories; the USDA/NRRL; the National Research Council; and the OSRD.[59]

With one eye on war, the U.S. government had taken its first significant step toward assuming control of the penicillin project. According to the official account of the work done at the OSRD, it would be second in importance only to the development of the atomic bomb.

2

With Operation Barbarossa, one blitz gave way to another as Hitler swapped Russia for England. The island nation survived but only just. The damage inflicted by eight months of Luftwaffe bombings—from Black Saturday until May 11, 1941—left cities shattered. Coventry. Bristol. Birmingham. Southampton. Manchester. Liverpool. London. British morale remained fragile, neither broken nor encouraged. The fact still remained: Great Britain had been savaged.

Meanwhile, Hitler's Wehrmacht continued its relentless eastward march into Soviet Russia, sweeping Red Army battalions aside like dust mites. Every hamlet in its path bent its knee. Riga. Vitebsk. Smolensk. Minsk.

The trail of dead continued to mount on both sides. Maimed soldiers bled through their bandages. They nursed deformities and mutilations. Sometimes their skin tore apart. Other times it ripped away from bone. The worst was when it melted, burned to a viscous mess. Sulfa drugs could only do so much against the onslaught of opportunistic microbes spilling into open wounds. For most of the conflict, the most effective protection against life-threatening complications involved the mechanical removal of affected tissue. Doctors sawed off mangled limbs and lopped off damaged skin. Anything to prevent infection. They learned to let wounds breathe. They used boric acid for wound debridement. In military terms, these soldiers would never return and needed to be replaced. The effect of an injured infantryman on the front filtered all the way home when new conscripts left their towns to ride the conveyor belt of dispensable soldiers. During a shooting war, armies were constantly trying to make up the difference caused by casualties.

The struggle against disease and infection represented a third, but unspoken, conflict being waged by the Allies and Axis. A good showing against the microbe world could mean the difference between victory and defeat in an actual shooting war. Students of European military history understood the devastation unchecked disease inflicted on physically powerful armies. In 1528 typhus inflicted so much damage on the French army laying siege to Naples during the struggle between Hapsburg Spain and Valois France that the French ended up retreating. It wouldn't be the last time microbes changed the course of history. In 1812 Napoleon's doomed Russian campaign failed as much due to crippling disease, the most notable being typhus, as it did due to inclement weather. The perils were undeniable.[1]

ON OCTOBER 8, 1941, a meeting was held with the Office of Scientific Research and Development, the Committee on Medical Research, the U.S. Department of Agriculture, and the pharmaceutical companies. On the government side, Vannevar Bush, A. N. Richards, and Charles Thom presented penicillin and discussed its potential. On the pharmaceutical side, H. T. Major (Merck), George A. Harris (E. R. Squibb & Sons), Jasper Kane (Chas. Pfizer), and Yellapragada Subbarow (Lederle) represented their respective companies. At the time, the only company that could be considered big was Lederle, a subsidiary of the chemicals conglomerate American Cyanamid.[2]

Pfizer was still a small Brooklyn-based business that revolved around the production of ascorbic acid by fermentation. Merck's status was slightly more complicated. It was founded in 1891 as the U.S. branch of one of Europe's oldest pharmaceutical companies, Merck KGaA. However, during World War I, the U.S. government's Office of Alien Property Custodian seized the American branch under the authority of the Trading with the Enemy Act. George Merck Sr. eventually bought the company back but maintained it as an entity independent of the German company.[3]

With the OSRD and the CMR barely a year old, Bush and Richards introduced their agencies, explaining their structure and organization. They stressed that the agencies did not conduct actual research;

they supervised and funded scientists engaged in a wide range of research interests. Next, Thom described the scientific aspects of penicillin and the work being done at the Northern Regional Research Laboratory: the compound's instability, its chemotherapeutic activity against gram-positive bacteria, and the difficulty of achieving meaningful yields. He also detailed the lab's pursuit of a more productive strain of *Penicillium notatum* than Fleming's.[4]

Even with the OSRD's explicit backing, the reactions of the private sector scientists to penicillin were mixed. At one end of the spectrum, Squibb and Lederle expressed reservations about its overall production at a laboratory scale, let alone an industrial one. They also hinted at corporate concerns. Merck and Pfizer assumed a contrary position. They were eager to join the nascent consortium and get to work. For now, things stood at an impasse.[5]

Meanwhile, the quest for increasing yields continued unabated at the NRRL. While the researchers had made undeniable inroads with the mold Florey and Heatley smuggled into the country when they fled to the United States, they had yet to solve the most perplexing problem of scaling up the penicillin production process. While the Chain-Heatley method solved the discouraging instability and extraction issues that had put off researchers from Alexander Fleming's work, a more efficient method needed to be devised, especially if penicillin was to be anything beyond a medical novelty.

Florey's group employed a method commonly referred to as surface fermentation. Visually, it resembled French onion soup with the melted cheese topping the piping hot broth. Picking up where Fleming left off, the researchers' approach entailed growing *Penicillium notatum* (melted cheese) on top of a medium (the soup itself) that provided all the nutrients necessary for growth. Heatley nurtured the mold in flat, bedpan-like ceramic containers. Five to ten days later, the "cheese" was taken off, exposing the "soup." The liquid that formed under the sheet of mold, called a mycelial mat, contained the antibiotic that, when treated, yielded solid versions of penicillin.

Each stage of the penicillin production process presented unique problems when scaling up. How would they wash and sterilize hundreds, if not thousands, of flasks used to grow the mold? Moreover, how would they ensure that each flask received the exact same amount of inoculum (in this case, the spores that grew into mold) while maintaining the same conditions in each flask? How would they ensure that not a single iota of contamination crept into the penicillin containers? What works in a small laboratory often fails when it meets the demands of mass production in a cavernous factory.[6]

The inefficiency of scaling up the surface method was on full display when American researchers at Columbia University attempted to grow and extract penicillin of their own for research purposes.

Soon after seeing the Oxford group's first *Lancet* paper regarding penicillin, Martin Henry Dawson reached out to Ernst Chain for a sample of the mold. After receiving it, Dawson—joined by Karl Meyer and Gladys Hobby—dedicated time to investigating penicillin's characteristics. They emulated Heatley's method with slight variations. They used two-liter Erlenmeyer flasks rather than the flat ones. They also relied on a different growth medium. In no time, Columbia's Microbiology Department was flooded with containers.[7] "Soon hundreds of two-liter flasks with *Penicillium notatum* growing on a modified Czapek-Dox medium lined every classroom laboratory bench at the Columbia University Medical School. We had no adequately large incubators and no space in our own small laboratory for such large numbers of flasks, but moved in and out of classrooms as the students moved in and out. . . . Eventually it was discovered that the flasks could be incubated under the seats of a two-story amphitheater."[8]

MUCH TO VANNEVAR BUSH'S and A. N. Richards's credit, they recognized the problem and realized the solution would most likely come from people who made a living solving the issues that scaling up entailed. It involved a different mind-set and approach to the problem. Producing meager amounts of penicillin in the lab using expensive materials was one thing; successful mass production entailed keeping costs down, sometimes by using cruder methods and materials. Private industry and academia subscribed to seemingly incompatible business models, and that was a good thing. Bush and Richards just needed to convince the pharmaceutical companies that they had something to gain.

A meeting with the four companies on November 13 showed how large a leap remained for everyone involved. It made the Columbia River Gorge look like a crack in the pavement. Nothing had changed. If anything, their positions became more entrenched. Merck and Pfizer continued to express their enthusiasm, while Squibb and Lederle remained unconvinced of penicillin's potential worth and of each other.[9]

Bush and Richards searched for some combination of incentives and inspiration that might sway everyone to agree. Nothing doing. Matters took a discouraging turn when Squibb insisted that the four companies present at the meeting should be the only ones to participate in the project from start to finish. It wanted guarantees that each of the four companies involved would make equal contributions and that significant commercial advantage would result from their efforts. When the meeting concluded, the only point everyone agreed on was the need to meet again.[10] The way things were going, Bush and Richards couldn't be blamed if they considered that a minor victory.

George W. Merck emerged as penicillin's early private sector champion. He personally telephoned Richards the following day to discuss the meeting and expressed frustration at Squibb's and Lederle's unwillingness to compromise. He suggested there might be more to their stances than just their uncertainty over penicillin. According to Richards, Merck suspected that "it is not impossible that bad feeling in the commercial field between Squibb and American Cyanamid Corporation [Lederle's parent company] extends into the scientific field; hence, if Lederle were not in, Squibb might play ball better." It was a long shot but worth considering. Meanwhile, Merck did not hesitate to remind Richards that two companies were ready to move forward immediately—his company and Pfizer.[11]

Perhaps sensing a chance to strategically exclude two competitors from sharing "first-mover" advantage, Merck insisted that with the NRRL, CMR, and OSRD handling the basic research on one side, his company and Pfizer could take care of the commercial side without Squibb's and Lederle's input.[12] Anyone with eyes could see that the nation's industrial sector had switched gears in recent months, cranking out airplanes and vehicles at a record clip. If anything represented a reliable tell, that did. War and production would be synonymous, and soon the pharmaceutical industry would be called upon to do its part. Whether he was prompted by patriotism, by a canny business acumen, or by being privy to inside information, Merck was well ahead of the curve.

Richards demurred. They needed to have at least one more meeting. Not only that, he had work to do. He needed to break the impasse. In his own words, "They all have the feeling that they don't quite know what the Government wants. . . . Apparently it is my business to find out or to formulate what the Government does want."[13]

For the time being, foot-dragging would hold the day. The massive strategic and health significance of penicillin had yet to be understood. In a month's time, the United States wouldn't have the luxury of adopting a wait-and-see approach. If the men had known about the true impact of the Oxford group's August 6 *Lancet* paper, their urgency would have bordered on panic.

EVERYONE FEARED THE GERMANS. They excelled at everything. At least, that's how it seemed. Whether crouching in a trench or sitting at a lab bench, their mythical efficiency, intellect, and technical prowess demanded respect. Opponents readily obliged. The sentiment extended into the scientific field as well. As master chemists, they were at the forefront of the nascent field of antibacterial drugs.

German scientists played important roles in the development of microbiology and bacteriology after Louis Pasteur's research resulted in his seminal germ theory of disease. In particular, Robert Koch's research—first with bacterial staining and microscopy, followed by his identification of the bacillus that caused tuberculosis (TB)—represented major contributions to understanding the role of germs in disease.[14]

On March 24, 1882, Koch presented his research on *Mycobacterium tuberculosis* at the Physiological Society in Berlin. He postulated objective rules, later known as Koch's postulates, that defined when a pathogen is involved in an infection and that are still used to this day. According to Koch, for an infection to be bacterial in nature:

(a) the bacterium must be present in every case of the infection,

(b) the agent must be isolated from the infection and purified by culture in a laboratory,

(c) the culture is then inoculated into a suitable experimental animal and causes a similar infection, and

(d) the infection must contain a significant amount of the infecting bacteria.[15]

A young researcher named Paul Ehrlich sat in the audience, transfixed by what he heard. He later recalled the moment as the most exciting experience of his life. It would also pave the way for the emergence of antibacterials.[16]

Initially, Ehrlich's attention focused on bacterial staining, and he worked closely with Koch. But he saw something else. His creative mind made the imaginative leap that often jump-starts discovery. Due to chemical differences in the cell walls between gram-negative and gram-positive bacteria, they possessed different affinities to dye stains. He realized that if microorganisms were able to be selectively stained—such as gram positive—then it should be possible, in theory, to develop a chemical that targeted them while leaving the host's tissue unaffected. Technically called selective toxicity, it came to be known by another name—Ehrlich's magic bullet. And although he never realized his vision completely, his work with dyes resulted in the production of the first compound to have antibacterial properties. It was called Salvarsan.[17]

Enter IG Farbenindustrie.

The industrial conglomerate and its numerous subsidiaries, which included Schering, Bayer AG, and BASF, played a major role in antibacterial research because of their position as market leaders in the manufacture of textile dyes. They recognized that a natural synergy existed between their core business and the antibacterial chemical research field. During the same year that Ehrlich was testing Salvarsan, IG Farbenindustrie created the first research laboratory dedicated to developing antibacterial pharmaceuticals. It was established at Bayer's Eberfeld location and was headed by Wilhelm Roehl, a scientist who had worked with Ehrlich on the selective binding of dyes. With the heft of one of the world's largest companies behind him, Roehl refined Ehrlich's discovery. He surmised that the dye itself was not the active ingredient since it was a mixture of chemicals, and he went on to isolate the molecule responsible for the dye's curative properties. The resulting chemical derivative, called Germanin, was the first effective cure for sleeping sickness.[18]

IG Farbenindustrie was not done yet. In 1927 the company poached a promising microbiologist named Gerhard Domagk from the University of Münster's Pathological Institute to work at the experimental lab Roehl headed. Domagk took inspiration from the tragedy of Roehl's sudden death due to a bacterial infection and focused on the strain responsible for it—*Streptococcus*. Together with the chemist Josef Klarer, Domagk developed the drug Prontosil rebrum, which succeeded in targeting streptococci. Unfortunately, it proved less effective against most other bacteria, but it represented a significant step forward in the development of what would later be known as antibiotics. By the time Hitler's tanks annexed Czechoslovakia in 1939, sulfathiazole, another one of Domagk's discoveries, demonstrated its effectiveness against the old enemy TB.[19]

In 1935 Domagk published the results of the clinical trials he conducted with Prontosil. Rather than singing his praise, the medical community greeted the news with skepticism. But word got around, and as the popular press reported news of the drug's effectiveness, patients pressured their doctors into administering it. Prontosil's use became widespread around the developed world. In the United States, it garnered headlines due to a very high-profile case when Franklin Delano Roosevelt Jr., the president's son, was treated with the new drug.

So with good reason, Allied scientists feared that the Nazis would pip them to the full development and production of penicillin. They even took it for granted that the Germans would eventually synthesize the antibiotic in the laboratory, doing away with the cumbersome fermentation process. Daily reports streaming across the ocean from Europe must have just made things worse. The battering that Nazi forces inflicted on their European opponents could only have reinforced the notion of the irrepressible German juggernaut.

Even George W. Merck harbored reservations. He also had been made aware that the CMR chief was toying with the idea of pulling in another pharmaceutical firm, Winthrop, which had expressed interest in joining the nascent consortium. Before hanging up with Richards, he offered words of advice: be careful.[20] The company's convoluted history made its ownership structure suspect. Up until the First World War, it had been a subsidiary of Bayer AG, and rumor had it the Germans still held a stake, despite technically losing ownership to the Office of Alien Property Custodian. Without a doubt, there was a danger that it would serve as a back channel for the Nazis to monitor the penicillin program, to procure strains for their own use, and, most important, to steal technical information in virtual real time.

Founded in 1901 as Neuralgyline Company in Wheeling West Virginia, the company rebranded with the name Sterling Drug. The outbreak of World War I provided the company with an opportunity to expand. Taking advantage of the Office of Alien Property Custodian, which essentially confiscated companies owned by enemy nations during wartime, Sterling Drug purchased the U.S. assets of the German drug firm Bayer AG for $5.3 million. When hostilities ceased, Sterling Drug entered into an agreement with Bayer AG that granted it the rights to adopt the "Bayer" brand and to sell aspirin. In turn, Bayer was able to reenter U.S. markets, which it had been forced to abandon during the war. In 1922 Sterling Drug merged with Winthrop Chemical to form a holding company that went by the name Winthrop.[21]

In the end, though, Winthrop was excluded from the consortium. Merck's suspicions reflected a more general concern, one first manifested when Florey fled Oxford with mold in his coat: were Hitler and the Nazis trying to develop penicillin of their own?

The answer was a clear yes, and while only an inkling, Florey knew this better than anyone at that point. In April 1941 he learned German scientists were making inquiries regarding penicillin. They hoped to acquire samples through Switzerland, specifically through the company Ciba.[22] Meanwhile, the pharmaceutical firm had also taken an interest in the mold—due in part to Fleming's old paper and Florey's most recent one—and had already dedicated resources to developing it. They turned to Ernst Gäumann of the Swiss Federal Institute of Technology for expertise.[23]

The news alarmed Florey and must have played a role in his decision to fly to the United States. He wasted no time contacting Alexander Fleming to inform him and warn of the consequences of the Nazis' procuring penicillin of their own. He also sought advice from Sir Edward Mellanby, the chairman of the United Kingdom's Medical Research Council that had partially funded the penicillin research, regarding the upcoming publication of the Oxford group's paper in the *Lancet*. In it, the group documented each step of its penicillin process including the growth conditions for *Penicillium notatum*, the detailed diagrams of Heatley's ceramic pan apparatus, and, most important, the unique method the group devised to extract penicillin from the broth containing the liquid.

Mellanby's analysis of the situation and subsequent advice would have far-reaching implications. "In his reply, Mellanby assured him [Florey] that he was miles ahead of any competition and that there was no point in suppressing publication on penicillin in the national interest because effective antibacterials—information on sulfanilamides—was widely available." On August 16, 1941, the *Lancet* published "Further Observations on Penicillin."[24] Clearly, Mellanby had no idea just how much more effective penicillin would be than the entire crop of sulfa drugs. He lacked the vision to comprehend what sat before him. He wasn't alone, but it doesn't make the decision to publish such vital information during wartime any less egregious.

The question whether Nazi scientists engaged in the development of penicillin and how they first learned about the antibiotic has been debated by historians. Gilbert Shama has published several papers investigating the path and timetable of penicillin research in the Third Reich. His work "Zone of Inhibition? The Transfer of Information Relating to Penicillin in Europe during World War II" offers a detailed picture of the various opportunities available to German scientists and their scientist-collaborators working in occupied countries.[25]

With Alexander Fleming's central and primary role in the discovery of *P. notatum*, he also became an important source of the mold for researchers around the world who were interested in exploring its properties. While he later claimed that he would not pass the mold to enemy countries, he admitted sending samples to other scientists. "During the past ten years, I have sent out a very large number of cultures of penicillium to all sorts of places, but as far as I can remember none have gone to Germany. In this country many people have (or had) cultures, including places like Burroughs Wellcome, Evans Leischer & Webb, May and Baker, Parke-Davis, and Boots."[26]

This information, which Florey received after requesting that penicillin not be provided to the Germans, must have been disconcerting. In particular, the phrase "have sent out a very large number of cultures of penicillium to all sorts of places" called to mind another wartime slogan, "Loose lips sink ships." As more evidence emerges, it becomes clear that Fleming's samples did in fact reach Germany, directly and indirectly.

According to British intelligence documents, a man referred to as "Dr. Schmidt" had been the recipient of Fleming's penicillin mold some time before the war. At that time, Schmidt worked at IG Behring in Marburg. When asked to culture and extract penicillin, he failed. The fickle mold refused to grow. Schmidt passed the sample to researchers at the pharmaceutical firm Schering, where it met a similar fate. Eventually, Schmidt's sample was abandoned because scientists assumed that the mold had been inactivated by improper storage.[27]

German researchers almost certainly worked from Florey's 1941 *Lancet* article, as a start point at least. While the normal channels that carried scientific information between the United Kingdom and Nazi Europe had been shut down, official and unofficial channels still existed. In 1939 the German government created a special operation with the sole objective of collecting foreign academic journals. Scientific attachés located in neutral countries were tasked with obtaining the desired publications and shipping them to Germany. They were then photocopied, placed on microfilm, and distributed to research institutions around the country as well as to local scientific journals. Private German industries had their own methods of acquiring information, and the larger companies often received criticism from smaller competitors for harvesting information and refusing to share it. Taken together, clearly opportunities existed for the Nazi science machine to work on penicillin.

According to declassified Allied documents, Florey's *Lancet* article was also widely disseminated by the summer of 1942.[28]

The race for penicillin had begun.

AS THE WAR IN Europe shifted toward the Soviet Union, the dam holding back casualties broke into pieces. Soldiers and civilians faced a grim reality that included corpse-strewn landscapes, shattered bodies, and food shortages. By September Hitler's troops had penetrated as far as the gates of Leningrad. On September 4 German artillery began shelling the city. On September 8 the Luftwaffe embarked on a brutal three-day shelling, dropping incendiary bombs, delayed-action bombs, and land mines.[29]

The citizens believed all was lost. "My eyes beheld a horrible sight. A dark room covered with frost, puddles of water on the floor. Lying across some chairs was the corpse of a fourteen-year-old-boy. In a baby carriage was a second corpse, that of a tiny infant. On the bed lay the owner of the room—dead. At her side, rubbing her chest with a towel, stood her eldest daughter."[30]

Soviet troops battled and refused to abandon the city. The Germans expected them to capitulate within a week. It did not happen. Instead, Stalin sent Gen. Georgy Zhukov to Leningrad to reorganize the defense of the city. It took him only three days. After that, the Nazis had no choice but to lay siege to Leningrad.

Other cities did not fare as well. Each time a city fell, the situation worsened. Large swaths of citizens became vulnerable to disease. While they could escape the Nazi onslaught by pushing eastward, outrunning microorganisms such as *Salmonella typhi* and *Yersinia pestis* wasn't an option. Throughout history, disease wielded its opportunistic sword during times of upheaval, particularly during times of war. This time was no different. As always, the noncombatants suffered the most for decisions thrust upon them.

The Soviet state of Georgia escaped much of the carnage. Shielded by the Caucasus on its northern border and cushioned between the Caspian Sea and Black Sea to the east and west, respectively, it managed to retain a semblance of normalcy while cities across the north burned. In this sense, its citizens were fortunate, especially since Hitler's intentions of reaching the oil-rich Caucuses region were clear from Operation Barbarossa's inception.

While the Nazi onslaught never materialized, the self-inflicted violence of the Great Purge festered like a boil. Perhaps nothing captured the destructive effect of Stalin's Great Purge on the antibacterial field than the case of the Georgian bacteriologist Georg Eliava.

When it came to fighting bacterial infections, the Soviet Union had options, unlike the American and British populations. During those early days of antibacterial chemotherapy, the scientific community pursued numerous research avenues. They turned to chemistry for sulfonamide and its derivatives, and while effective to a degree, its side effects proved too toxic for many patients. What's more, it spawned resistance at a furious rate. It worked, though, and soldiers on both sides carried it in their first aid kits. Penicillin relied on the organic world of mycology, and while promising, it was nothing more than fairy dust in those early days, as the pharmaceutical industry's ambivalence proved. It was still a long away from being useful on the battleground. A third path, however, whose tradition stretched back at least as far as the sulfa drugs, was also being investigated at the time. It was called phage therapy and turned to the murky world of live viruses for its power.

Bacteriophages first appeared in the scientific discourse when Frederick Twort, a British microbiologist, discovered them in 1915. However, it wasn't until their subsequent "rediscovery" two years later by the French-Canadian Félix d'Hérelle that their therapeutic potential became evident.[31]

Phages come in various shapes and sizes. One common type is shaped similar to the Apollo 11 moon lander, *Eagle*, only with longer legs. Phages attack by latching onto target bacteria, piercing the cell wall, and injecting phage DNA into it. The invading genetic material then becomes incorporated into the host's genome. Once this happens, it's over for the bacteria, as the phage hijacks the host's cellular machinery to spawn more phages. This cycle is repeated over and over until the bacteria is overwhelmed, dies, and bursts open like a balloon, unleashing a mini army of new and lethal phages.

Bacteriophages would make the ideal antibiotic if their collective power can be harnessed. They kill bacteria and are highly specific to individual strains. What's more, they would presumably adapt with their targets as resistance emerged. Unfortunately, this also makes bacteriophage therapy wildly unpredictable because there's no telling how the viruses might change. Finally, phages represent one of the key ways in which bacterial DNA is transferred between bacteria, a process called transduction. In a worst-case scenario, phage therapy has the potential of causing more harm than helping, especially if current technology is unable to control the process.

Early in the twentieth century, scientists around the world jumped at the opportunity to put phages to the test, although the quality of their experiments varied. D'Hérelle tested the effectiveness of the new therapy around the world, fighting bubonic plague in Southeast Asia and dysentery in Europe. In India doctors administered a cocktail of phages to people suffering from cholera and noted the treatment eased the symptoms of the disease. In Russia scientists employed phages topically to infected wounds and lesions. After the October Revolution, the Soviet Union would become the center of bacteriophage therapy research and production.[32]

Centers dedicated to bacteriophage research cropped up all over the Soviet Union during the 1920s. Taking their inspiration from the great Ukrainian microbiologist Il'ia Mechnikov, young scientists accepted the challenge the microbial world offered. Phages played a significant role in the new science, and many people weighed in on the subject. In particular, Lev Zil'ber, Leopold Peretts, and Magdalina Pokrovskaia championed and studied the role of phages in the environment and as a possible therapy. However, one man, with his passion for bacteriophages and his very close link to d'Hérelle and the Pasteur Institute, stood out.

Georg Eliava grew up in Sachkhere, Georgia, and was a contemporary of Josef Stalin's but traveled in altogether different social circles. As a youth, his interests lay in the arts, but he eventually fell under science's spell. He studied at Imperial Novorossiysk University in Odessa and then at Moscow University, where he graduated in 1916. Two years later, he left Georgia for a position at the prestigious Pasteur Institute in Paris. There he attended a lecture by d'Hérelle about bacteriophage therapy. It captured Eliava's imagination. The two eventually became collaborators in the field.

Eliava returned to his homeland, carrying the flame of phage therapy with him. He set out to establish the world's first research center dedicated to bacteriophage therapy and through sheer determination succeeded. The Eliava Institute was established in the Georgian capital, Tbilisi. He even managed to get d'Hérelle to join him in the venture, and the Canadian took a central role in the research center's formation.[33]

Showing great confidence in phage therapy, Eliava introduced it to the Soviet public, taking it out of the laboratory and into the field. According to Nina Chanishvili, a researcher and historian at the Eliava Institute, he used his cocktails of bacteriophages to treat members of the Red Army. While working with the military, he also was involved in vaccination programs for Soviet soldiers.[34]

At some point in 1939, Lavrenti Beria entered the picture. Formerly the first secretary of the Georgian Communist Party—a prestigious position considering the state was Stalin's birthplace—he had just risen to power the year before in Moscow as the minister of internal affairs of the Soviet Union. As such, he controlled the People's Commissariat for Internal Affairs (Narodnyy Komissariat Vnutrennikh Del [NKVD], the secret police agency), succeeding Nikolai Yezhov, who had implemented the Great Purge (perhaps too well since he eventually fell victim to it). Until Stalin's death, Beria served as one of the premier's most trusted subordinates.[35]

The exact reasons for Eliava's coming to Beria's attention as an "enemy of the people" remain murky, but there are several possible reasons. One theory suggests that Eliava's active participation in inoculating soldiers against dysentery backfired. Caused by either bacterial, viral, or parasitic infection, the disease was particularly present in crowded military conditions where sanitation and hygiene were often compromised. However, when two soldiers became sick after being vaccinated, authorities suspected Eliava bore responsibility. When they ended up dying, Beria had the scientist arrested and eventually executed as an enemy of the people.[36]

The second theory claims that Eliava actively sought to damage members of the Soviet population. It's a highly suspect story, particularly when he had spent the better part of his life trying to devise ways to save people from disease.[37]

Still another theory is more of an urban legend featuring a love triangle between Eliava, a young woman who worked in his laboratory, and Beria. According to this narrative, Lavrenti Beria was smitten by the woman. When he learned that Eliava and his employee were often seen spending time together, he reacted by using his power as head of the NKVD to eliminate Eliava from the equation and had him arrested.[38]

One final possibility revolves more around the political circumstances of the time as opposed to speculative mythmaking. At about this time, two forces came together to act as catalysts for Eliava's incarceration. His arrest occurred just as the Lysenkoism campaign against Nikolai Vavilov and other geneticists kicked into high gear. Political and scientific denunciations were being flung around recklessly. Immediately after Beria's ascension to his powerful post as minister of the interior and command of the NKVD, he embarked on a determined purge of intellectuals from a variety of fields. That one of the country's leading bacteriologists should be swept up in Beria's dragnet should come as no surprise.

About the time of Eliava's arrest, a young aspiring scientist name Nikolai Mikhailovich Borodin was traveling through Transcaucasia on his way to Baku, Azerbaijan. Moscow had asked him to consult with local authorities regarding an outbreak of a highly infectious disease among livestock. On his way, he stopped in Tbilisi, Georgia, and while there befriended Eliava, who was about twenty years his senior. The friendship was one of mentor and student, with the worldly, multilingual Georgian recounting his past experiences as a scientist in France. No doubt the young scientist was interested in Eliava's experiences with bacteriophage therapy since their fields of research overlapped. Indeed, Borodin would soon head antibacterial research of his own.[39]

According to Borodin's memoir, Eliava came from old Georgian nobility, something rendered less than meaningless by the Bolshevik Revolution. "He was an influential man and had important contacts in the Party and Government. He was a Party member himself and a very ambitious scientist who wanted, and had a chance, to be a great man. He obtained large Government subsidies for building a State research institute in Tbilisi for experimenting on Bacteriophage . . . and was appointed director of the new institute."[40]

Borodin recalled that Eliava viewed "the liquidation of State enemies" a necessary evil, similar to clearing weeds from a garden. His memoir also charges that Eliava played an active role in having some of the "weeds" arrested, only to fall victim to the same fate. After the scientist's death, Moscow claimed that Eliava "together with the famous spy d'Herrelle were hired by a foreign intelligence service and were acting in the interests of international capitalists to turn back the wheels of history and destroy the Soviet Union." Specious claims indeed.

In the end, while it is difficult to speculate how the field of phage therapy would have developed had Eliava lived and continued to collaborate with d'Hérelle at the institute, it's not a stretch to say that antibacterial research lost a singular mind and a passionate champion.

After Eliava's passing, Soviet, Japanese, and, ironically, Nazi soldiers often carried vials of bacteriophage cocktails into battle during World War II. Their doctors relied on phage therapy in combat hospitals. It was another tool in their arsenal that complemented the use of prevalent sulfa drugs.[41]

IN LATE NOVEMBER, THE situation could not have looked worse for the penicillin project. The more Bush and Richards pushed the pharmaceutical companies, the more entrenched their positions became. Even though George W. Merck continued trying to persuade the OSRD to proceed without Lederle and Squibb, by November negotiations remained at a standstill. The U.S. war machine, however, did not.

From the moment Howard Florey and Norman Heatley set foot on U.S. soil, the issues facing the penicillin project mirrored Roosevelt's industrial problems. Scaling up production became a paramount concern, especially once the drug's efficacy had been proven in clinical conditions. Florey wanted more for research purposes. The U.S. government wanted more for strategic reasons. The pharmaceutical companies wanted more for pure profit motives. Fortunately, everyone's interests overlapped. Initially, the cumbersome fermentation process posed the biggest problem. By the end of the summer of 1941, this was no longer the case.

When the Oxford team arrived at the NRRL, the men brought a raw product that was still miles away from being ready for army medics' kits or pharmacy shelves. It was more a proof of concept than anything else. The heavy lifting still lay ahead, and it started with improving the yields of the penicillin process. Only after they solved that puzzle could they move on to questions of mass production.

Heatley and A. J. Moyer were charged with the task of reproducing and improving the surface fermentation method. The Englishman divulged every ounce of knowledge he gained during his trial-and-error period in Oxford. His contribution cannot be underestimated. The information he shared saved American researchers considerable time and effort. Moyer did not squander the head start.[42]

Looking back, a serendipitous inevitability seemed to bless the development of penicillin at different stages. The first was Alexander Fleming's observation that the contaminated petri dishes he would discard under normal circumstances contained an antibacterial element. The second was Florey's decision to leave the United Kingdom for the United States, as discussed earlier. The third was the moment they arrived at the Northern Region Research Laboratory's front door.

One of the research center's primary missions as dictated by the Food and Drug Administration involved finding uses for corn steep liquor. Thanks to advances in hybrid corn technology that genetically modified the plant's DNA, making it sturdier and easier to grow, the United States was corn country. There was an abundance of it and its by-products.

During the processing of corn, sodium sulfate is used to remove the hard kernel encasing the corn. The resulting effluent—mostly composed of the kernels and starch—is then processed further, and the water is taken out. What remains is the corn steep liquor, which has a thick, viscous property and a slight blue color. Since maize was one of the country's primary crops, there was more corn steep liquor than processors knew what to do with. Normally, they disposed of it. If it could be done productively, all the better. And that's where the NRRL came in. The researchers basically used corn steep liquor in every process they tested to see if it worked. In the case of penicillin, it worked wonders and represented a key development in the process. Over a decade later, Robert Coghill recalled that the NRRL was the only laboratory using corn steep in its research. It was routine.[43]

"We tried corn steep liquor in every fermentation problem we ever studied. The discovery of its place in a penicillin medium was foreordained and inevitable once the problem was assigned to our Fermentation Division."[44]

The corn by-product increased the amount of penicillin that could be grown compared with the Czapek-Dox medium the Oxford group used. The mold ate it up. It was like adding fertilizer to a field of crops. It performed even better after Moyer incorporated lactose, essentially more sugars, that supercharged the growing process. It would differentiate the penicillin produced in the United States with the antibiotic produced in other countries such as the United Kingdom.[45]

The actual fermentation method offered another area that could be improved, and the Peoria lab, being experts at fermentation, did just that. After establishing that corn steep liquor supplemented by lactose was the medium of choice, the researchers discarded the Oxford group's unwieldy surface fermentation method of growing *Penicillium* mold one flask at a time. They replaced it with a method called deep fermentation that involved submerging spores in a deep drum of medium, mixing it constantly at slow speeds, and providing a steady flow of sterile oxygen. It amounted to a multi-surface fermentation method that improved the process's efficiency.[46]

Unfortunately, Florey's strain of *P. notatum* refused to grow when submerged. Moyer took it upon himself to search for a better strain of mold that would grow under those conditions. He combed the NRRL's culture collection until settling on a different strain of *P. notatum* called NRRL 832, but because the lab's collection was so limited, it proved a red herring. Rather than give up, the NRRL enlisted the aid of the U.S. Army Air Forces. Wherever their planes touched down, personnel took soil samples. Soon, the NRRL's collection included mold from all around the world. Chungking. Calcutta. North Africa. The best strain, however, ended up coming from a rotten cantaloupe sitting in a nearby Peoria fruit market. Officially labeled NRRL 1951, it came to be known as the cantaloupe strain. It turned out to be perfect and produced a thousand times more penicillin than Fleming's original mold.[47]

With the fermentation problem seemingly solved, the OSRD needed the private sector's know-how and dexterity more than ever. Producing small amounts of penicillin was tricky enough for research labs. Mass production was a different ball game and involved skills researchers did not possess.

On December 8, 1941, the Japanese bombed Pearl Harbor, dragging the United States into an actual shooting war, albeit one they had been fighting economically for well over a year. The following day, Germany declared war on the United States, and Italy followed suit. The industrial pieces Roosevelt had been preparing finally came into play. Now the successful production of penicillin assumed a new level of urgency.

3

Howard Florey's return to Oxford from the United States in October 1941 restarted British penicillin activity. While there were pockets of weakness with respect to the essential fermentation process, industry banded together to combine knowledge and efforts. This time, for whatever reason, Florey found more receptive ears.

Florey returned to the Dunn School of Pathology and resumed his research on penicillin with the help of Ernst Chain and the rest of the lab. Much to his chagrin, only meager amounts of the substance were available to him. Production had not improved much in his absence. He'd traveled thousands of miles, shaken dozens of hands, and imparted invaluable knowledge to strangers but had nothing to show for it. His goal had been to acquire enough penicillin to conduct clinical trials. As far as he could see, he'd come up well short of his goal. He'd have to produce as much as possible in his lab. And he did. Unfortunately, the Heatley-Chain process would never produce adequate amounts of penicillin in so small a space.[1]

Noticeable movement took a few months to materialize, and when it did, it came from Florey's side of the Atlantic. In February 1942 London-based Kemball, Bishop and Co.'s joint managing director J. E. Whitehall contacted Florey regarding the Heatley-Chain process. Sir Robert Robertson, an Oxford organic chemist and soon to be a key player in the penicillin story, had informed him that Florey would teach Kemball, Bishop scientists how to produce penicillin and supply them with a sample culture.[2]

Florey readily obliged. Given the realities of producing penicillin in wartime Britain once again, shortages and rationing made even the simplest tasks challenging. Proper equipment was still difficult to find, forcing would-be producers to rely on improvisation as much as inspiration. Limits on gasoline forced shipments between Oxford and London to travel a more circuitous route—a car to the station, a train between cities, and a car from pickup point—that added countless opportunities to mishandle unstable chemicals. Even something as basic as feeding the lab mice necessary to conduct simple tests ended up needing governmental intervention. But that's how it was and why the development of penicillin was anything but a preordained conclusion.[3]

At about the same time Kemball, Bishop made its approach, Imperial Chemical Industries offered its services to play an early role in the British penicillin project. However, at that point, the company's skill set did not immediately match the situation's needs. While it was the largest chemical corporation in the United Kingdom, it lacked experience in the field of fermentation and could not constructively address the issue of scaling up production. However, by 1942, the company managed to set up a small pilot plant that supplied Florey with modest amounts of penicillin.

Meanwhile, the British pharmaceutical industry waded into the antibiotic scrum with tepid commitments to the development of penicillin. In a move mirroring that of the U.S. Office of Scientific Research and Development consortium, British firms—including Boots, Glaxo Laboratories, May and Baker, and the Wellcome Trust—signed an agreement to share information with each other, but it would take another year before any significant movement occurred. Even the British government took a stake in the development of penicillin. The Medical Research Council decided that better results could be achieved through coordination with its American counterparts at the OSRD and its Committee on Medical Research.[4]

The British approach to scientific openness bears some mentioning, especially since it ran contrary to U.S. attempts at stifling the flow of information regarding strategically significant technologies. At the time, the scientific culture in most of Europe, certainly in England but to a lesser degree in Germany, functioned according to an unspoken commitment to scientific openness. This applied not only to the transfer of information but also to ownership. Guarding discoveries did not happen, and patenting discoveries was frowned upon. That sentiment certainly played a role when Mellanby advised Florey to publish the Oxford group's fermentation process. During most of World War II, British scientists—Florey included—continued to publish articles documenting their work with penicillin. This is not to suggest that all of the research made it into Axis hands; wartime controls between combatants still posed a significant barrier. As we have seen with Florey's 1941 *Lancet* article, however, the barrier was porous. Neutral countries often functioned as conduits for procuring otherwise prohibited materials.

Florey remained determined to demonstrate penicillin's capabilities. Using what little penicillin he had at his disposal, he and his wife Ethel embarked on limited clinical trials with the product Kemball, Bishop and Imperial Chemical Industries provided him.[5] He did not go far. However, his choice of hospitals indicated that he had one eye fixed on distant battlefields either in Europe or, most likely, North Africa.

Patients were selected at the Radcliffe Infirmary, the Wingfield-Morris Orthopaedic Hospital, the 101st General Hospital of the Royal Army Medical Corps, and the Princess Mary's Royal Air Force Hospital. The goals of the trials varied.[6] First and foremost establishing continued proof that penicillin's safety and efficacy superseded everything. Up until this point, the drug was only applied topically or intravenously. In the real world, that type of administration would hamper its use and adoption. The ultimate goal lay in treating deep infections orally. People preferred pills.

They also needed to establish the proper dosage of penicillin. To this point, they administered penicillin according to one overriding principle: how much they had available to them. Guesswork, in other words. That was fine for establishing that the drug worked, but in moving forward, it would never do. By determining the exact amounts of penicillin necessary to treat various types of infections, they could begin to project how much they needed to produce and how much it might cost to manufacture it. At this point, making penicillin entailed a lengthy and labor-intensive process. It cost a lot. Giving a patient more than he or she needed amounted to a significant loss of money.

In all they treated over 200 patients: 15 received doses systemically—meaning they took it by mouth or injection—and 172 received local treatment on their wounds. The infections ranged from periorbital cellulitis (an infection of the eye socket that leads to blindness or death) to chronic osteomyelitis (a bone infection that leads to loss of limbs) to mastoid infections (similar to those found in war wounds). Every infection, if left untreated, resulted in death. This time, everyone survived after receiving injections of 15,000 Oxford units every three hours. It was a stunning success.[7] In particular, one individual sparked the first spectacular media rush of the young antibiotic era.

The subject was a fifty-two-year-old man with a suspected case of bacterial meningitis. What made him different was that he was also a close friend of Alexander Fleming's family. At first, Fleming treated him with sulfapyridine. The patient's symptoms—frontal headache, vomiting, and drowsiness—worsened. A violent case of hiccups preceded the patient's falling into a coma. At a loss, Fleming sampled spinal fluid to determine what was causing the infection, something he had failed at a few days earlier. This time he met with success and determined that the culprit was nonhemolytic streptococci, a bacterium resistant to sulfa drugs but sensitive to penicillin.[8]

On August 5 Fleming wasted little time in contacting Florey. He needed help. He needed penicillin. Without hesitation, the Australian supplied what little he had in his possession—a total of 1.3 million units stored in his refrigerator at the Dunn School—and only asked that data accumulated during the case be included in his case notes. With instructions from Florey, Fleming administered the drug intravenously. For six days, very little improvement was observed. That's when Fleming took a drastic measure and injected penicillin into his friend's spine, a clinical first. After 125,000 Oxford units, the patient showed signs of getting better. He recovered fully.

When news got out, the Fleet Street press corps ran with the miraculous story of a wonder drug that pulls patients from the grip of death. It caused an immediate sensation. Much to Florey's and Oxford's chagrin, news reports credited Fleming and St. Mary's Hospital for developing and testing penicillin, a factual error the latter failed to correct.[9] It would be the start of a long-running narrative that celebrated Fleming for much of Florey's work.

All things considered, everything looked positive for Florey on the penicillin front; however, he still had not received the supply of penicillin he had hoped for. He'd have to wait for his kilogram of penicillin. Nothing came from his contacts in the States, and the same could be said for his British sources. He had to know that forces were now moving without him. Less and less information trickled his way from government and corporate sources. The process had started while he was in the United States. He no longer viewed the challenge of production as his primary undertaking. Now, he was out to prove penicillin's clinical effectiveness in the hospital or on the battlefield.

GERMAN TROOPS WERE ENGAGED in ferocious battles on both their eastern and southern fronts. Casualties were mounting on all sides. Battalions and brigades met bullets and bombs head-on. Diseases ravaged bodies. Insects and rodents nibbled through uniforms, transmitting debilitating bacteria in their saliva. Then there were the sexually transmitted diseases such as syphilis and gonorrhea. More than any form of explosive, they weakened an army's manpower to the point of crisis.

They could have used some penicillin.

Everything they needed lay right under their noses. The world's premier collection of mold. The most modern laboratories. World-class bacteriologists. Groundbreaking fermentation experts. Knowledge of the Chain-Heatley surface fermentation method. The mass production of German penicillin shouldn't have been a question of if but when. History being what it is, the ifs won the day. As it turned out, actual production was going all the while.

On May 10, 1940, the Wehrmacht marched into the Netherlands, and fierce fighting ruled the day. But on the fourth day, the Dutch surrendered to Hitler's war machine, and the Nazis took possession of the nation's riches.

The Dutch had a long tradition in the history of microbiology, dating all the way to Antonie van Leeuwenhoek in the seventeenth century. Industry and academia maintained close ties, and academic scientists often went on to become industrial microbiologists. The Nederlandsche Gist-en Spiritsufabriek (Netherlands Yeast and Spirits Factory), located in Delft, was a major research center. More important, it was one of the oldest fermentation companies in the world. In 1869 Jacques C. Van Marken had founded the company to produce baker's yeast.[10]

Over the course of sixteen months till the end of European hostilities, scientists at the factory embarked on the production of penicillin independent from American or British efforts. While definitive proof about the program's origins is still lacking, archival documents indicate that Dutch scientists had referenced Fleming's 1929 paper and a 1943 German journal that published papers by Florey's lab regarding penicillin. From there, the Delft researchers turned to their mold collection—the largest in the world—and began screening for bacteriostatic activity. They found the best strain to be *Penicillium baculatum* Westling. They called the antibiotic substance bacinol. By not calling it penicillin, the Delft group kept it secret from the Germans.[11]

As with Florey's lab in Oxford, wartime shortages forced the Dutch to improvise. They used hundreds of milk bottles to ferment the mold. During the brutal winter of 1944–45, they continued to fine-tune their process. In April 1945 the Germans allowed the Allies to airdrop food and supplies into the Netherlands. Penicillin was included, thus allowing the Delft group to compare its bacinol with American penicillin. Laboratory analysis confirmed that the researchers were, in fact, producing the antibiotic.[12]

STALIN HAD BEEN BEGGING for a western front in Europe; instead, he got a southwestern front in Africa. It wasn't what he wanted or needed to relieve the pressure from the Germans' push into Soviet land. Nevertheless, the Red Army and Russian population dug in their heels and resisted. Winter gave them a chance. Room to breathe. An opportunity to believe again. But by August 1942 the war had reverted to past form, and Soviet Russia was on the defensive again.

German forces continued marching deeper into the Soviet Union, pushing the fluid front to the east and south. Though never ideal, the Wehrmacht forces were split in two. Army Group A, led by Field Marshal Wilhelm List, included the Seventeenth and First Panzer Armies. Their objective was to secure the rich oil fields in the Caucasus region to the south. Army Group B was under the command of Field Marshal Fedor von Bock.[13]

The Nazi's Sixth Army carried an air of invincibility. Its exploits preceded it, having conquered every force it had ever met. The army trampled over Poland's armies and exemplified the word "blitzkrieg." It pounded the British Expeditionary Force at Dunkirk, pushing its troops back across the channel. When Hitler sent the army to Yugoslavia, it had the country on bended knee in weeks. According to the führer, the vaunted Sixth Army could storm the heavens.[14] In this case, all it had to do was march to the Volga and sack Stalingrad in the process. Compared to storming heaven, taking the industrial city must have seemed like a cakewalk.

The Red Army did what it could. The vozhd insisted on it. Implored his troops. Threatened his generals. Swapped officers like replaceable action figures. Occasional Soviet counterattacks interrupted hasty, often chaotic retreats. Every little bit counted, though. Even in defeat, each enemy casualty or neutralized tank represented a small gain that would eventually accumulate into a strategic advantage.

The Luftwaffe pounded Stalingrad and its inhabitants for nearly a week. The onslaught reduced factories to rubble. Residential buildings that escaped collapse burned until only an empty shell remained. The city's inhabitants fled in droves. Those who remained, who didn't want to abandon their homes, resigned themselves to uncertain fates. By the time the bombing ended and the Sixth Army's infantry entered the city, nearly forty thousand civilians had died. It was only the beginning.[15]

Archival footage of the Battle of Stalingrad provides glimpses of the devastation that the German attack and the Soviet response inflicted on the city. Troops combed the streets in small packs, moving in short bursts, one after another, scraping against walls for cover, eyes roaming high and low, rifle nozzles ready to fire. They scaled mounds of rubble in empty lots where buildings once stood. Steel and glass and concrete—all shattered—made any movement a challenge. Someone was bound to fall. Lose his footing. Twist an ankle. Get taken out by a sniper. Diving on the ground to avoid gunfire, that was when wounds happened. Soft flesh tore in an instant when it scraped against sharp edges. Even the slightest, most insignificant scratch was an opportunity for infection to set in. In the preantibiotic age when resistance was rendering sulfonamides useless, it was a game of roulette. Whether by bullet or bacteria, the result was the same—one more soldier down.

Soviet doctors had choices, though. They possessed multiple drugs that they could use against infection. If sulfa drugs failed, they had phage therapy. If phage therapy did not work, they had another alternative, gramicidin S, which is an antibiotic in the penicillin sense of the word.

Ever since d'Hérelle's groundbreaking work with bacteriophages as treatments for dysentery, cocktails made from the virus were used for similar purposes, especially in the Soviet Union and Eastern Europe. Phage therapy also proved useful in treating various conditions including staphylococcal skin infections, abscesses, vaginitis, chronic and acute respiratory infections, and mastoid infections. Its efficacy emerged as a point of contention, particularly in the West. In fact, phage therapy encountered numerous problems that the technology at the time was unable to resolve. No doubt, Soviet and Eastern European scientists and doctors encountered the same issues as their Western counterparts.[16]

The first significant problem facing phage therapy during the first half of the twentieth century resulted from the bacteriophage's limited host range. Because a virus's activity was so specific, health care providers needed to know exactly what bacteria and strain were present.[17] Diagnostics of the time made this essential step longer than ideal. When faced with a quickly deteriorating patient, phage therapy's specificity—central to its power in a twenty-first-century setting—made treatments more of a guessing game.

Another very serious problem that confronted phage therapy in the early twentieth century had to do with impurities in the bacteriophage cocktail preparations—in particular, the presence of bacterial debris. Even the minutest presence of endotoxins or other bacterial artifacts proved fatal, especially if administered intrathecally. At the time, most phage preparations were crude lysates mixed together, and patients often fell ill and died due to the impurities before the phages could cure the initial condition.[18]

In addition to bacterial debris, the presence of actual bacteria in the phage cocktails was another problem. To address this, researchers at the time used mercurials and/or oxidizing agents to remove unwanted bacteria from the preparations. Unbeknownst to everyone involved, the chemicals destroyed the coating of the bacteriophages, rendering them inactive. This resulted in failed therapies in hospitals and false negatives in research laboratories.[19]

The patient's own defenses also posed hurdles to bacteriophage therapy efficacy. The first problem was somewhat to be expected with knowledge of the human immune system. Antibodies created specifically to combat intrusions by bacteriophages often hindered the ability of therapeutic phages to perform. Luckily, this phenomenon tended to occur in chronic treatments that lasted months. Acute conditions that resolved within a couple of weeks tended to be more successful.[20]

Rapid clearance of phages was not known at the time and was only proven in 1973. When confronted with foreign proteins, the spleen, liver, and other filtering organs cleared the phages from the patient's system. At first this neutralizing effect was thought to have been due to antiphage antibodies attacking the virus; however, it turned out to be yet another attack on the phage by the human body's defenses.[21]

Doctors and public health officials were not limited to using phages as treatments. Many scientists, particularly in France, Germany, and the Soviet Union, explored the possibility of using the viruses as a preventative solution. Starting with d'Hérelle, teams of researchers could be found tending to wells in dusty countrysides and conflict-scarred hamlets in Egypt, India, or Afghanistan. They understood that only real-world success could validate a potential new treatment. A million test tubes of cleared bacteria could never match a single successful clinical trial.

Between 1929 and 1935, a team of bacteriophage scientists from the Kharkov Mechnikov Institute conducted frequent trips to its neighboring territory, Donbass. Dysentery outbreaks were frequent occurrences there and around the world, particularly in impoverished areas. The researchers seized the opportunity to test the effectiveness of using bacteriophages on patients and in the environment. It was believed that exposing the public to bacteriophages would cause them to be infected, so to speak. Once the dysentery-specific phages were incorporated into a host's body, the scientists thought the phages, along with the immune system, would protect against the dysentery bacteria. During an outbreak, this would serve to keep new infections in check.

Not until the early twenty-first century would scientific technology reach a point where the hurdles of phage therapy could be cleared without problems. Meanwhile, technology of the early twentieth century hadn't caught up to the theoretical cure, leading most scientists to conclude that phage therapy was ineffective. With the development of penicillin, the most logical course was to switch to the novel chemotherapeutic drug that had minor side effects and such powerful antibacterial effects.

During World War II, Soviet scientists worked diligently to understand and produce penicillin in the Soviet Union. Institutions doing basic research on penicillin included the Academy of Sciences (Moscow), the All-Union Institute of Experimental Medicine (Moscow), and the Central Laboratory of the Leningrad Meat Combine. Manufacture of penicillin took place at Moscow's Central Laboratory of Penicillin at the Mikoyan Meat Combine . However, it was the Medical Products Factory in Baku, Azerbaijan, that conducted the lion's share of the applied science research and production. The program was run by Nikolai Borodin, the man who had befriended Georg Eliava years before. Despite the researchers' best efforts, meaningful progress eluded them.[22]

Gramicidin S stood as a triumph of Soviet microbiology, so much so that the fate of Georgyi Frantsevitch Gause, the man who discovered it, was the complete opposite of that of his compatriot Georg Eliava. Originally, he was a Darwinian evolutionary biologist. While geneticists such as Nikolai Vavilov were being targeted by Trofim Lysenko and his scientists, Gause was fortunate enough to have pivoted out of genetics and into microbiology. So where one man was murdered, the other was feted. The randomness of their fortunes reflected the capriciousness of Stalin's purge or, perhaps, the value of antibiotics.

Identified in 1939 by René Dubos, a microbiologist at what was then called the Rockefeller Institute for Medical Research in New York City, gramicidin (not to be confused with gramicidin S) was one of the first antibiotics discovered. He made his discovery by cultivating a sample of New Jersey peat. He found that bacteria in the soil, *Bacillus brevis*, actually secreted a bactericidal substance. It killed most gram-positive bacteria by destroying their cell walls, making them susceptible to immune attacks. He called the substance tyrothricin, and it was the first antibiotic produced commercially. Unfortunately, tyrothricin also caused red blood cells to rupture, a process called hemolysis, so its toxicity limited the antibiotic to topical uses. In the end, tyrothricin was found to be composed of two chemicals, gramicidin and tyrocidine, both of which proved effective topical antibacterials.

When the Second World War erupted in Europe, Gause went to work for the Soviet Union's national defense. He worked with the Disinfection Unit with the aim of defending against biological warfare. While working in government, he used his connections to convince the minister of public health and academician Petr G. Sergiev that establishing a special laboratory dedicated to antibiotics was in the country's best interest. He made a strong point, and not only was the lab opened but he was also appointed its head. Together with his wife, Maria Brazhnikova, a trained chemist, Gause scoured Soviet soil for leads. Their goal was to replicate the production of tyrothricin that Dubos had achieved a few years earlier. While they failed to find the exact strain, they found a related strain of *Bacillus brevis* that also secreted an antibacterial substance. In this case, the bacteria only secreted gramicidin and in a form that possessed different properties, reinforcing their hunch that their discovery was an entirely new substance. In 1942, only two years after the antibiotics lab opened, Gause and Brazhnikova had developed a new antibiotic that he called Soviet gramicidin, or gramicidin S.[23]

Within months, the novel antibiotic made its way to military medical hospitals to treat soldiers injured while fighting the Nazi invaders. Gause and Brazhnikova conducted clinical trials, immediately testing its efficacy in war wounds. Unfortunately, like Dubos's tyrothricin, gramicidin S's toxicity prevented it from being administered orally. The two substances were so similar that they had identical median toxic doses at 15–20 milligrams in lab mice.[24]

The first group they tested consisted of soldiers with infected gunshot wounds in their hips; burns to the stomach, chest, and hands;

and abscesses to the lining of their stomachs. Gramicidin S acted quickly, and before long, clinicians observed the "rapid disappearance of bacteria in the wound."[25] The antibiotic stabilized a wound enough to allow surgeons to prepare it for surgical procedures. It was all they could ask for, really—a chance for doctors to do their jobs.

Gause and Brazhnikova tested gramicidin S in three more groups consisting of septic gunshot wounds to the upper body, infected compound fractures due to blunt force trauma (osteomyelitis), and severe cases of wounds with excessive pus formation (empyemas). In a total of 573 documented cases, the results were overwhelmingly positive. Their findings were published in Russian in a monograph titled "Soviet Gramicidin and Wound Healing," and on December 2, 1944, they introduced gramicidin S to the West in the journal *Nature*.[26]

The Soviet antibiotic had an immediate impact. Where sulfathiazole failed because of sulfa drug resistance, gramicidin S picked up the slack. It seemed the perfect complement for the treatment of local infections. A year later, medics at the front carried gramicidin S. It saved Soviet lives and spared countless limbs. Gause was a hero, and after the war, his status was confirmed by the country's leader. For the discovery of gramicidin S, G. F. Gause was awarded the Stalin Prize for Medicine in 1946.[27]

With the ability to treat wounds, the Red Army could stand its ground against the Wehrmacht. As we shall see to a greater degree with penicillin, the ability to fight infections meant that soldiers did not need to be replaced as often; instead, they healed and returned to battle. Inexperienced troops were given a little more time to learn. Not only that, morale improved. Net-net, the introduction of antibiotics to the war effort resulted in an increase in active troops without having to add more personnel. It was a minor military miracle.

THE MOMENT HAD ARRIVED for the British Eighth Army; 220,000 soldiers from across the commonwealth awaited word from one man, Lt. Gen. Bernard Law "Monty" Montgomery. The Spartan general. Their leader. When the signal was transmitted, they would slide out from their trenches, camouflaged by the crisp, desert night air. They knew their orders. Crawl on your bellies. Keep your head down all the way to the enemy line. Then wait again. Let the artillery soften the German underbelly a bit. When the time came, the soldiers brushed aside their nerves and just got on with it. The distance must have seemed endless, and when they reached their destination, the wait forever. At this point, everybody knew what was coming, especially the 102,000 German and Italian soldiers on the other side.[28]

At 9:40 p.m. on October 23, 1942, Allied artillery announced their intentions, shattering the uneasy quiet. The barrage deafened. It destroyed. With 750 heavy guns beating down on a single target, shells fell out of the sky onto Axis positions like hellfire, howling their warnings only seconds before impact. The Germans responded in kind.

One of Montgomery's infantrymen recalled artillery coming in. "There was a terrific explosion, and something flew past my head. It was a leg with a boot on it. A round of HE [High Explosive] had taken Chalky White's leg off. He was looking at me with astonishment and pointing to the raw, bleeding stump with the white bone sticking through."[29]

Forty minutes later, the Eighth Army infantrymen, spectators up until this point, stood up, clutching their rifles for dear life, and began the perilous and lonely march toward the Panzerarmee Afrika. They formed columns under the moonlight. Searchlights scraped paths across the sand. Bagpipes rang out in support of the Scottish Brigade. Land mines speckled the terrain, any trace of their presence made invisible by the night, the noise, and the commotion. Behind the soldiers, the stretcher-bearers were tasked with cleaning up the wreckage and delivering the wounded to medics waiting in the rear.

A stretcher-bearer recalled, "One of the casualties had both legs and an arm blown off. While I stand there, he regains consciousness and starts pleading, 'Kill me, God, please kill me.' I find I am incapable, and with tears in my eyes cover the body with a greatcoat, thinking how small he looks."[30]

Another soldier described the impact of the S mines. "When a foot trod on the detonator there were two distinct explosions. The first flung the mine up in the air and the second explosion was at waist height and it spewed out hundreds of ball bearings horizontally."[31]

Still another infantryman reinforced the chaos. "A bullet smashed into my hand causing me to drop my rifle. I felt something boring into my shoulder and a taste of blood in my mouth. Nearly everyone seemed dead or dying, and I ran away from the senseless slaughter, unable and unwilling to stay and let myself be shot full of holes like a colander."[32]

Vernon Scannell, a corporal in the Argyll and Sutherland Highlanders, had anguished memories of "the voices of those who'd been badly wounded, their voices raised in terror and pain. I can remember one particular sergeant who'd always seemed to me almost a kind of father figure . . . he was badly wounded and hearing his voice sort of sobbing and calling for his mother seemed to be so demeaning and humiliating and dreadful."[33]

The Battle of El Alamein would last for another thirteen days. All said, Axis soldiers suffered somewhere between thirty thousand to sixty thousand casualties. Allied soldiers took nearly fifteen thousand.

Fortune swung in the Allies' favor after Montgomery's victory in El Alamein. The humiliation had ended. Prime Minister Churchill summed up the sentiment: "Before Alamein we never had a victory. After Alamein, we never had a defeat."[34]

Churchill's North African crusade divided Roosevelt's cabinet from the beginning. Roosevelt's chief of staff, Gen. George C. Marshall, and Adm. Ernest King of the Joint Chiefs of Staff argued against taking part in the British North African Campaign. Their priorities lay in Europe, and, like Hitler, they viewed combat in Africa as a sideshow. They pressed Roosevelt for a cross-channel invasion of Europe by 1943 at the latest. Their plan entailed the immediate buildup of troops in England so they could begin the invasion from there. They presented their argument to Churchill and the Allied combined chiefs of staff during meetings and were rebuffed.[35]

The first joint venture of Allied forces, known as Operation Torch, involved an amphibious landing on the north coast of Africa, with two groups in Algeria and one in Morocco. Much of the terrain where they were set to land was some of the most inhospitable. The mission's objective would have been ambitious even for seasoned soldiers, but as it was the Americans' first foray against Axis forces, it bordered on masochism. They were expected to seize nine important locations along a thousand-mile stretch of the North African coast from Casablanca to Algiers and Oran. Once that was achieved—

and nothing was certain at this point—the Allied forces were under orders to push into Tunisia and capture Bizerte and Tunis before Axis soldiers could. Making matters worse, the troops were poorly trained, and the planning, while perfect on paper, was found wanting. Maj. Gen. Lucien K. Truscott, who later commanded the Third Infantry Division in Africa, called Torch "a hit-and-miss affair that would have spelled disaster against a well-armed enemy intent on resistance." Gen. Dwight Eisenhower, who commanded the entire operation, later admitted to praying as he'd never prayed before.[36]

The invasion was plagued by mistakes. Faulty communications. Mechanical failures. Missed targets. It took nothing short of a miracle to land troops. The dry run for the later invasion of Europe ended up a debacle, highlighting how unprepared the Allies were for performing a cross-channel invasion. The British insistence on fighting in North Africa first was the correct call. They would have been slaughtered if they had landed in France. As it stood, they suffered heavy casualties.[37]

Allied forces continued carrying out the planned drive toward Tunisia. Every step of the way, the Germans further vindicated the British assessment of the U.S. forces. The U.S. Army bungled its way through those initial confrontations with the enemy. Fleeing American troops, overrun by German forces, were a common site. Humiliating defeats mounted. Faid, Sidi Bou Zid, Kasserine Pass. It earned the U.S. command derision from the British, and American troops began to get relegated to minor supporting roles during planning. The Tommies even started referring to GIs as "Alice."[38]

It took months for the Americans to find their footing, stretching well into 1943. But they eventually did. President Roosevelt's instincts about getting American troops experience proved salient. The U.S. military had a steep learning curve to overcome, and that was particularly true for the leadership, from Eisenhower at the top (and Gen. Douglas MacArthur in the Pacific) to the battalion level. Yet through all the setbacks and near disasters, the Allies—particularly the Americans—always kept one eye on the ultimate goal. And with one amphibious landing under their belts and a (successful) Sicilian landing on the horizon, their goal slowly began to become a reality. With Stalin and the Red Army's tenacious defense of Stalingrad and after that of Kursk, the Axis powers' strength diminished by increments. Hitler was fighting a full-on war on two fronts now, and even when he won, he lost. If the Allies ever opened the third front, which everyone knew was coming, it would signal the end. It didn't take a military mastermind to grasp that point. And that's why everything the Americans did from Operation Torch onward was with the cross-channel invasion in mind. That goal held true at home as well.

IN EARLY 1942 THE penicillin project had bifurcated, thanks to Howard Florey's return to Oxford. For the time being, neither the Americans nor the British had produced enough to make a difference in the war efforts. They didn't even have enough in their possession to move forward with large-scale clinical trials. Establishing its effectiveness in combat situations, however, was of paramount importance. That much was clear. It mattered in the war effort and in terms of funding. Nobody, especially governments, wanted to waste precious wartime funds on a dead end.

American scientists still struggled to produce adequate quantities of penicillin. Unlike their British counterparts, they hadn't settled on a proper way to produce penicillin, let alone embark on any clinical testing. The inefficiencies of the Chain-Heatley surface fermentation technique made it a nonstarter in the long run, especially not if they wanted penicillin to play a role in the war. The size, scale, and logistics of it ran contrary to their scientific instincts. Deep fermentation, where a single massive tank could equal dozens of Chain-Heatley containers, provided a more elegant solution to the problem. And that's what modern science and mathematics are about—elegant solutions. It was also more economical and allowed for the cost-effective mass production of penicillin. Unfortunately, there was a problem. A big one.

From day 1, the Northern Regional Research Laboratory understood that deep fermentation provided the only option in the long run, and not adopting it for short-term expediency would be a mistake. It was akin to using a mortar and pestle to make pesto when a food processor sat a few feet away; the difference was that stark. One major thing standing in the way was consistency. Their results were all over the place. The hurdle must have seemed immense. A. N. Richards, the man who single-handedly moved the penicillin project forward in the United States, doubted that penicillin would be ready in time to make a difference during the current war.

That's where the pharmaceutical industry's role provided an invaluable service. Its raison d'être lay in scaling up processes originally devised in laboratories. The associated companies had the perfect skill set for the moment. The problem for them, beyond the scientific, came down to finances. If they were going to reap the spoils of penicillin production, it would be on their own dime. Their R&D efforts and future profits would not be subsidized by the American taxpayer.

Vannevar Bush recognized that pharmaceutical companies would need to be incentivized if they were to be effective. The OSRD addressed the problem creatively and facilitated the private sector efforts in numerous ways. First, it shared all the data and methods developed at the NRRL lab in Peoria, preventing any time- and money-wasting duplication of efforts. Second, any techniques individual companies developed in the process of working on penicillin would be patentable, and exclusive ownership of the technique would belong to them. Third, the OSRD and War Production Board (WPB) would ensure the private companies could circumvent the strict wartime rationing limits on key machinery, chemicals, and raw materials by providing them with "certificates of necessity" that placed them at the top of the list for supplies. Finally, the companies would also be granted tax breaks to cushion their financial risk.[39]

Giving credit where credit is due, Pfizer staked its future on penicillin. The company stood to lose the most but was uniquely positioned to gain the most and in the shortest time. Its expertise in using a submerged fermentation process in the production of citric acid informed how its researchers approached the problem of growing penicillin cultures. They knew a more efficient method was possible; it was just a matter of adjusting the process to fit. In all, Pfizer invested millions of dollars of its own money in the penicillin program. As it turned out, its deep fermentation process and its lactose solution emerged as the best of the lot. Merck and E. R. Squibb simply tweaked the process in search of increased yields.

Companies relied on Pfizer's proprietary lactose solution in their fermentation process.

Producing enough penicillin for every American soldier involved in the invasion of Normandy became the latest goal. To achieve it, responsibility for constructing and running penicillin plants fell on the War Production Board. The OSRD remained responsible for basic research and overseeing extended clinical trials.

IN AN APRIL 1942 meeting of the War Wounds Committee of the Medical Research Council, Florey offered Maj. Gen. L. T. Poole, the director of pathology at the War Office, a sample of penicillin to be used for a small trial in North Africa. The offer was accepted. A few months later, while Montgomery's Eighth Army was seizing the initiative at the battle of El Alamein, a doctor named Robert Pulvertaft at the Fifteenth Scottish General Hospital in Cairo administered penicillin to an unidentified soldier. It was the first time penicillin was used on an Allied soldier in a war zone, a monumental landmark in the brief history of the antibiotic.[40]

The subject had suffered two broken legs in a road accident. After two weeks of sulfanilamide treatment, the New Zealand sergeant's legs had not healed. Just the opposite, his pus-filled wounds and bacteria-soaked bandages reeked. Pulvertaft washed the infected wounds and sprinkled penicillin powder on them. The doctor recorded the outcome in his case notes: "Complete recovery. Streps [streptococci] disappeared from injuries twenty-four hours after start of treatment."[41] Considering that Pulvertaft had received a deliberately weak penicillin due to the limited amount available to Florey, it represented a convincing outcome.

The first soldier on active duty to receive penicillin treatment was a member of the vaunted Eighth Army. He was gravely ill after German shrapnel tore through his hips. Pulvertaft did not record whether he lived or died. However, his notes indicate that the doctor intended on testing the effects of penicillin on the bacteria plaguing his wounds: "17th August, 1942: Not suitable for treatment since probable duration of illness would absorb all available penicillin; case used as a test of action on organisms."[42]

Pulvertaft washed the wounds with a solution composed of 0.01

milligrams of penicillin. As was so often the case, improvement was almost immediate. He noted, "Patient and his friends commented on the alteration of smell. Discharge less; smell less offensive." However, when treatment with the solution was terminated, the pus and smell returned. When penicillin was applied again, improvement occurred.[43] He used the remaining penicillin to treat a few more cases. What he saw impressed him. Clearly, the antibiotic performed in the battlefield.

The results galvanized Florey. Years of work had paid off. Like any good researcher worth his salt, he wanted to conduct the trials himself and see the results with his own eyes. He immediately began planning a trip to North Africa. That would be his proving ground, where he'd stake his claim to history.

After discussions with Whitehall, Florey received permission to move forward with his clinical trials in the war zone. He was offered an officer's position, but he wasn't interested. He preferred doing his work as a civilian. The government did not provide him with a date, unfortunately. With a war going on and the Allied push to take Tunisia stalled for the winter, there was no telling when it would be safe for Florey to head to North Africa. All he could do was wait. In the meantime, he took advantage of the situation and produced as much penicillin as his Dunn School setup allowed.[44]

DISASTER STRUCK BOSTON, MASSACHUSETTS, on a Friday night at the end of November 1942. Christmas season had officially started for Americans only a day before. Technically, it was still Thanksgiving weekend, a time when Americans celebrated the transition from one joyous occasion to another. People from across the social spectrum spent the night at the Cocoanut Grove nightclub. Husbands and wives. Friends extending a day that started at an afternoon football game between Boston College and Holy Cross College at nearby Fenway Park. An unusual number of servicemen were in attendance, having been given furlough for the long holiday weekend. They brought girlfriends and siblings and childhood buddies.[45]

At about 10:30 p.m., a parking attendant kept close watch over patrons' cars. A few minutes earlier, he'd heard Mickey Alpert's Cocoanut Grove Orchestra swinging through a rendition of "Happy

Birthday." Some guy named Jimmy. There must have been dozens of Jimmies partying that night. The music died down for a moment, and the night fell quiet. That's when he heard screams. Lots of them. In unison. Something must have happened. Some kind of a joke.

But the screams kept coming, louder and more desperate.

Inside the club, eyewitnesses recalled seeing Stanley Tomaszewski, a busboy working in the basement dance floor called the Melody Lounge, struggling to find a light socket. A patron had requested he change a bulb. Unable to see properly in the dimly lit room, he lit a match. The faux tropical decorations—nothing more than tinsel, paper, and wood—caught fire like acetate film. Within seconds, aggressive flames enveloped the entire ceiling. More than one witness recalled that the conflagration spread as if someone had poured gasoline.[46]

Dark smoke filtered upstairs, followed by a sudden rush of screaming people. Flames rushed to the main floor behind the panic. Within minutes, it was impossible to see, and people ran in hopeless circles, struggling to find an exit, inhaling carbon monoxide and soot, and banging into each other full stride. They'd fall to the floor, clutching their throats, scratching their eyes, overcome by the smoke and heat. Corpses piled up everywhere, dunes of dead revelers.

All around the building, exits had been locked shut by the owners earlier in the evening. Only a handful were open. Bodies clogged doorways. The crush stuffed patrons together at the exits ten at a time, blocking the only way out. They cried for help. They gesticulated toward people chatting on sidewalks. Inches more, they'd be safe, but that final inch might as well have been a mile. Groups of firemen banded together to muster the strength to yank a man free to unclog the passageway and allow people to stream into the fresh air. It also allowed them to enter.

The carnage inside the nightclub beggared belief.

Nina Underwood, a twenty-year-old Red Cross nurse, recalled, "Unless people were covered when they got into the air, their skin fell off." For many of the dead, the terror and desperation were recorded on their faces and their bodies. According to Underwood, "In many cases before getting people into ambulances we found that rigor mortis had set in when we tried to cross their arms."

Ambulances tore through Boston's streets, delivering burn victims to emergency rooms across the city. Doctors and nurses did what they could to stabilize their patients.[47]

A scientific report written by Oliver Cope, a doctor at Massachusetts General Hospital, provided a vivid description of what the medical staff endured. "The burns were sooty and shaggy, with unruptured blebs. Many were cherry-red color from carbon monoxide poisoning. Some of them looked clean, others grossly dirty. Many of the patients had been crawling on the floor at the fire, others had been dragged out from piles of lead. Many of the dead, and some of the unconscious who lived had been incontinent of both urine and feces."[48] After assessing the severity of the burns, the staff applied boric ointment and gauze and then covered the wounds. Significantly, they broke with the consensus procedure of cleaning and debridement, opting to leave any patch of undamaged skin intact. None of the wounds were cleaned. It would become the accepted way to treat burns soon afterward.[49]

After treating the burn, warding off opportunistic infection represented a major concern. A combination of topical and intravenous sulfathiazole was administered, with most cases falling toward the latter. Because sulfa drugs could reach toxic levels quickly, internal administration made it easier to control.

Merck shipped thirteen gallons of penicillin fermentation liquor from Rahway, New Jersey, to Massachusetts General Hospital. The still experimental drug was administered internally to nineteen individuals.[50] While it is difficult to make an objective assessment of how the drug performed, especially considering the chaos, generally the staff agreed that it saved the lives of those people fortunate enough to have been treated with it.

When the news about the mysterious new drug began to trickle from the media, it was often the first time Americans heard about penicillin. They liked what they heard, and they wanted some.

EVEN WITH EACH SIDE of the Anglo-American partnership developing penicillin its own way—the British opted for surface fermentation while the Americans chose submerged fermentation—both reached similar milestones at roughly the same time. The British had already tested penicillin's effectiveness in the field with Major Pulvertaft, and with Florey at the helm, they would conduct more extensive clinical trials once the weather and the war allowed them to fly to North Africa. On the American side, researchers saw its effectiveness in almost warlike conditions at the Cocoanut Grove fire. Their similar paths would end in 1943.

Early that year, Pfizer applied its knowledge of submerged fermentation to producing penicillin on a large scale. It had converted the tanks used for citric acid production, its bread and butter, into penicillin fermentation vats.[51] The company was all in now. If the antibiotic turned out to be a dud, the company might not recover.

Turned out it had nothing to worry about. The deep fermentation process, albeit on a limited industrial scale, was a revelation. The researchers achieved yields in one batch that the surface method would need an entire factory to produce. The modest citric acid operation had leapfrogged Merck and Squibb, much to their chagrin. Because of these results, the companies wasted no time committing their resources to deep fermentation. Once they did, it was as if a dam had crumbled, and penicillin came flooding out.

News of the mysterious drug that had been used to treat the Cocoanut Grove burn victims percolated in the American subconscious. Story after story created a mythology. As Gladys Hobby recalled, "By mid-1943, penicillin's value as a chemotherapeutic agent for control of infection was known to virtually everyone in England and the United States."[52] And that meant one thing—civilian inquiries. Where can I find some? Why can't my condition be treated with it? The requests poured in. It was all futile, however, because the War Production Bureau already had strict guidelines for the who, what, and where of penicillin treatment. Until the foreseeable future, the drug remained for military use only and specifically for testing. As long as production levels remained at the middling levels currently in place, the civilians would have to make do with their toxic, semi-effective sulfa drugs.

Military hospitals across the country, including Halloran, Walter Reed, Percy Jones, Ashford, Kennedy, Valley Forge, Bushnell, McCloskey, Letterman, and Barnes, received supplies of penicillin. Each hospital was manned by a medical officer who received special training regarding penicillin storage and administration.[53]

Unfortunately, the results reflected the controlled conditions within the confines of hospitals in the zone of the interior. Would the drug perform as solidly in less ideal situations?

THAT SAME QUESTION MUST have burned in Florey's head as he sat on board the hospital ship HMHS *Newfoundland* headed to Algiers in May. It would be his first chance to observe the effects of penicillin in the field.

Most of Florey's research team arrived before he did and included Lt. Col. Ian Fraser, a surgeon, and Maj. Scott Thompson, a bacteriologist. They were under strict orders from Florey not to waste penicillin on conditions that had already been fully researched—for example, osteomyelitis, malignant endocarditis, or venereal disease. In the end, Florey left the decision to his team's clinical judgment. The penicillin team followed the Allied forces as they swept across Africa and up into Sicily for invasion.[54]

The initial situation in Algiers had improved and enough time had passed that all of the cases consisted of long-standing sepsis. They represented hopeless cases, beyond penicillin's reach. A disappointed Florey must have recalled telling doctors back in Oxford, "Send me your cases early, I cannot resurrect a corpse."[55]

He also found most army surgeons placed their faith in sulfonamides, though one suspects that was because they were the only antibacterials available for regular use. Writing to his wife Ethel, Florey observed that "all surgeons have their opinions [about sulphonamides], ranging from being no use to they are the goods."[56] This sharp division must have reflected the development of resistance among bacteria. On the rare occasions sulfa drugs worked completely, nobody complained. Of course, bacteria had exhibited resistance since the 1930s, so complete recovery from infection was becoming harder to achieve.

Florey requested that his team move closer to the front in Tripoli. Recently wounded patients there were better suited for clinical trial needs but only just. Once again, the team pushed closer to the front in Sicily, but this time only Fraser and Thompson went. They sailed on board a hospital boat and returned with wounded soldiers. The two would return to Sicily one more time and conduct their studies there.[57]

In all over a hundred casualties received penicillin. Most of them recovered. The team observed how the drug performed on a variety of wounds common to combat situations. Chronic septic wounds. Recent soft tissue wounds. Fractures. Gas gangrene. Head wounds. Gonorrhea. Burns. All of the data pointed to one conclusion: penicillin was of strategic importance. Whoever possessed it would have a significant advantage.

Florey's work had paid off. The evidence vindicated him.

IN JUNE 1943 THE War Production Board set production goals at 200 billion units of penicillin per month. A sign Albert Elder had on his desk at the time summed up the WPB's and OSRD's objective in terms of the venereal diseases it treated: "The goal—to make penicillin so cheaply that it costs less to cure it than to get it."[58] They were stockpiling whatever was not being sent to hospitals for clinical testing. Considering that only a year and a half had passed since the companies had agreed to work together and struggled to manufacture the ten thousand liters of culture fluid Florey had asked for, the WPB's request was enormous for the time. At that point, Merck, Squibb, Pfizer, Abbott Laboratories, and Winthrop produced all the penicillin in the United States. Clearly they would not be able to meet the WPB's target alone, so the board selected seventeen new companies to join the effort.[59]

A. N. Richards summarized the situation in a memo to Vannevar Bush. Projected production for the fall was at 3.4 billion units. By February 1944, Richards forecast 18 billion units being produced by thirteen companies. As for how much penicillin would be needed, Richards estimated the following: "Army says 5000 million units a month; Navy 2000; U.S. Public Health (my guess), 500 million; OSRD investigators, 400 million."[60]

He went on to add that Great Britain was said to be making 20 million units a week and that it expected to produce around 60 million units in three months. Canada had yet to produce any significant amounts of penicillin. Clearly the surface fermentation method that British industry utilized was proving to be a hindrance.

Could American industry meet the challenge?

AMERICAN AND BRITISH OFFICIALS harbored similar reservations. That's why they must have viewed a 1943 Soviet request for a scientific exchange program warily. However, as wartime allies, their options were limited, and the meeting between scientists took place in Moscow the following year. The American side was headed by Vannevar Bush; Baird Hastings, who represented the National Research Council during early penicillin meetings; and Michael B. Shimkin, a scientist who was fluent in Russian. On the British side, Howard Florey was accompanied by A. G. Sanders.[61] It was clear that someone, somewhere in the Soviet Union had made the specific request for information about the wonder drug that had been developed.

For years, reports of scientific wonders filtered out of the Soviet Union through the handful of Western reporters allowed into the country. Naturally, members of the U.S. scientific community were anxious to learn about the almost fabulous achievements of Communist science. According to Shimkin, "These wonders included the resuscitation of dead dogs; the grafting of extra heads on dogs; use of cadaver bloom for transfusion; a rejuvenation serum, ACS [anti-reticular cytotoxic serum]; and a cancer remedy, KR [Kliueva-Roskin], derived from trypanosomes. We were hoping to be the first of scientific exchanges that would open the doors between our countries following the victorious conclusion of the war."[62]

The American delegation arrived a week before their British counterparts. Their first official meeting was with Vice Commissar Vasilii V. Parin, who was responsible for medical research and education at the People's Commissariat of Public Health. He immediately brought up the topic of penicillin research and informed his guests that Soviet scientists had made some progress with the mold even without access to Western scientific journals. Unfortunately, in what by now was commonplace among all scientists outside of the United States and, to a lesser degree, the United Kingdom, they had little success producing significant quantities of the drug. Their output was limited to whatever meager amount they mustered in the laboratory. For the time being, the only antibiotic being made in significant quantities was Gause's gramicidin S.[63]

After being delayed in Cairo due to illness, Florey arrived in Moscow on February 24, 1944, with a suitcase full of penicillin vials and scientific reports describing the production and use of the drug. In addition, he brought footage of home movies he had shot while in North Africa that documented how the antibiotic performed in the battlefield. In the spirit of openness among the Allies, he shared everything he knew about the clinical aspects of penicillin, while Sanders was responsible for the part the Russians probably wanted most—the production and assaying of the antibiotic.[64]

The visiting delegation toured the Department of Biochemistry of Microbes and Immunity located in the Institute of Biological Prophylactics of Infection. There they were greeted by Professor Zinaida V. Ermol'eva who, by both American and British accounts, was a "charming vivacious Cossack woman in her forties, with a ready smile, good sense of humor, and better understanding of English than she would admit."[65] She must have been a welcome change from her more formal counterparts. Ermol'eva explained the work being done in the department and showed them around the old stone building, which had previously been the residence of a wealthy merchant.[66]

Ermol'eva emerged as a significant player in the Soviet Union's antimicrobial scene and in the microbiology community in general. In 1939 she pushed the Scientific Council of the Soviet Narkomzdrav to invest more resources in the Soviet bacteriophage research and production program. She filed an extensive report to the council breaking down the promise and limitations of phage therapy as it stood. She also placed her support behind the endeavor and "emphasized the successes of phage therapy, noting that 'phage therapy of dysentery gained recognition among physicians.'"[67]

Ermol'eva backed her words with actions. She established a new laboratory at the All-Union Institute of Experimental Medicine (VIEM) dedicated to phage biochemistry. From there she oversaw the production of phages in Moscow and Tbilisi, paying particular attention to improving the quality of the production process. She was particularly concerned with the prospect of falling behind the rest of Europe in the industrial production of phages.[68] When it came to antimicrobial information, the Allied delegation had one of the Soviet Union's top minds at its disposal.

The Department of Biochemistry of Microbes and Immunity focused on the intracellular metabolism of microorganisms. Specifically, its researchers focused on lysis, or the way microbes were attacked and destroyed, much as Alexander Fleming, Howard Florey, and Ernst Chain had. Their interests naturally led them on an experimental path that started with bacteriophages, through gramicidin S, and finally to *Penicillium notatum*.[69] In addition to bacteriophages, Ermol'eva oversaw the research end of the Soviet penicillin program.

Ultimately, the exchange did not result in any meaningful improvement in the Soviets' capability to produce penicillin. Florey had suggested that a Soviet delegation embark on a tour of Oxford's science facilities so that the scientists could see the penicillin process firsthand. Ultimately, the realities of postwar international politics proved that proposition nearly impossible.[70]

During the scientific exchange visit, Ermol'eva showed Florey a selection of the bacteriophage program at VIEM. He was less than convinced by what he saw and later concluded, "It is impossible to estimate what this phage work amounts to. Much of it, I feel, belongs to the 'Impressionist' school of science."[71] Members of the Medical Research Council in the United Kingdom shared his skepticism when they read his report. They concluded that until they had more facts about the Soviet bacteriophages at their disposal, undertaking similar research was an essential nonstarter.[72]

Ermol'eva also presented Florey with her research into the Soviet scientists' version of penicillin called krustozin. Early trials conducted on wounded soldiers indicated that it performed better than penicillin. Ermol'eva went so far as to have a friendly competition between Soviet and Western penicillins. Depending on whose version is consulted, their versions won. However, in the long run it was pointless. Soviet scientists were unable to scale up production and had to eventually settle for Western penicillin.[73]

The Allied delegation's visit proved an invaluable source of intelligence information regarding the state of Soviet microbiology as well as the conditions in which they conducted their research. Considering the circumstances, Soviet laboratories were not much different than those in other European countries. Wartime shortages limited supplies. The laboratories were housed in "old" buildings, a common practice all across Europe, where even during peacetime existing structures were retrofitted for whatever purpose was needed. They found hospitals overcrowded. Libraries were relatively up to date in terms of foreign scientific journals, one of the enormous benefits of Stalin's brief thawing of relations with the West.[74]

Unfortunately, the dramatic Soviet achievements the American delegation looked forward to seeing turned out to be letdowns. The rejuvenation serum was a variation of connective-tissue stimulators and purely experimental. The same went for the cancer cure KR. The Americans considered the double-headed and resurrected dogs nothing more than laboratory tricks. Soviet science, it turned out, wasn't much different from that of their Western counterparts.

PENICILLIN PRODUCTION EXPLODED AFTER the inclusion of new companies. By March 1944 there was no doubt that enough penicillin could be produced to meet Eisenhower's army for D-Day. However, to be safe, the WPB requested that Wyeth construct a factory utilizing the surface fermentation method in case the submerged fermentation plants failed for whatever reason.

Robert Coghill later recalled, "Our prime goal was to have ample stocks on hand for General Eisenhower's invasion of Europe in the spring of 1944. . . . Whatever course we were to take, we had to be sure of that D-Day supply."[75]

In the laboratory and the hospital, a fuller picture of penicillin's capabilities and shortcomings developed. In early 1944 Coghill toured Pfizer's new plant in Brooklyn, the first dedicated penicillin plant in the United States. The NRRL man so impressed that it convinced him that the conflict would soon be over. He later recalled, "I stood at the end of the finishing line and saw 100,000-unit vials coming out faster than I could count them. It was then that I knew the battle had been won and victory was ours."[76]

On June 6, 1944, Allied forces crossed the English Channel and began the long-awaited invasion of Normandy. Medics continued to rely on sulfa drugs to address the wounded, but now surgeons manning battlefield hospitals had a new and powerful weapon in their arsenal. It would save untold numbers of lives.

4

Yoshida Katsuji struggled to open his eyes. His lids were heavy. He slipped in and out of consciousness. Blink. His clothing clung to his body. His hair was wet. How could that be? Impossible. Blink. He remembered walking with his friends. Blink. Returning to school after a routine air raid drill. Blink. The Nagasaki Prefecture Technical School. Blink. None of the shelters allowed them to stay. No space. Find somewhere else. Blink. So Yoshida and his friends did just that. They marched off school grounds and into the nearby forest-covered mountains. Blink. They waited there until the sirens died out, and the trilling birds, unseen, signaled the time to return.

That's when they saw them.[1]

Overhead, beyond the reach of Japanese antiaircraft guns, a pair of enemy B-29s drifted toward the city. They were so high, they didn't even whisper. As the planes passed over the city, they released their payload. Parachutes. Drifting gently. The city must have breathed a sigh of relief. No incendiaries this time.

Then it happened.

A flash of light as bright as the sun.

The spark in the sky delivered a morsel of the stars to the earth. A nuclear reaction catalyzed by human ingenuity and deployed by cruelty. Atomic particles battered and split so many times in less than a second. The blast released energy equivalent to over twenty thousand tons of TNT. Its effects spread out in concentric circles from the hypocenter. Everything incinerated instantly. The farther the circles the subtler the effects.[2]

Within seconds, the streets of Nagasaki reached 7,200 degrees Fahrenheit. The vertical blast pressure reduced temples, churches, office buildings, schools, and storefronts to smoldering ash. Waves of thermal energy incinerated the people unfortunate enough to be under the bomb, reducing them to carbon. The hurricane-force winds generated by the chain reaction swept away their memories, dispersing their ashes all over the Japanese countryside. The massive gusts followed the outward concentric trajectory of the explosion and converted pieces of the shattered metropolis into lethal projectiles.

A kilometer from the epicenter, humans and animals melted into heaps of bubbling flesh, scorched internal organs, and scorched bones. The force ripped heads from necks. Arms and legs, attached to bodies by mere cartilage, were strewn along country roads and in overgrown fields and even dangled from leafless trees. However, unlike in the immediate blast circle, here the carnage varied, depending on which direction victims faced and whether anything was in their path to shield them.

The distant blast knocked Yoshida unconscious, hurling him into a nearby rice paddy. That's where he remained while his entire world burned. When he finally opened his eyes, he searched for his friends, but nobody seemed to be around him. But other people were, and Yoshida struggled to process what he saw. Then he checked his own body. The skin had fallen off his face. Sunlight from the cloudless sky seared as if alcohol washed over his exposed flesh. In a panic only pain could produce, he grabbed leaves from the ground and tried to cover himself to block the sun. Later back at his school, when his mother went to claim him, she could not recognize him from all the other bodies on the floor also waiting to be claimed. Only by calling his name—Katsuji! Katsuji!—was she able to find him.[3]

His convalescence involved grafts and surgeries and meticulous efforts to keep the open wound that his body represented free from infection. Doctors took skin from his thigh and used it to replace his face. He survived. Antibiotics played a central role in staving off infections, just as it did for the victims of the Cocoanut Grove fire two years before. Yoshida Katsuji was thirteen. Only pure luck saved him the day the bomb fell. Whether he was lucky to have been saved was a different question for another time.[4]

Yoshida's story wasn't unique for that day in that place for that event. Tens of thousands of his compatriots suffered some variation of his torture. Three days earlier, over one hundred thousand people—including noncombatant women, children, and the elderly—fell victim to the bomb in Hiroshima. The carnage of the day was as indiscriminate as it was complete. The scale of the atrocity in Nagasaki would have been almost unimaginable had it not been the coda to the bomb dropped earlier in the week.

The human wreckage continued long after the final fires were extinguished in Japan. It took the form of a "mystery illness" that afflicted citizens of Hiroshima and Nagasaki. Uninjured people started to die. Their sickness started with vomiting and diarrhea. Doctors thought it was dysentery. Wounds failed to heal. Then a smattering of purple spots appeared. Later, the ominous dots would symbolize a pending death, the same way blotches of Kaposi's sarcoma would decades later during the AIDS crisis.[5] In this case, it was radiation poisoning, and it would continue the barbarity of those two days in August.

The historical record suggests that the atomic bombs were meant to prove a point, though to whom remains a matter of debate. The Japanese hard-liners? The Soviet Union? The entire world? Certainly the Americans were eager to control the narrative surrounding the atomic bombs. The occupation forces did everything in their power to stifle stories such as Yoshida's. The concerted effort at whitewashing the devastation and suppressing news about the radiation poisoning indicated that they had perhaps proven their point too well.[6] That President Harry Truman refused to consider bombing a third city because the thought of killing more children bothered him speaks volumes.[7] It represented a stark contradiction to his declaration—"This is the greatest thing in history"—upon hearing of the successful detonation of the first atomic bomb in Hiroshima.[8]

Taken in tandem, using atomic weapons on a civilian population represented a singular event in history. It would shape international policy for half a century. In the immediate postwar years, it always lurked in the background of daily discourse. In fact, after V-J Day, the world woke up to a morning where apocalyptic weapons, real and imagined, threatened to wipe out wide swaths of humanity in a single blow. Did the Americans come to the realization that by putting the bomb in play, they had inadvertently painted a bull's-eye on their backs? What was certain was that the United States of America had introduced a new world order that broke down into two columns: the haves and have-nots. The criteria: atomic bombs, biological weapons, and antibiotics.

DURING THE CLOSING STAGES of the war, penicillin was the worst-kept secret in American history (not to mention that information about it was public knowledge in the United Kingdom). What started as a trickle of passing mentions with the Cocoanut Grove disaster dripped and dripped until the Office of Scientific Research and Development decided to control the narrative, granting the press access to key figures such as A. N. Richards, A. J. Moyer, and Robert Coghill.

The media coverage transformed penicillin into the hottest commodity around the world. Everyone wanted some, and especially governments were eager to join the penicillin club. The symbolism behind its curative powers was not lost on politicians at the mercy of fickle electorates. Preferably, they wanted to produce it on their own. If it needed to be imported, so be it.

With the horrors of the battlefield fresh in government officials' minds, penicillin took on an added significance. Of course, it served the national interest by keeping troops disease free and preventing already-serious wounds from worsening. It was like doubling the number of available troops without actually drafting new recruits. But there was more.

By minimizing the human costs of war, penicillin allowed politicians in combatant countries to soften the perception of the conflict. Consciously or not, it had a very real effect because few indicators communicated how a war was going than the way dead soldiers did. Increases in casualties would lead to decreasing national support of a war and its leaders. On an individual level, increases or decreases in casualties would influence elections nationally and locally. They altered social and political discourse. Minimizing casualties, which penicillin achieved, kept the home front supporting the war.[9]

Letters flooded into the OSRD offices from governments around the world. At the same time, Washington felt it necessary to track any work with penicillin. American eyes kept tabs on the state of penicillin research and production attempts in other countries. The respective embassies reported on three questions: Is penicillin being manufactured? Are there any plans to manufacture penicillin in the future? Is there any research being undertaken or completed in connection with the use of penicillin?

That a number of countries maintained active programs should not have come as a surprise. Ever since Howard Florey's initial papers describing penicillin's chemotherapeutic aspects and later the Heatley-Chain fermentation technique, the information about the antibiotic had circulated in the public. Anyone who wanted to investigate it was free to pick up a copy of the *Lancet*. Turns out, many did. Their engagement with the fickle *Penicillium notatum* met with limited success.

The most impressive results belonged to an East German microbiologist named Hans Knöll working at the Institute of Microbiology in Jena. His path toward penicillin followed the same trajectory as other scientists' the world over, with Fleming's 1929 paper and Florey's 1939 *Lancet* article documenting the isolation of penicillin. When the outbreak of war halted overt international cooperation between scientists, Knöll and his colleagues turned to their immediate environment in their search for a local analog to Fleming's strain of *P. notatum*. His efforts received a considerable boost after Schott-Glass and Carl Zeiss, two local industrial giants, took an interest in the search for antibiotics. With their backing, Knöll was able to regain access to international scientific journals and locate a promising strain of *Penicillium*. By 1942 his laboratory was producing limited amounts of the antibiotic. That same year, a small clinical trial took place when penicillin was applied to an injured factory worker. The results were as immediate as they were striking. Knöll and his team felt confident that they had reproduced the same antibiotic that they had read about years earlier. Knöll embarked on the quest to mass produce penicillin. In 1944 the Bacteriological Laboratory was renamed the Institute of Microbiology (Schott-Zeiss Institute). Three years later, it would be renamed again, taking on its final name, Jenapharm.[10]

Around the world, efforts to scale up production of penicillin suffered from similar setbacks. Relying on surface fermentation methods, contamination, low yields, and questionable potency plagued the production process. Moreover, most research attempts relied on *P. notatum* rather than on exploring alternative species or modifying the strains in their possession. In other words, using a similar roadmap, European scientists drove full speed toward the same roadblock that had bedeviled researchers from Fleming forward. While their apparatus and setups may have been fine, the fermentation process was more an art than an exact science. An instruction manual, which is what Florey's 1941 *Lancet* paper was, only communicated the basics under ideal conditions. It did not take into account the countless variables in producing penicillin. How could it?

While a number of countries submitted requests to Washington for help setting up penicillin plants of their own, the government displayed a wariness in giving the green light, whether it entailed its own agencies or private pharmaceutical firms entering partnership agreements with foreign entities. Mexico's desire to produce the antibiotic and its subsequent approaches toward pharmaceutical industries provides some insight.

Early efforts at obtaining penicillin included the formation of the Mexican Penicillin Committee in December 1943. A presidential decree dated February 16, 1944, prioritized the manufacture, importation, and sale of penicillin in Mexico. That the U.S. government refused to grant permission for sharing information with South American countries undoubtedly played a role as well. Mexico would essentially serve as the primary supplier of the antibiotic due to its geographic proximity. It attacked the problem from various fronts.

First, the researchers attempted the obvious, researching and developing homegrown methods for the fermentation and isolation of penicillin, albeit based on the Heatley-Chain technique. One company in particular, Acidos Organicos S. A., held promise and enjoyed the confidence of the Mexican government. While the company's progress may have been encouraging, it still needed help from someone with intricate knowledge of the penicillin production process. As a result, Acidos Organicos sought the release of technical information from the United States. The company also lobbied the U.S. Embassy in Mexico City to have Albert Elder from the War Production Board visit the firm's plant. His observations and feedback would prove invaluable.[11]

Ultimately, the Department of State declined the request, stating, "At the present time, the War Production Board has limited personnel concerned with the production of penicillin. It is felt that this personnel can be best utilized for the purpose of increasing penicillin production in the United States to meet military and other essential requirements. The Penicillin Program is in a critical stage, and our primary responsibility is to assist domestic producers."[12]

Another route entailed querying pharmaceutical companies engaged in penicillin production. In November 1943 the Mexican-American Commission for Economic Cooperation received an application from Sons de Mexico S.A., a local pharmaceutical company, that proposed a strategic partnership with E. R. Squibb & Sons. Under the terms of the agreement, Squibb would oversee the construction of a penicillin plant, presumably in exchange for a percentage of future sales. Most of the equipment would have been sourced from the United States and paid for by the company.[13]

Again Washington declined permission, stating, "Although the American section is inclined to believe that this industry might be a desirable one for Mexico, over the longer term, it has considerable doubts as to the advisability of giving any encouragement to the project at this time. . . . No action with regard to this project will be taken until the viewpoint of our government has been received."[14]

The indecision regarding the transfer of technology was on full display three months later when Wyeth was granted permission to enter a strategic partnership with another Mexican company, Laboratorio Stille, S. A. A senior economic analyst at the U.S. Embassy in Mexico concluded, "The Embassy believes that, unless the authorities in Washington perceive some objection, this new enterprise should be supported to the extent of supply assistance for the few items of equipment which may be necessary and for the materials needed in the production of penicillin."[15]

Ultimately the production of antibiotics in Mexico commenced in 1944.[16] The episode captured issues that would continue to crop up for the next twenty years. Washington DC would exercise its newfound political influence to control as much of the worldwide antibiotic industry as possible. The task bedeviled American politicians and policy makers because with Florey's publication of the Heatley-Chain process, at least one method of producing penicillin was in the public domain. Even if it lacked the efficiency of the patent-protected submerged fermentation methods developed by the OSRD consortium, it still provided a foundation from which others could work.

The State Department's unwillingness to allow American experts to consult with foreign firms eager to produce penicillin of their own foreshadowed the only strategy at its disposal. If it could not control the flow of information about the research and production of the antibiotic, it could still thwart efforts by withholding the various proprietary production techniques developed by the U.S. pharmaceutical companies, as well as the intangible know-how that could only be acquired by working with the fickle *P. notatum*. It also became clear that the mechanical technology necessary for the most up-to-date methods could only be acquired in the United States.

WHEN THE GUNS FINALLY fell silent around the world, sacrifices continued. The gulf between soldiers and their loved ones back home remained torturous. Suspicions between former enemies lingered. And the wretched plight of civilians, displaced and hungry, showed no signs of abating. If anything, former war zones from Tokyo to Berlin and from Tripoli to Warsaw entered a new phase of existence that was every bit as chaotic and challenging as the war years.

As the haze began to lift, new, artificially imposed borders partitioned entire swaths of land in Europe and Asia without anyone consulting the citizens living there. Germany was split into two sovereign nations, eastern and western, while Berlin was partitioned into four quadrants under the supervision of France, Great Britain, the United States, and the Soviet Union. Eastern European countries were technically sovereign but ultimately answered to Moscow, with Soviet control over Poland proving much more resilient. In Asia, Japan fell under U.S. control, while the Soviet Union controlled Manchuria, undoubtedly much to the chagrin of Chiang-Kai Shek and Mao Zedong (yet even that couldn't unite them). Meanwhile, Korea was split into north and south along the thirty-eighth parallel, using a *National Geographic* pullout map and no other criteria beyond expediency.

The postwar occupations—real and de facto—that emerged presented unique opportunities for the occupying nations, particularly the United States and the Soviet Union. In their cases, with proper planning, their respective spheres of influence represented both outlets for their products and sources of raw materials for their industry. In terms of geopolitics, the occupations provided opportunities to establish sympathetic governments that shared a worldview, crudely breaking down along capitalist-democracy and Communist-authoritarian lines. The occupations also served as exhibitions for their ideologies and what was achievable under each system. Materialism and idealism battled head to head.

But they also encountered a not-so-minor problem. For all the war booty, economic promises, and political opportunities dangling from tree limbs and light posts, something stood in their way—the civilian population. Millions of human beings. Conquered and compliant but only just. Military men understood that under stressful, life-threatening conditions, people were unpredictable and prone to form mobs bound together by a sense of injustice. There were times that called for tanks and guns, and there were times for bread and medicine. For the time being, stemming civil unrest entailed the latter, although in Germany's case, it was anything but an open-and-shut case.

Allied planning for the various occupations started late. It did not begin in earnest until the 1943 meeting between Roosevelt, Churchill, and Stalin in Casablanca. That was when it became clear that Germany's borders would be redrawn. In addition, regardless of whether countries were friendly or hostile, military governments would be installed to facilitate the reconstruction process. The question of punishment became a major point of contention when Secretary of the Treasury Henry Morgenthau Jr. submitted his plan for postwar Germany.[17]

The Morgenthau Plan argued that simply focusing on reconstruction and denazification did not go far enough and was, in fact, doomed to fail. Factories converted to peacetime production by the occupiers would simply be reconverted when situations dictated. Meanwhile, purging Nazis would simply drive them underground. After being involved in two world wars, Germany could not be allowed to start a third. Instead, Morgenthau proposed setting the Germans back hundreds of years by returning them to a pure agrarian society. Their entire industrial sector would be subjected to a systematic deconstruction, and in many cases, entire factories were to be torn down, transported to victorious countries, and reassembled as a form of reparations.[18]

The plan dictated that the Allies abstain from providing any economic aid in any form to Germany, nor should it be involved in any postwar planning beyond what was necessary for the military governments to perform their duties. To put it bluntly, the Germans should not be allowed to enjoy better conditions than those of their shattered neighbors, who were struggling to rebuild after Nazi aggression. It would be a common sentiment during most of the reconstruction years.

While the Morgenthau Plan eventually lost support in Washington after initially having Roosevelt's backing, many of its points were adopted after the war. In particular, the quality of life for ordinary Germans was reframed and considered an extension of the Nazi war machine. This clearly punitive measure meant that the health and well-being of noncombatants were now negotiable. From that point forward, the notion of a "hard peace" would hold sway, and the civilian population would be provided with the bare minimum to survive. A Joint Chiefs of Staff directive (JCS 1067) to General Eisenhower formalized the government's stance, stating, "You will estimate the requirement of supplies necessary to prevent starvation or widespread disease or such civil unrest as would endanger the occupying forces. You will take no action that would tend to support basic living conditions in Germany on a higher level than that existing in any one of the neighboring United Nations."[19]

Unsanitary conditions prevailed in Berlin, a city that had experienced incessant bombings followed by fierce urban warfare. The city's critical infrastructure barely functioned. The specter of communicable disease lurked in buckets of stale water and behind closed doors where Berliners shared cramped quarters.

Public health officials working in the Civilian Affairs Division were under orders to prevent epidemics as infectious diseases threatened occupying armies just as much as they did civilians. An operational health plan produced by a U.S. detachment in April 1945 laid out the concern about disease: "In the event of danger of spread of communicable disease beyond the borders of Germany, emergency measures beyond those prescribed by the International Sanitary Convention may be taken." However, in nonemergency conditions, the role of occupation medical teams would be limited to "control of communicable diseases among civilians which might affect the health of Allied troops."[20]

Of course, it was easier said than done.

To begin with, there was always the punishment problem, particularly in Allied occupation zones. Policy makers and the top military men wanted to drive home a point. They were the victors, and the vanquished needed to pay their debts. Supplying them with food when other non-aggressor nations were struggling to rebuild and feed their populations made little sense. In the case of public health, providing former enemies with antibiotics—so-called miracle drugs—that were still in short supply for everyone other than the United States was practically rewarding them for bad behavior.

A striking degree of uniformity existed between the immediate postwar needs in Germany and Japan that demanded solutions from the Allied occupiers. That's because toward the end of hostilities in both countries, Allied bombers—B-29s, B-17s—unleashed torrents of incendiaries like the world had never seen, and the inhumanity of which remains unmatched to this day. While the atomic bombs Little Boy and Fat Man receive the lion's share of fanfare and notoriety, the firebombings of cities such as Dresden, Tokyo, and Nagoya are also often cited by historians and war buffs (a perverse fascination if ever there was one). The attacks are often presented in tandem, usually to convey the destruction, if not the barbarity, of the firebombings. While Little Boy and Fat Man wreaked their devastation in an instant, the carpet-bombing campaigns were accomplished over the course of hours and saw frenzied citizens scurrying out of burning buildings and houses, and spilling into the streets filled with corpses. The futility of their flight is encapsulated by the image of Japanese civilians jumping into rivers only to find out what the dead failed to communicate: the water temperature was boiling. The floating bodies had been boiled to death, their bodies bestowed with the ultimate indignity of having been slow cooked like cheap cuts of meat.

The victorious armies marched into cities of rubble. Electricity, running water, sanitation, food, and housing were nonexistent. Writing in the *Observer*, George Orwell observed that "[as] the advance into Germany continues and more and more of the devastation wrought by the Allied bombing planes is laid bare, there are three comments that almost every observer finds himself making. The first is: 'The people at home have no conception of this.' The second is: 'It's a miracle that they've gone on fighting.' And the third is: 'Just think of the work of building this all up again!'"[21]

From a military standpoint, civil unrest had to be contained if not actively stifled. Politically, Nazi and imperial loyalists needed to lose their positions of prominence and authority. Economically, industry needed to be rehabilitated. Socially, rebuilding the housing, health care, and sanitation infrastructure was most important. Then there was the question of food. People needed to eat enough calories. Malnourished bodies were vulnerable to disease. In many ways, all of the Allied postwar plans hinged on maintaining stability. That meant keeping citizens fed and healthy.

Like most of the Allied occupation, rebuilding the health care infrastructure depended on finding the sweet spot, not more than a sliver, where punishment and compassion overlap. As alluded to earlier by Eisenhower's directive, the conquered could not be seen living in better conditions than the people in noncombatant countries had. What's more, in the case of medical issues, the victors simply could not be seen serving the conquered. Ideally, local doctors and nurses would bear the weight of treating their compatriots while under the direction of occupation authorities. As W. H. Boucher, the director of the British Control Commission's Public Health Branch, put it when addressing his officers, "Our job is to control them, not to do the work for them."[22] Unfortunately, the process of denazification and demilitarization left hospitals and doctors' offices dangerously understaffed, so much so that Nazis often managed to hold onto their positions.

The policy U.S. and British occupation armies maintained even trickled down to the dispensation of medicine. Penicillin represented a particularly extreme example, and its manipulation reflected the priorities of the respective governments and crystallized the radical change antibiotics created for military operations that exist to this very day.

THE JAPANESE GREETED THE arrival of American troops in their country with suspicion. For years they were told that the hairy and burly foreigners would stop at nothing to destroy their way of life. If that meant killing or castrating their men, so be it. If it meant enslaving their children, so be it. If it meant raping and inseminating their women, so be it. The Westerner was nothing so much as a monster. Now, the GI was their conqueror and by extension their superior. For a society that valued obedience from the top down, the internal conflict must have bordered on maddening.

Time changed all that. Interactions between the military and civilian populations relaxed, the tension dissipating into smiles and Hershey bars. One likes to think that a mutual respect emerged, though an uneven relationship favoring the American GI was more likely the reality due.

During the early days of the Allied occupation of Germany and Japan, planners zeroed in on something that had the potential to severely hamper the ability of their soldiers to carry out orders—sex. It wasn't so much the act itself but rather the aftereffects in the form of syphilis or gonorrhea or, for the truly unlucky, both.

Working together, military and local health officials first tried to change troops' behavior by force. Fraternization with the civilian population was strictly forbidden. The military men didn't stop there. As if acknowledging the uphill battle they were engaged in, occupation authorities established that under the Rules of War, "if a soldier failed to take a prophylaxis following exposure and contracted a venereal disease, he was subject to two penalties: He lost his pay while he was under treatment. . . . He had also violated an order in failing to take a prophylaxis and was tried by court martial for such a violation." On other occasions, commanding officers were relieved from their companies due to high rates of venereal disease.

It was useless, though.[23] They had to know that when it came to soldiers, fraternization, and sexually transmitted diseases (STDs), history was not on their side.

During the pre-antibiotic era, venereal diseases represented major public health threats. Syphilis and gonorrhea—often grouped together under the ambiguous term "venereal disease"—represented a real threat to military forces everywhere. Caused by bacteria, gonorrhea resulted in urethritis and cervicitis in women and significant penile discharge in men. If left untreated, it caused pelvic inflammatory disease, sterility, and general discomfort. Syphilis was more serious, and lifelong infection was the norm. As the disease progressed through its four stages—primary, secondary, latent, and tertiary—it presented a variety of symptoms from genital sores on the point of infection during primary infection to skin rashes and swollen lymph nodes during secondary infection. Left untreated, syphilis spread to the nervous system and skeletal system, often resulting in deformation and ultimately death.[24] Before World War II, it ranked fourth in overall causes of death behind tuberculosis, pneumonia, and cancer.[25]

Morbidity and mortality that resulted from infections posed serious threats to waging successful campaigns. In plain English, soldiers infected with gonorrhea or syphilis required hospitalization, and obviously even the best soldiers are useless while lain up in bed. Nobody wanted a repeat of World War I when STDs resulted in the loss of more than 7 million person days and ten thousand discharges from service. Those figures didn't even factor in troops who died as their infections progressed.[26] That they were unofficially labeled "noneffectives" tells you everything you need to know about how they were viewed in the military.

Nothing seemed to stem the tide of soldiers picking up unwanted "luggage." When Hitler's tanks rolled into Poland, syphilis and gonorrhea continued to plague armies, often staking claim to their victims even before embarking from their ports of call. The mighty freedom-fighting American heroes likewise never stood a chance against the dual assault from their libidos and the local brothel.[27] When they arrived overseas, things only got worse. Brig. Gen. Crawford F. Sams, the head of the Public Health and Welfare Section under General MacArthur's command, recalled, "Venereal disease has always been a major problem in military forces. Healthy young men are removed from normal contacts with the female sex. . . . They are removed from their home environments into a barracks environment. Whether they be in training camps, combat areas, or overseas theaters, they frequently find that it is impossible to establish normal social relations in the neighborhood of their camps or military installations, so many of them are limited to contacts with prostitutes and women who may not be professional prostitutes but who are promiscuous."[28]

The war and subsequent occupations presented unique situations for soldiers and citizens. The temporary breakdown of social norms and the forced interaction between visiting and host cultures were explosive ingredients. Right or wrong, the need for sexual release usually won the day. Making matters worse, the testosterone-filled military culture celebrated the virile male and often went out of the way to cater to his needs. Gen. George Patton distilled the reasoning and justification for soldiers' seeking out sex in his famous quip that "if they don't fuck, they don't fight."[29]

The cavalier attitude toward sex was perfectly encapsulated in 1944 at the Blue and Gray Corral. For five hours on September 10, American GIs lined up outside of a battered country house in the Brittany countryside. The building had been requisitioned by the Twenty-Ninth Infantry under Maj. Gen. Charles Gerhardt for purposes he deemed necessary to combat the Nazis. Fresh off the storming of Normandy, his boys deserved it. A sign hung over the door: "The Blue and Gray Corral Riding Lessons 100 Francs." It was one of many U.S. Army–run brothels that popped up as the Allies swept through France toward Germany.

Inside, four sickly French women did their best to accommodate the enthusiastic American libido. Earlier that morning, the acting division surgeon, Maj. Gerald A. Logrippo, paid a visit to the Blue and Gray Corral before its doors opened. Under orders, he conducted a cursory medical examination of the recruits.[30]

According to Logrippo's testimony, the women's health was already compromised. "Two of the women had bad tonsils, one had a bad ovarian tube, and one had rales on the left chest (a sign of lung disease). In general, he concluded, the women were already physically stressed and in poor health."[31] His rushed diagnosis did little to temper the waiting soldiers' enthusiasm. No surprise there.

Much to the American GIs' dismay, the Blue and Gray Corral's run ended by late afternoon. The constant complaints from the infantry chaplain—again, no surprise there—put a decisive end to General Gerhardt's five-hour stint as an army pimp and a less than glorious chapter in the annals of U.S. military history.[32]

As expected, the incident did not go over well with the general's superiors when word got out. A full investigation was conducted, and everyone involved was questioned, including General Gerhardt. While he remained coy about the Blue and Gray Corral's origins, he settled on a single line of defense he knew would strike a chord. "Boys being boys," Gerhardt had opened the brothel for the good of the American army's fight against Nazi Germany. The general claimed that he did it for health reasons.[33]

Prior to the advent of penicillin, treating a single case of syphilis entailed months of treatment with uncertain outcomes. The most common medicinal regiment came in the form of mercury injections.[34] A simple infection could take a soldier out of action for months at a time. Even the discovery of beta-lactam antibiotics could not get treatment time to less than a month. Multiply that by the total number of soldiers infected, and you get a considerable amount of man-hours lost unnecessarily. This was what General Gerhardt intimated he wanted to avoid by opening his own whorehouse. At least he could control the quality of women his boys had sex with, or so the argument went. The army seemed to agree and let Gerhardt off with a slap on the wrist (though after the war he would be demoted to the rank of colonel, only to rise to major general before his death).

The high incidence of venereal diseases among soldiers illustrates that during a war, keeping soldiers and civilians segregated was impossible. Preventing soldiers' contact with the local population was like jumping into a swimming pool and trying not to get wet. Moreover, the suffering that accompanied outbreaks of disease often found expression in the form of civil unrest. The presence of diseases among noncombatants thus presented a direct threat to the conduct of military operations.

When the need for sexual gratification mixed with the desire for revenge, indulgence often manifested in the form of rape. This proved particularly true for soldiers whose countries suffered the direct effects of war, with the most famous case being the Red Army soldiers as they swept westward toward Berlin.

In the past, treating STDs—in particular syphilis—meant painful remedies such as weekly arsenic injections that seldom resulted in cures. The discovery of sulfonamides went some way toward alleviating the torturous therapy and actually reduced the infection. Unfortunately, bacteria developed resistance to sulfa drugs quickly, and the drugs' toxicity made it impossible to simply increase the dosage administered. Penicillin changed everything.

From a very early point in penicillin's development, it had been tested against syphilis and gonorrhea with promising results. When initial clinical trials were being conducted at military hospitals, special consideration was paid to venereal diseases. Entire allotments of antibiotics were set aside for research on the effectiveness of penicillin on syphilis and gonorrhea. The results did not disappoint. Normally a single dose did the trick. The military advantage penicillin provided was inestimable.

THE CRUSH OF HUMANITY that emerged from behind shattered walls when the cease-fires took effect shouldn't have taken anybody by surprise. But it did, despite the world having fought a massive world war only twenty-seven years before. Families shuffled from behind crushed brick walls in broken buildings. Widows crawled out of underground shelters, shading their eyes from the sun. Decommissioned soldiers crisscrossed the world, eager to reunite with loved ones but also uncertain whether civilian life still suited them. Liberated prisoners of war searched for familiar uniforms and common accents. Concentration camp survivors approached freedom and a semblance of life with measured steps. The vast inhabitants of countries who had been uprooted from their homes by the Nazis packed up and headed home, uncertain whether anything from their past still existed. They found life. They found death. Most of all, they found disease.

To a certain degree, diseases are predictable. The pathogens that cause them require certain conditions to thrive and spread and not burn out. They follow distinct paths toward infection. Once they anchor themselves in the body, microbes elicit immune responses that present themselves on the surface as symptoms and begin the process of destroying its host.

War and the destruction left in its wake created conditions ripe for the outbreak of certain diseases. The aerial bombings, artillery barrages, and urban warfare decimated sanitation systems. In particular, the proper disposal of fecal matter presented a significant challenge, one that wasn't always solved hygienically. Contaminated drinking water became sources of diarrhea, dysentery, typhoid fever. The dearth of housing increased the density of people dwelling together, creating the perfect environment for diseases of crowds—TB, influenza, smallpox, measles, and plague—to take hold. The danger of uncontrollable outbreaks forced officials' hands when it came to repairing the sanitation infrastructure, providing housing, and feeding the populace.

Postwar Japan provides a perfect example of how quickly disease could take hold and the efforts public health officials took to address the problem. In the months after the war ended, the country suffered major outbreaks of typhus and TB that threatened to destabilize an already volatile situation.

Caused by the gram-negative bacteria *Rickettsia prowazekii*, typhus had been the scourge of armies around the world since the sixteenth century. It spread via lice, which took advantage of the unwashed bodies of soldiers and civilians. As much as the brutal winter stifled Napoleon's ill-advised invasion of Russia, the case can be made that an outbreak of typhus inflicted irreparable damage to the emperor's armies even before they fired a shot. More recently, *Rickettsia prowazekii* tormented Lenin and the Bolsheviks while fighting the tsar's armies, causing the founder of the Soviet Union to exclaim, "Either the lice will defeat socialism or socialism will defeat the lice!"[35]

During World War I, an estimated 10 million deaths were attributed to typhus epidemics in Europe. According to Brigadier

General Sams, between September 1945 and July 1, 1946, 33,500 cases occurred with roughly 30,000 cases taking root between January and July 1946.[36] Because penicillin, the only antibiotic available at the time, was not effective against the bacteria, the military was as helpless as Lenin was.

That same year, a major tuberculosis outbreak occurred. Since 1932 the so-called white plague had been the leading cause of death in Japan. Each year, the death rate climbed higher than the previous one. By the time the Americans' occupation started, TB was responsible for 280 deaths per 100,000 people. The figure wasn't surprising, considering the deteriorating state of Japanese cities after constant bombing campaigns. Chronic overcrowding and poor nutrition exacerbated the situation.[37]

While there's no denying that penicillin proved the perfect fit for a world enveloped by warfare, its limits became evident during the ensuing peace. It lived up to its billing as a miracle drug when treating gram-positive bacteria such as *Staphylococcus aureus* that caused so many infections of open wounds. Without a doubt, it became synonymous with the powerful new class of antimicrobials. Yet, when faced with the grim realities of postwar societies, it proved wanting, particularly when combating what Sams referred to as "wildfire diseases" such as typhus and dysentery. It was impotent against scourges like TB. Fortunately, a newer antibiotic emerged that would compensate for the beta-lactam's chemotherapeutic shortcomings. Its name was streptomycin.

ASSIGNING CREDIT FOR THE discovery of antibiotics can be messy, and in the rush to assign an accessible and logical narrative, the Fleming-Florey-Chain version of events became the official one. Unfortunately, it ignores the fact that antibiotic activity had been observed and commented on long before Fleming's 1929 paper. Moreover, the first mass-produced antibiotic was not, in fact, penicillin; it was the previously discussed gramicidin. René Dubos's work with tyrothricin/gramicidin in 1939 provided a clear proof of concept that chemicals with antibacterial properties can be derived from certain strains of actinomycete bacteria.[38] At the same time, Florey's Oxford lab had undertaken the study of *Penicillin notatum*'s baceteriostatic properties.

While fungi tend to stand out as the original source of antibiotics—specifically *P. notatum* and its country cousin, *P. chrysogenum*—bacteria called actinomycetes played a much more significant role in the history of antibiotics. Primarily found naturally in the soil, it is a general term for a host of bacterial genuses, many of which exhibit antibiotic properties (although some are pathogenic). Colonies form fuzzy microorganisms with fringes that resemble a head with a grown-out crewcut.

Selman Waksman, a microbiologist at Rutgers University, knew all about actinomycetes and worked with them throughout his career. His initial research into the bacteria started in 1915 when he observed the antibiotic activity of *Actinomycetes griseus* in soil. It would not be the last time he'd encounter naturally occurring antibacterial activity. Between 1932 and 1935, Waksman conducted experiments with *Mycobacterium tuberculosis* in soil. He arrived at numerous conclusions based on his observations that should have tipped him off to the bacteria's potential. According to his research, *M. tuberculosis* died out when placed in raw sewage or ordinary potable water. Moreover, protozoa present in soil ingested the pathogen. When he compared the growth of *M. tuberculosis* in sterile soil with the bacteria in ordinary soil, he found that the bacteria grew in the clean soil but were inhibited in the "dirty" batch. Finally, he observed that certain strains of fungi were also able to inhibit the growth of *M. tuberculosis*. All of this plus previously published material by various scientists dating to the late 1800s should have been enough to at least pique his curiosity. Alas, it didn't, and he simply moved on to his next experiment.[39]

Why did Waksman miss such obvious clues? Most likely it was because Waksman's original interest lay in soil microbiology and the role of saprophytic bacteria in the decomposition of organic materials into humus. As is often the case in any form of research, he failed to see the obvious simply because he was looking for something else. Something as simple as the term he used to describe the bacteria he was studying—in this case "saprophytic," meaning it derives energy from dead or decaying organic matter—meant that he'd be asking all the wrong questions. Had he been focused on isolating antibacterial substances, he would have been credited with discovering antibiotics before Dubos and Florey and possibly even before Fleming. In retrospect, he had enough evidence at his disposal to have made the leap. But that's the difference between Waksman and Fleming and why the latter deserved his Nobel Prize regardless of whether he was able to bring penicillin further than he did.

After witnessing the success Dubos, a former student, had achieved with gramicidin and the flurry of scientific interest after Florey's 1939 paper documenting penicillin's effects, Waksman's research took a drastic turn.[40] He joined the rush of scientists determined to discover the next antibiotic, though reading his recollections, clearly he was loathe to concede that he hadn't considered antibiotic research through his own volition. As a result, he started asking the right questions and found that the answers had been under his nose all along.

By 1939 Waksman's lab embarked on an ambitious drive to find the next antibiotic, a term he would coin. While he later referred to the process as a "comprehensive screening program of various groups and species of soil inhabiting microbes that had the capacity to inhibit the growth of certain bacteria," it mostly entailed grabbing samples of soil from different locations, isolating the microorganisms present, and testing whether they showed any promise by using susceptibility tests. It was like casting a wide net and trawling the ocean floor rather than fishing with a bait and pole for a specific fish. It also required more than a little luck, something Waksman himself conceded. His lab isolated and tested hundreds of microorganisms. It worked, though. Two of the first antibiotics—actinomycin (1939) and streptothricin (1943)—came from *Streptomyces parvulus* and *Actinomyces lavendulae*, respectively, but were too toxic to be administered parenterally. The wildly inefficient process proved effective and went on to become one of the primary techniques for locating potential antibiotics.[41]

In 1943 the third time proved the proverbial charm when Albert Schatz, a researcher in Waksman's laboratory who took the initiative and worked with the bacteria that causes TB, identified an actinomycete that produced a substance that worked on gram-negative bacteria. In other words, it worked against bacteria unaffected by penicillin. Its significance wasn't lost on Waksman, particularly when it was effective against *Mycobacterium tuberculosis*. In 1944 Waksman published the first of many papers dealing with streptomycin.[42]

At the time, Waksman received a significant portion of funding from Merck and Company. In addition to its financial support for the development of new drugs, the Rahway, New Jersey, company made its chemists available to Waksman, provided the use of its testing facility at the Merck Institute, and made the implicit agreement that a pilot plant would be available when the time came to scale up production. Waksman's lab managed to make only enough streptomycin to conduct initial efficacy tests. To have enough to test, the fermentation process ran around the clock, forcing Waksman's staff to sleep in the office. (Presumably, the principal investigator had a good night's sleep.) Once the researchers proved and published a paper detailing the nature of the new antibiotic, it was time to pass the production baton to the people at Merck.[43]

By this time, Merck had already acquired a vast amount of experience with the temperamental manufacturing process that produced penicillin. Its scientists understood the importance of the growth medium and how it influences the end product. They had already worked out the most efficient ways of extracting the active chemical. Most important, the surface fermentation method had already been shown wanting. Producing streptomycin came down to tweaking each step as opposed to starting from scratch and in the dark. It was this knowledge, the so-called technological know-how, that proved invaluable and nearly impossible to re-create without help. It gave the United States—the experts on antibiotic deep fermentation methods—a considerable advantage that surpassed even its closest allies, Canada and the United Kingdom.

When the time came to conduct tests on animals, Waksman relied on Merck's patronage and was not let down. The chemists at the company produced enough for limited testing. When physicians at the Mayo Clinic then agreed to conduct clinical trials there using streptomycin, Merck supplied it on demand.[44] The ease of bringing streptomycin to the market owed everything to the rocky path Howard Florey had cleared for penicillin and the vital lessons learned by the OSRD consortium, particularly from a production standpoint. That streptomycin proved chemically more stable than penicillin and therefore less prone to degradation and contamination helped as well.

Streptomycin seemed to pick up where penicillin left off. Most of its activity took place on the gram-negative end of the spectrum. All forms of the disease tularemia were susceptible. At the time, streptomycin was the primary chemotherapeutic agent used against the highly contagious disease. It proved mildly effective against cholera and very effective against urinary tract infections since gram-negative bacteria played outsized roles in its development. In a more general sense, the antibiotic performed well in most cases where gram-negative bacteria were involved.

The most important role of the new antibiotic, however, was in the treatment of TB. In vitro and in vivo, it performed well against *M. tuberculosis*. Considering the damage the so-called white plague or consumption played in history, it's hard to argue against the fact that streptomycin continued the medical revolution penicillin started and perhaps even surpassed it in global importance.

5

For years, George W. Merck was privy to some of Washington DC's darkest secrets. Under his direction, scientists embarked on the first coordinated, interagency effort to develop biological warfare capabilities in American history. Plague, anthrax, smallpox, cholera, botulism—everything was fair play as long as the threat of an attack remained. And all of the research conducted on American soil proceeded under the guise of defensive readiness as opposed to first-strike capabilities. When the war ended, Merck compiled a comprehensive study of the U.S. biological warfare (BW) program and analysis of German and Japanese capabilities at the behest of Secretary of War Henry Stimson. His analysis and recommendations would influence the path America's BW program would take for years to come, even after he had left the program and returned exclusively to civilian service.

On January 3, 1946, the U.S. Army called a press conference about the in-depth investigation Merck conducted regarding the clandestine BW program and his concluding correspondence with Secretary of War Stimson.[1] The army wanted to seize the initiative and present his findings to the public. It was the perfect way to avert the possibility of leaked information that may or may not have been factually correct. It allowed the military to control the narrative. By bringing general information of the program out into the public, the army gave the illusion of transparency. Meanwhile, not a single specific detail about the program's research was shared. In essence, the army had transformed its existence from an explosive and potentially damaging secret to an opaque piece of common knowledge.

The question of biological warfare had vexed military and government officials from logistical, theoretical, and ethical standpoints.

Everyone understood disease and the suffering that resulted from it. Weaponizing the physical suffering elicited a visceral response, even among people "in the business." While making the case for a BW program to President Roosevelt, Stimson went so far as to admit, "Biological Warfare is, of course, 'dirty business' but . . . we must be prepared."[2]

Early on, controlling infections emerged as a major logistical concern, particularly when dealing with infectious diseases. There was simply no way of preventing the spread of disease to civilian populations. That also meant that there was no guarantee that American soldiers could avoid being infected. As a result, BW always received tepid support. A niggling uncertainty persisted among policy makers, particularly from a defensive standpoint.

In October 1941 Stimson turned to the National Academy of Sciences and requested that it investigate the potential of BW. The resulting committee was called the War Bureau of Consultants. It consisted of members of the Office of Scientific Research and Development, the Chemical Warfare Service, the Office of the Surgeon General, the Department of Agriculture, the U.S. Public Health Service, and the National Academy of Sciences.[3]

Five months later, the committee reported its findings. The offensive deployment of biological weapons by foreign states was indeed feasible, and, by extension, defensive measures needed to be developed with some urgency. Stimson acted on the committee's recommendations immediately and approached the president about creating a civilian agency to oversee the nascent BW program. By August 1942 the War Research Service (WRS) was created under the Federal Security Agency with George W. Merck recruited to serve as its director. In addition, a committee of prominent scientists, called the ABC Committee, was formed by the National Academy of Sciences and the National Research Council that would provide expert advice to the WRS.[4]

Under Merck's direction, the WRS began to lay the groundwork for "the organization of a program of research and development to extend the boundaries of knowledge concerning the use of pathogenic agents as a weapon of war and as a means of protection against enemy use of these agents." Every disease-causing pathogen was studied and tested for its potential as a weapon. Microbes that showed promise were assigned to a network of university and private research laboratories for further evaluation. Each agent was tested for its lethal properties and means of production and for how the agent could be defended against. One of the main objectives of the BW program was to test the effectiveness of antibiotics against potential BW agents.[5]

Eventually, the Chemical Warfare Service was asked to assume responsibility for a larger-scale program of research and development. Fort Detrick became the heart of the BW program. However, as it ballooned in size, the War Department stepped in and assumed full responsibility for research and development. Merck was named chairman of the U.S. Biological Warfare Committee. In this role, he would act as an adviser to Secretary of War Stimson and as a liaison between the United States and representatives of British and Canadian BW programs.[6]

Safety remained a daily concern for researchers and policy makers. Many of the microorganisms researchers handled were dangerous in their natural state. The weaponization of pathogens for BW use entailed not only identifying the best candidates but also engineering them with the aim of increasing their virulence and contagiousness. According to the Merck report, there were "only sixty cases of proven infection caused by accidental exposure to virulent biological warfare agents which required treatment." At the time of the press conference, fifty-two had recovered fully, while the remaining eight were still being treated. In addition, 159 accidental exposures were reported with only one person actually falling sick.[7]

One passage in particular deserves attention: "Obviously none of these cases were brought about intentionally, and were not, therefore, 'controlled' experiments, but in any event certain valuable information was obtained from their treatment, particularly with regard to new antibiotics, chemotherapeutic agents, and immunizing procedures, which, but for these cases of accidental infection, could otherwise have been tested only in animals. Considering the variety of highly pathogenic agents handled, the scale of operations employed, and the relatively large number of people involved, the safety record of our biological warfare program is truly remarkable."[8]

The paragraph highlights the importance antibiotics played in the program and, by extension, the primary role they would play in defending the United States in the event of a biological attack. Antibiotics provided a safety net in case something went terribly wrong. Unfortunately, the wonder drugs served a more sinister role in the hands of industrious scientists as it also provided them with a model to improve their weapons. BW scientists designed bacteria with resistant characteristics, rendering antibiotics useless.[9]

Merck's statement also highlights one of the unintended benefits of having workers infected by mistake. It was one of the rare occasions when scientists actually possessed experimental data that included humans, albeit acquired in less than ideal conditions.

What was left unsaid but very much implied in that same paragraph represented the single-most significant hurdle that faced the BW program and one that lingers to this day—human experimentation. It was a moral quandary that vexed the development of modern biological weapons because there were no simple solutions to such a straightforward question. For obvious reasons, testing fatal pathogens on people was a nonstarter. Dead bodies on the scale needed for proper experimentation would be hard to hide, much less explain. Yet, without testing the effectiveness of a biological agent and the ability to deliver the pathogenic payload without compromising its potency, there were few ways to gauge a weapon's effectiveness. It was similar to developing a drug to fight dengue fever without ever testing to see whether it worked.

By the end of World War II, official public accounts of the U.S. biological warfare program indicate that the only microorganism researchers produced in large quantities was a harmless, black-pigmented bacterium previously called *Bacillus globigii* but is known today as *Bacillus atrophaeus*. Under normal circumstances, researchers rely on *B. globigii* as an indicator strain for various decontamination processes; however, its most prominent use is as a BW simulant, specifically as a stand-in bacterium for *B. anthracis*, the bacteria responsible for anthrax. During BW testing—for example, determining scatter patterns of aerosolized pathogens—*B. globigii* serves as a surrogate. In addition, certain strains developed at Fort Detrick were selected because they exhibited high sporulation rates, a trait valued by BW scientists.[10]

The report hinted that at least five countries possessed active biological warfare programs: the United States, Canada, Great Britain, Japan, and Germany. The glaring omission was obviously the Soviet Union.

Merck concluded his report with a warning: the work done in the BW field by the United States, the United Kingdom, and Canada indicated other countries could duplicate it and establish BW programs of their own. "It is important to note that, unlike the development of the atomic bomb and other secret weapons during the war, the development of agents for biological warfare is possible in many countries, large and small, without vast expenditures of money or the construction of huge production facilities. It is clear that the development of biological warfare could very well proceed in many countries, perhaps under the guise of legitimate medical or bacteriological research."[11]

That last sentence highlighted profound implications for the global antibiotic industry and the Cold War, ones that would play a supporting role in the rapid emergence of resistance.

GEN. ISHII SHIRO DESERVED to hang. At the least, he deserved to spend the rest of his life in prison, atoning for the barbarity his men inflicted in his name. Instead, he enjoyed the protection of one of the world's newest superpowers. Not only that, he felt confident enough in his relationship with his American interrogators to set the conditions for his cooperation: Ishii wanted full immunity from war crimes prosecution and nothing less. In the backdrop, the International Military Tribunal for the Far East crept toward public trials with armies of translators, investigators, military policemen, intelligence officers, and lawyers working around the clock preparing legal cases against suspected war criminals. Members of the emperor's armies languished in prisons from Russia to Japan. But not Ishii. He was special. He had information the U.S. government desperately wanted to own and no doubt believed, as one of the victors, it was entitled to possess.[12]

For years, rumors about Japan's biological warfare program, Unit 731, and its leader, Ishii Shiro, made their way to Washington. During the Pacific war, the Chinese government accused the Japanese Imperial Army of developing weaponized strains of cholera and bubonic plague in its primary research center at Pingfan, China, and then deploying them among residents in surrounding areas. Japan denied the accusations, and most Western experts doubted the Asian country's ability to succeed in an area they'd so far failed to crack.[13]

As the conflict progressed, that view began to change, thanks to a number of events. First, intelligence confirmed that plague had indeed occurred in areas of Manchuria where there had been no record of prior outbreaks. Taken with China's repeated accusations, it raised concerns among Allied military officials.[14] As the war continued, captured Japanese documents went a step further in confirming the rumors by indicating the primary locations of research facilities and revealing that the BW centers functioned under the aegis of Water Supply and Purification units. They also detailed how Japanese planes dropped allegedly infected cargo consisting of wheat and fleas into cities that soon afterward experienced outbreaks of plague. The documents reinforced the findings of Allied intelligence data. They also included reports indicating that local livestock had been deliberately infected with glanders, an animal disease caused by the bacterium *Burkholderia mallei* that had the potential to infect humans. The name "Ishii Shiro" also emerged as the head of Japan's BW efforts.[15]

By 1944 Allied intelligence began filling in the blanks regarding the Japanese BW program and firmly established Ishii's role. A larger, intricately linked operation that connected facilities in Pingfan, Mukden, and Harbin to research universities across Japan proved that initial conclusions regarding Japan's technological ability to develop biological weapons sorely underestimated the threat. At the same time, documents show that Washington grew particularly concerned that Japan would launch a biological attack as a last measure of desperation.[16] That the phenomenon of kamikaze pilots emerged as a means of combat indicated that Japanese military officials viewed victory as an increasingly remote outcome. BW could not be far off, or at least that was how the logic went, and a barrage of mysterious hot air balloons from Japan that landed in the United States increased the paranoia. American officials went from underestimating the Japanese BW program to grossly overestimating its capabilities.

Perhaps the most striking aspects of the information trickling out of Manchuria were indications that Unit 731 researchers had experimented on Chinese and Allied prisoners of war. As a result, President Roosevelt went so far as to warn the Japanese that if their activities were not halted, the military would inflict retaliation on the Imperial Army "in full measure." Unfortunately, the indignation and moral outrage expressed did not extend to the scientists and their research findings. In other words, U.S. and Allied governments objected to the policy of forced human experimentation but not to the practice. The postwar coddling of General Ishii proved a prime example.[17]

For the former Allied powers—France, Great Britain, the United States, and the Soviet Union—payback didn't end with casualties in the millions, cratered sidewalks, rampant disease, and rolling waves of rape. Articles of surrender only formalized defeat. Humiliation came later. It was a lesson dispensed with palpable venom and satisfaction. Whether the people of Germany and Japan liked it or not, payback had just begun.

Reparations assumed various forms. Contrary to popular belief, monetary compensation played a minimal role. Requisitioning factories and industry in occupied territories offered much greater returns in the long run. Entire buildings were carefully taken apart in East Germany and transplanted to the Soviet Union. If allowed to remain, much of their output made its way to Moscow either free of charge or at a significant discount, echoing the imperialist trade that formed between colonies and their colonizers.

Payback also appeared in the form of what historian John Gimbel referred to as intellectual reparations, consisting of the forced technological transfer of confidential trade and manufacturing secrets. In other words, there was more to war booty than treasure chests and confiscated weapons. A much more lucrative and long-lasting reparation entailed the seizure of industrial know-how. In the case of the production of penicillin, it would have meant the difference between miraculous success and abject failure. The parties engaged in the Unit 731 horse race believed it held true in the field of biological weapons as well. At worst, the troves of data that resulted from Unit 731's work provided researchers with unprecedented information regarding potential methods of infecting victims, how the human body reacted to different diseases, and which microorganisms made the most promising biological weapons. They could avoid investigative dead ends and, in the process, save valuable funding. The information also provided insights regarding how to defend against a biological attack, since the Japanese were equally interested in protection. There was no way to quantify the actual value of Unit 731's trove of data.

Immediately after the war, experts from Camp Detrick landed in Japan tasked with a single goal—tracking down Ishii. Col. Murray Sanders was initially assigned to lead the manhunt, though he would later be replaced by another Detrick scientist, Lt. Col. Arvo Thompson, who in turn was replaced by Dr. Norbert Fell. The hunt was also high on Douglas MacArthur's list, with him purportedly asking, "Where is Ishii?" upon landing at Atsugi Airport for the first time. From that point forward, the supreme commander for the Allied powers (SCAP) followed the investigators' efforts carefully, often meeting with them for personal updates, offering advice, and signing off on offers of immunity to former Unit 731 members in exchange for information leading to Ishii. Once they had the general in custody, SCAP kept him in isolation, going so far as rebuffing Soviet requests to extradite him so he could go on trial for crimes against humanity during war crimes trials in Khabarosk. Ultimately, Moscow issued muted protests since thirty-five Unit 731 scientists would eventually join the Soviet BW program and avoid extended prison sentences.[18]

Interrogations of Unit 731 members and limited access to documents described a program with striking similarities to the U.S. program hinted at in the Merck report. Japanese researchers investigated *Salmonella typhi* (typhoid fever), *Salmonella enterica* (paratyphoid fever), *Vibrio cholerae* (cholera), *Shigella* (dysentery), *Yersinia pestis* (bubonic plague), and *Burkholderia mallei* (glanders), to name a few. As with the U.S. efforts, the Japanese ran the gamut of infectious pathogens to see which ones held the most potential. According to interrogated scientists, they conducted field trials with mainly nonpathogenic organisms, the same way the U.S. program relied on *B. globigii*. They did admit to live testing anthrax and glanders pathogens.[19]

Unit 731 also focused on methods of dissemination since creating virulent strains of contagious organisms was useless unless a reliable means of delivering them existed. They attempted to use bombs dropped from airplanes, artillery shells, aerosol sprays from airplanes, and human delivery. Of all the methods they explored, bombs held their attention most. It was also probably the trickiest to perfect since bombs—which tend to explode at some point—usually ended up destroying their disease-causing payloads. (You don't boil water to purify it for nothing.) Extreme heat ended the campaign before it began. Non-exploding bombs posed a different problem. While their payloads remained intact and viable, the pathogens often failed to spread and, given time, would eventually die without a host. Other times, the blowback from the biological attack would cause infections among Japanese troops as well.[20] Perhaps because of the Japanese struggles, American BW scientists invested heavily on aerosolized delivery methods.

Once SCAP investigators gained access to most of Unit 731's documents, they realized that the Japanese had actually conducted experiments on live human beings. They infected Chinese prisoners of war with glanders, anthrax, and plague, to name a few. They also tested various methods of dissemination from exploding bombs to porcelain containers.[21] While they may not have devised a working model yet, they had significant data documenting what did not work.

The Americans' pursuit and protection of General Ishii and many of his Unit 731 scientists was a perfect example of the forced transfer of technology. Up until end of World War II, Japan had one of the biggest, if not the biggest, BW programs in the world. The United States, meanwhile, had just launched its program. Unit 731's data gave the American researchers a head start. It was as if they were running the fifty-yard dash and starting from the twenty-five-yard line.

MERCK'S REPORT SIGNALED A significant policy shift in Washington, one that saw government officials abandon self-enforced silence and embrace disingenuous openness. It was also reflected in British and Canadian media coverage of the topic. The specter of biological warfare never faded far from the spotlight. Newspaper headlines made sure of that: "Scientists See U.S. Very Vulnerable to Germ Warfare," "Congressmen Reveal Germ Weapon Can Wipe out City at Single Blow," "Destruction by Disease Looms as Rival to Atomic Bombs and Gases," and "Bacteria Put above A-Bomb as Weapon."[22] By 1949 there were rumors of a biological superweapon, forcing Secretary of Defense James Forrestal to break a three-year enforced military silence and go on the record with the sole purpose of dispelling the rumors.[23]

One of the ironies of the secret Japanese BW program SCAP and Fort Detrick investigators frantically chased was that it wasn't that much of a secret. They only had to take the ominous Chinese reports, subsequently repeated by government officials, at their word. Considering the contemporary colonial attitudes in place at the start of the war—most of Asia still "belonged" to Western countries—that Chinese exhortations were dismissed as "Oriental hysterics" is not surprising. Media coverage was minimal. However, one science writer did take them at their word and served one of the most incendiary, worst-written, and misinformed accounts of biological warfare in history. And its publication caused panic among American policy makers.

Published in July 1944, *Japan's Secret Weapon* claimed to be a tell-all exposé documenting the capabilities of the Japanese biological warfare program and the U.S. Army's inability to deal with an attack by unconventional weapons. The book's author, Barclay Moon Newman, used the accusations made by the Chinese Embassy as his start point. He singled out Miyagawa Oneji from the University of Tokyo as the head of Japan's BW program. He was wrong, of course. Moreover, he failed to even mention Unit 731 once.[24]

By sheer coincidence, Capt. Saul Jarcho, a member of the Medical Intelligence Division of the Surgeon General's Office, came across an advertisement for the book in the *New York Times* and immediately looked for it in local bookstores. Unable to locate a copy, he went straight to its publisher, Current Publishing Company, in search of answers.[25]

News of Newman's book sped through the top secret channels involved in the BW program as well as the Counterintelligence Corps,

Chemical Warfare Service, U.S. Army Intelligence (G-2), and Office of Public Information. It also came to George W. Merck's attention. Together with his executive officer, Lt. Cdr. William B. Sarles, a bacteriologist at the University of Wisconsin, they played a central role in the analyzing the book and developing a strategy to address it. According to Roger B. Jeans Jr., "Merck and Sarles moved swiftly. The very next day, they reported back to Special Assistant to the Secretary of War Harvey Bundy that the book was 'an emotional and inflammatory piece of writing and its publication is to be regretted.'"[26]

As a work of scholarship, *Japan's Secret Weapon* fell far short of a home run, and as far as facts go, it barely landed in foul territory. Newman's book lacked any concrete information about Japan's BW program. Instead, he relied on hysterical declarations about Miyagawa, unfairly characterizing him as the evil villain driving the program forward. He also used innuendo in the place of a rational argument. The alarmist tone betrayed Newman's likely goal when he set out to write *Japan's Secret Weapon*: he wanted to make a name for himself by using the only tools at his disposal—unabashed scaremongering and sensationalism.

The few book reviewers who did notice Newman's book tended to take him to task for his faulty polemics, if not for his intellectual slothfulness. Everyone, however, recognized the importance of the book's publication, regardless of the disparaging criticisms.

The significance of *Japan's Secret Weapon* lay in the potential interest it might trigger among the public and the elected officials representing them in Congress. The last thing elected officials and the military wanted was to answer questions regarding their covert and morally questionable research into yet another means of killing and the unfounded accusation that the government had been delinquent in its responsibility to protect the American people. They grappled with whether to suppress or ignore the book, wary of the unintended consequences of whatever action they adopted. On the one hand, ignoring the book ran the risk of allowing Newman's false facts to go unchallenged. On the other hand, attacking the book would only serve to call more attention to the book than it warranted. After all, wasn't all press good press?

After weeks of debate, Merck and other people involved in the

BW program settled on a strategy tailor made to address the problems Newman's work posed. First, they adopted a wait-and-see attitude toward the book. They closely monitored press coverage of the book and mentions of biological warfare and ensured that a sense of panic did not take hold of the public. Merck and Sarles agreed with the running consensus that suppressing the book would be counterproductive. They went on to suggest discrediting the book, whether it be through negative book reviews or requests that news sources ignore it. "If means were available to prevent reviews and ensure that all references to the book be eliminated from newspapers and magazines, and above all 'digest prevented' it would be very desirable." They also suggested *Japan's Secret Weapon* would open up the Office of the Surgeon General and the navy to attacks in the press. They advised drafting a public statement, "should the book arouse more than passing interest and result in apprehension on the part of sufficient members of the public." It would explain that the dangers were known and that defensive measures were in place and "constantly being improved." Moreover, they would inform the public that the government was taking active steps to develop defenses against a BW attack.[27]

After the Merck report, U.S. officials implemented the strategy of acknowledging the BW program in the most opaque manner possible while pivoting toward a discussion of the country's defensive readiness. While officials would affirm the presence of an offensive BW program, they stressed that the primary concern was building an adequate defensive response to attack. The argument would eventually evolve into the standard explanation given by governments across the world: the need to develop a defensive BW program entailed first creating pathogens on steroids and ways of disseminating them so that government scientists could develop defenses against them. After all, they could not defend against a weapon that did not exist.

The Americans had little choice but to embrace the existence of their biological warfare program. The preparations for the various war crimes trials indicated that the subject would inevitably arise. No matter how much they wanted to keep it under wraps, they could not. What really mattered at that moment was diverting attention from the Japanese program as much as possible.

THE DISCOVERY OF STREPTOMYCIN revolutionized tuberculosis treatment around the world. One of the first places to experience the antibiotic's benefits was occupied Japan. However, by itself, the antibiotic could only do so much. The SCAP Public Health and Welfare (PH&W) Section, headed by Brig. Gen. Crawford Sams, and the Japanese Ministry of Health and Welfare combined forces to implement a full-scale holistic approach to attacking the TB problem.

When the occupation began, the first thing the PH&W program did was to make sure each city's sanitation and hygiene infrastructure was rebuilt. Teams of workers went out literally to clean the city. They cleared rubble, collected trash, and cleared drains. Engineers repaired the water supply systems so that clean potable water was available to everyone. They also engaged in pest eradication so that disease vectors such as rats and mosquitoes were greatly reduced.[28]

Rehabilitating the public health system presented a major challenge due to the abject state of every hospital. Private hospitals usually consisted of nothing more than straw mats and rudimentary medical equipment. They were poorly staffed and lacked any centralized standards. Public hospitals received funding from the government and were better, though by the end of the war when the funding had dried up, the standard of care had fallen precipitously. Only the military hospitals that catered to officers in the Imperial Army still retained any semblance of being health care facilities.[29]

General Sams took a personal interest in fixing the country's hospitals and sanatoriums. He visited many of them during the first few months of his time with the PH&W Section. He found many of their beds empty. In fact, only 25 percent were occupied. Some of this phenomenon was because of shortages in food and medical supplies, but it was also the result of the Japanese tendency to avoid disclosing TB in the family. The stigma attached to the disease effectively crippled efforts to control it from the outset. Increasing the number of beds and occupancy rates remained a major focus of the PH&W Section.[30]

Staffing the hospitals presented another problem. At first, the PH&W Section was faced with a dual problem. It felt that the level of training, particularly in terms of tuberculosis care, was not adequate. Additionally, most of the doctors had been part of the imperial war machine, and SCAP wanted them purged from practicing medicine. To solve this, a new crop of Japanese doctors and nurses was trained according to U.S. standards. Eventually, the new doctors filled the hospitals and sanatoriums, pushing out the older ones.[31]

While the PH&W Section was tending to restoring basic health and hygiene services, the officials also set out to collect the most up-to-date data. Even though the Japanese had carried out surveys and other forms of data collection, their records were incomplete, particularly on TB data. Most likely, it was due to the fact that toward the end of the war as cities suffered repeated bombings, social services broke down. Armed with new statistics for disease morbidities, food supplies, and locations of indigent populations, the PH&W Section and the Ministry of Health and Welfare set out to inoculate the civilian population with the bacille Calmette-Guérin vaccine. Statistics showed that during the early years of the occupation, TB mortality rates were highest among young children (younger than ten years of age) and young adults (twenty-five years of age).[32] To attack the problem in young children, the first school lunch program was established nationwide as well. An improved, higher-quality caloric diet served as an additional preventative measure. Better-fed children had stronger immune systems for the most part.[33]

Finally, the PH&W Section launched an ambitious drive to treat people suffering from TB with streptomycin and to administer it to people who were simply asymptomatic carriers since they were still contagious. The task was complicated by the stigma and discrimination that TB carried. Many believed the condition was the result of a genetic disorder, so families were wary of sending loved ones to hospitals or sanatoriums for treatment. The health workers did their best to encourage people with the disease to come forward for treatment in either hospitals or sanatoriums. Part of this effort entailed public education campaigns in the media and public places. Eventually, the PH&W's and the ministry's determination won out. Citizens came around to a better understanding of tuberculosis, its origins, its prevention, and, most important, how and where to get treatment. Streptomycin allowed a stigmatized and deadly disease to be cured.[34]

The concerted efforts of SCAP's Public Health and Welfare Section and the Japanese Ministry of Health and Welfare resulted in a 79 percent drop in TB morbidity rates between 1945 and 1948. The mortality rate dropped from 280 deaths per 100,000 to 181 per 100,000 in 1948. Morbidity and mortality continued to fall for the length of the occupation and even after the last of the U.S. occupation forces departed. Armed with streptomycin, the U.S. anti-TB campaign represented an early and successful example of medical diplomacy, made possible thanks to antibiotics.[35]

U.S. COMPANIES ALSO ENJOYED the fruits that the end of World War II made available. The lifting of rations and the increasing demand for penicillin from the civilian population allowed antibiotic manufacturers to invest more money into production facilities. The six production plants that had been built using public money during the war were now sold at a steep discount to the original firms responsible for the antibiotic. In turn, the companies reinvested much of their money to modernize the equipment since most still utilized the single-flask Heatley-Chain method of fermentation.[36]

Even non-penicillin production plants constructed during the war were made available to opportunistic manufacturers. Eli Lilly purchased part of Plancor 44, an airplane propeller plant that the government had spent $5,941,968 to build, for $2.5 million. Merck purchased a portion of the Cherokee Ordnance Works plant in Danville, Pennsylvania, for $862,500, again at a discount. Pfizer purchased a navy plant in Groton, Connecticut, for $919,500 that had cost $5,285,538 to build.[37]

Of particular interest was an agreement between Pfizer and the U.S. government to lease what was officially identified as a surplus ammunition loading plant. The massive operation in Terre Haute was called the Vigo Ordnance Plant, and under the terms of the contract, the pharmaceutical company paid $200,000 annually. However, it wasn't the business end of the deal that made it significant. It was the fact that, beneath its drab manufacturing exterior, the Vigo Ordnance Plant was one of the U.S. military's original biological warfare centers where anthrax and *B. globigii* were mass produced. What it demonstrated firsthand was what George W. Merck had alluded to in his report to Secretary of War Stimson: much of the science, know-how, and equipment used to produce antibiotics was considered dual use. In other words, the stainless steel vats and fermenters could also be used to produce biological weapons.[38] Unwittingly or not, Pfizer provided a crystal-clear, unambiguous proof of concept.

Research labs and R&D departments also enjoyed significant boosts, thanks to the geyser-like flow of cash. If the discovery of penicillin represented a glorious blueprint, the discovery of streptomycin provided researchers and scientific home hobbyists worldwide with a methodology for hunting down antibacterial substances. They searched for novel sources of antibiotics in exotic locations such as the Sardinian coast (albeit at a sewage outlet) and mundane spaces such as a poor doctor's backyard in the Philippines. While efforts did not always meet with success, probability dictated that they occasionally would. The ranks of antibiotics soon doubled from two to four when bacitracin was discovered at Columbia University in 1945 and when dihydrostreptomycin, a less toxic version of streptomycin that was able to be administered orally, was developed the following year.[39]

Yet problems persisted, even when it came to the seemingly well-oiled penicillin machine. Sure, the companies had met their D-Day demands with mold to spare. Yes, the United States was the center of the antibiotic universe. Of course, the penicillin surplus proved to the world that when pushed into a corner, capitalism could solve any problem with a healthy dose of government intervention. American scientists knew a lot, but they certainly didn't know everything. That much was evident soon enough.

During the early penicillin years, unbeknownst to the scientific community, two different types of penicillin were in circulation. Penicillin G represented the primary output of collective U.S. efforts, while penicillin F was produced in England.[40] While the chemotherapeutic activity of both forms was roughly similar, the same could not be said for their chemical stability. As it turned out, penicillin G contained a slight chemical variation that minimized the antibiotic's notorious instability. Once again, the Americans' penicillin effort benefited from the fortuitous fact that thanks to hybridization, the country produced more corn than other countries in the world at the time. Using corn steep liquor to essentially feed the *Penicillium* mold allowed it to incorporate a different, more active side group.[41]

Eventually, both penicillins were crystallized, their exact structures determined, and their names bestowed. With the mystery solved and the nature of their differences established, pharmaceutical companies returned to their fermenters and resumed the game of increasing yields. Manipulating the process by various means, including radiation, X-rays, or chemically induced mutations to generate different strains of mold, allowed companies to differentiate their penicillins ever so slightly. Changing the contents of the fermentation medium the mold grew on was another way of manipulating penicillin production. One of the earliest new versions of penicillin was known as penicillin K.

In 1945 pharmaceutical companies adopted a new strain of *P. chrysogenum* known as Q. 176. When grown in submerged culture, it produced more penicillin than previously used strains. This strain was extremely sensitive to the nutrients present in the medium it was grown on and resulted in the production of a different penicillin, labeled K. As it turned out, this type of penicillin was also produced with previous strains, only in smaller amounts.[42]

In vitro, it was a beast, killing up to 90 percent of bacteria, surpassing its brethren by superhero leaps and bounds. Pharmaceutical companies began mixing different percentages of penicillins as if they were grape varieties. It allowed them to brand each new combination as a new product. Eventually, penicillin K made up the lion's share of the antibiotic. But then something interesting happened.[43]

Doctors treating patients for routine infections that were normally easily cured by penicillin began to notice a pattern forming. To properly attack their patients' ailments, they needed to administer more and more antibiotic. Former doses no longer worked. If anything, their patients' conditions worsened. It became obvious something was wrong, and the popular press picked up on the brewing crisis.[44]

A *Saturday Evening Post* article described one case out of many. "The doctors kept shooting penicillin into the thin young man's veins and muscles, but the more they poured in, the more tenaciously the green streps clung to the edges of his heart valves. . . .

Endocarditis had been changed through the miracle of penicillin, from a sure killer to one from which you had better than an even chance of recovering. But in Robert's case, the streps, after a year's treatment with a total of 90,000,000 units of penicillin, were tougher than ever—forty times tougher than at the beginning of treatment, to be exact."[45]

Clinics across the United States reported the problem extended to treating pneumonia and osteomyelitis. Military hospitals reported either being unable to treat syphilis and gonorrhea or experiencing a sudden uptick of relapses. Soon newspaper headlines documented cases with a greater frequency. There were whispers that the miracle drug was already obsolete. While nothing had been proven scientifically, the anecdotal evidence worried scientists, particularly those involved in the budding field of antibiotics. For the first time, the specter of antibiotic resistance, initially documented in a 1940 paper by Edward Abraham and Ernst Chain on penicillinase, reared its head.[46]

Scientists leaped into action. The National Research Council formed a special venereal disease study committee tasked with pinpointing the problem with the penicillin in circulation. Headed by Dr. Joseph Earle Moore of Johns Hopkins Medical School, it played a central role in enlisting investigators, organizing findings, and directing future lines of inquiry.[47]

Results came back to Moore's office at a brisk pace. The first promising clue came from the dean of Johns Hopkins Medical School, Dr. Alan Chesney. He had been assigned the task of testing the purified K strain of penicillin against rabbits infected with syphilis. The results would indicate if any one of the four types displayed decreased performance against syphilis. When Chesney injected the standard dosage into the rabbit, nothing happened. He waited six more weeks then injected double the amount. Still nothing. He repeated the process until he was administering ten times the standard amount of penicillin. The rabbit never improved.[48]

The next step was to determine what was happening to penicillin K inside the body. To test this, a different team measured the level of penicillin K in the rabbit's blood an hour after injection and then compared it with levels of penicillin G during a similar time frame. The results were startling. Only one-eleventh of penicillin K remained compared to penicillin G. During subsequent tests in humans, it was shown that K disappeared four times as fast as other penicillins. Somehow, something was causing precipitous drops in penicillin.[49]

This point in the investigation must have been where the researchers held their collective breath. If it was in fact, the obvious—penicillinase in action—then they were in trouble. The end might actually have been near. It would have been only a matter of time until the other penicillins fell victim because part of what made the enzyme effective was that it attacked the beta-lactam ring that formed the backbone of all penicillins. The scientists had seen this happen before when resistance rendered once-effective sulfa drugs useless. Nobody wanted to see that repeated.

As it turned out, penicillinase was not the primary culprit in the destruction of penicillin K. Something more benign, but still not harmless, caused the antibiotic to disappear. Once the molecule entered the bloodstream, it essentially self-destructed until it lost its effectiveness.[50]

Since penicillin K comprised such a large portion of the latest batches, the other drugs would only meet effective levels after extremely large dosages. For example, if 0.10 penicillin G was in 1 Oxford unit, it would take ten doses to reach that amount, since the effect of penicillin K was almost negligible.

While their livelihoods were still intact, penicillin manufacturers had considerable cleaning up to do. Because the mold that produced penicillin K supplied the highest yields, the weak penicillin made up a considerable portion of the penicillin distributed during the winter of 1945 and 1946. On top of that, because of its performance in vitro, many manufacturers tweaked their products by further increasing the percentage of penicillin K in the mistaken belief it would make their drugs more potent.

Even with all the damage control pharmaceutical companies had to do, they all must have felt relieved. While the general consensus was that antibiotic resistance played a minor role in the penicillin K fiasco, it was not the primary cause. For the time being, they got off easy. That would not always be the case.

6

In early 1948 Nikolai Mikhailovich Borodin trudged through Manhattan with a single goal in mind—buy a penicillin plant for the Soviet Union from Merck.[1] If that proved impossible, blueprints would do. It didn't matter who sold it. He didn't care how he procured it, legally or illegally, bought or stolen. And he damn well didn't care whether it had the latest and the greatest in fermentation technology. He just wanted an efficient manufacturing plant that produced pure, if not perfect, penicillin. As he marched in and out of Amtorg's headquarters in the Garment District empty-handed, he must have worried how much time he had left. Failure carried dire consequences, and so far he had nothing to show for all his efforts.

Amtorg was the Soviet Union's official trade entity in the United States. Every deal between the two countries passed through its doors. When the Soviet Union wanted to purchase machinery, Amtorg made it happen. When the Americans wanted to buy furs, they knew where to go. It played the dealmaker and arranged meetings between interested parties.[2] Amtorg would have set up Borodin's meeting with Merck officials.

The organization's office, located at 210 Madison Avenue, served another purpose: it was home base for just about every Soviet spy involved in industrial espionage. Some of it was real cloak-and-dagger stuff. Handlers ran their sources and agents. All of the stolen Manhattan Project documents went through there. Harry Gold. Ethel and Julius Rosenberg. David Greenglass.[3] Other times, the spy business resembled a bungling sitcom more than it did James Bond's intelligence service. The spies lived off their photocopy machines, copying information they received through mail-order catalogues, and by writing companies and asking for specific information or even for personal tours of their factories. Companies usually obliged since the requests were made with a stated intention to make major purchases, which normally ended up falling through conveniently enough.

For years Borodin's fate depended on one thing—penicillin. He was one of the Soviet Union's top officials in charge of producing the miracle drug and answered directly to members of the Politburo. As the world became more familiar with the antibiotic and its curative capabilities, it continued to figure more prominently in the Communist Party's plans. Stalin was personally signing off on the construction of manufacturing plants. No doubt he was monitoring the progress of production. That's how important it was.

Soviet scientists, led by Zinaida Ermol'eva, engaged in basic research, probing penicillin and searching for newer antibiotics. They promised that their findings would result in more efficient methods to produce penicillin, which they had proclaimed had been discovered in the Union of Soviet Socialist Republics (USSR). They had the mold to prove it; it was found on Soviet soil.[4] Whether there was any veracity to their boasts, though, was irrelevant. They still struggled to produce the antibiotic. Surface fermentation provided modest amounts of impure drugs in liquid solution. They hadn't even managed to produce it in dried form yet.

Borodin oversaw the Medical Products Factory located in the Meat and Dairy Combine in Baku, one of the main penicillin production centers in the Soviet Union. Unlike his counterparts in Moscow, he had a little bit of experience with fermentation problems.[5] Using Florey's *Lancet* articles as his guide, he set up facilities designed to produce penicillin. Unfortunately, they weren't anywhere close to the level needed to work with such a temperamental mold. He had just enough knowledge to appreciate how bad things were going.

During the summer of 1945, the minister of meat and dairy industry, Pavel Vasiliyevich Smirnov, summoned Borodin to Moscow. Smirnov oversaw the entire penicillin production program and was at wits' end, watching the failures accumulate.[6] When the Kremlin called him and ordered a supply of penicillin, even though the plant still hadn't produced an ampule of the antibiotic, he probably panicked. And that's how Borodin ended up on a nearly three-year quest to uncover the secrets of penicillin production.

Borodin received instructions to fly to Oxford. From there, he was to spend time in Howard Florey's lab and learn as much as he could about the British fermentation techniques.[7] The arrangement had already been agreed upon, thanks to Florey's invitation to the Russians during his visit in 1944. Borodin was instructed to remain silent regarding the state of Soviet production other than to claim it was exactly the same as theirs.

For a year, Nikolai Borodin was welcomed into Florey's Dunn School laboratory. He worked side by side with Florey and Ernst Chain. He investigated different strains of *Penicillium* and tested for antibiotic activity.[8] He was even the lead author on a 1946 paper with Florey titled "An Antibiotic from *Penicillium tardum*."[9]

When Borodin returned to the Soviet Union in 1946, he reported to Smirnov and Vice Premier of the Council of Ministers Anastas Mikoyan and submitted all of the printed information he had procured while in England. He did not have good news. While he engaged in considerable basic research into antibiotics, he was not exposed to much of the industrial setups used in British penicillin plants. When he did visit them, he was impressed by how far behind Soviet production techniques were. Since nobody in the USSR possessed the necessary knowledge about fermentation and setting up a factory, he suggested what he saw as the only solution—buying a plant as well as the technological knowledge to run the plant.[10]

That was how he ended up in New York City and why he was visiting pharmaceutical companies. Luck and timing were working against him unfortunately. Tensions between the United States and Russia rose by the day. Moreover, previous Soviet agents had been caught trying to smuggle atomic research equipment out of the country the previous year. As a result, U.S. Customs Service officials imposed stringent restrictions on exports, especially on products deemed necessary for national security. Antibiotics and the equipment used in its production fell under this category.[11]

Initially Merck entered a tentative agreement with Borodin. When that fell through, probably due to government pressure, the Kremlin recognized that conditions were not conducive to progress. Borodin was recalled immediately. He did not go to Russia, however; he returned instead to England to try his luck there.

IN 1947 AN ARTICLE by "X" appeared in *Foreign Affairs* that defined the Soviet Union's outlook and motivations from a Western point of view and suggested actions that might be taken regarding the country's rise. Authored by George Kennan, who had written the so-called Long Telegram while stationed at the U.S. Embassy in Moscow, it played an influential role in defining Washington's approach to U.S.-Soviet relations. In particular, it laid the groundwork for the conclusions in the National Security Council (NSC) paper NSC-68, which outlined the Truman administration's theory of containment. It codified the deterioration of relations between the two countries that started during the final days of World War II and accelerated after Winston Churchill's "Iron Curtain" speech in Missouri in 1946.[12]

In his Long Telegram, Kennan made the case that much of the Soviet Union's actions were driven by history. In particular, Soviet leaders believed that they were living "in antagonistic 'capitalist encirclement' with which in the long run there can be no permanent peaceful coexistence." He predicted a battle for command of the world's economy between capitalist and Communist power centers. The siege mentality was the modern manifestation of a longstanding historical paranoia. "At bottom of Kremlin's neurotic view of world affairs is traditional and instinctive Russian sense of insecurity. Originally, this was insecurity of a peaceful agricultural people trying to live on vast exposed plain in neighborhood of fierce nomadic peoples. To this was added, as Russia came into contact with economically advanced West, fear of more competent, more powerful, more highly organized societies in that area."[13]

The Long Telegram went on to predict the Soviet Union would continue to build up its military and economic strength and would project its influence outward in a limited but significant way. The U.S. government had little stomach for a full-on confrontation with the USSR with the aims of regime change; however, working to prevent the expansion of Communism appeared more plausible. The strategy came to be known as containment and was codified in NSC-68.

By the time Kennan's "X" article was published, Eastern Europe had fallen under Moscow's yoke. The Communist Party held power in countries such as Czechoslovakia, Poland, Yugoslavia, and Belarus. Whether the isolation of the Soviet Union and its satellites from the

West was the result of Soviet intentions or a self-fulfilling prophecy, Churchill's metaphoric iron curtain did in fact descend across Europe.

Domestically, Stalin retrenched. Intellectually, politically, and philosophically, no matter the price, Soviet Russia needed to turn its back on Western influence. Nationalism replaced rationalism, and Stalin's endorsement of Lysenko's sketchy evolutionary claims simply reflected the natural extension of state-sanctioned meddling in the scientific realm. After the summer 1948 meeting of the Lenin All-Union Academy of Agricultural Science (LAAAS) in Moscow, a complete purging of genetics from academia and educational syllabi finalized the transition and formalized Lysenko's erroneous thinking.[14]

After the war ended, Trofim Lysenko reemerged, ready to complete the purge of genetics he had started before Hitler's invasion. During the war, theoretical arguments—therefore, political in this instance—were put aside in the interest of applied science. Lysenko wasted little time afterward in shifting the scientific community's focus back to Soviet creative Darwinism.

On November 5, 1945, during a course for workers in state breeding stations, Lysenko presented a paper in which he denied the existence of competition between members of the same species. In other words, different animals—say, foxes and wolves—competed with each other for resources, but foxes never competed with other foxes. A blissful equal distribution of food must have existed. This, of course, went against a central tenet in evolutionary theory, and when Lysenko invited criticism from a well-known botanist, his paper received a withering critique that was subsequently published under the title "Darwinism in a Distorting Mirror."[15]

Lysenko went on the offensive, where he functioned best. Rather than publishing his reply in a scientific journal, he turned to *Pravda*, the official Communist Party mouthpiece, and penned an attack titled "Do Not Get into Another One's Sledge." Taking a cue from their leader, Lysenko's followers began publishing abusive articles in journals.[16]

Lysenkoism's initial ascendancy and subsequent resurgence could not have come at a worse time, scientifically speaking. The field of genetics was on the verge of transforming the way the most basic questions were investigated in the biological sciences. The gene lay at the core of modern science, and creative Darwinism's denial of its existence threatened to cripple Soviet life sciences.

The American development of penicillin would have been impossible without the implicit acknowledgment that genes do, in fact, exist and play a large role in defining an organism's traits. While the researchers at the Northern Regional Research Laboratory went on their famous search around the world for the ideal mold, eventually finding it on a local cantaloupe, that was not the end of the story. Once they located their candidate, scientists with the Office of Scientific Research and Development attempted to tease more out of it by bombarding it with radiation and ultraviolet rays. It resulted in genetic mutations, some of which generated less productive strains, but others were more productive. The researchers created hundreds of new strains of *P. chrysogenum* and tested each one until they found the best strain possible. Without acknowledging that genes existed and could be manipulated, the process simply could not take place.

Records indicate that early Soviet efforts to scale up production of penicillin were severely hampered by the strains of *Penicillium* at their disposal and stifled by the Lysenkoists' denial of genetics, which never completely went away during the war.[17] Making matters worse, Soviet scientists lacked the fermentation skills and knowledge to move past the inefficient surface technique most early penicillin programs used. While it's doubtful Soviet-aligned scientists would have been granted access to pharmaceutical companies' proprietary technologies, their isolation from the West most certainly did not help. It ended up forcing the Soviet scientific community to rely on alternative methods to supplement laboratory-based inquiries.

When World War II ended, the restrictions on scientific publishing loosened. Much of the data that was deemed classified or top secret was published in the appropriate journals. In fact, four years' worth of frantic, top-quality research flooded from behind the censorship dam and out into the public. The preferred ideal of scientific openness returned to a great degree, and for a brief time, even Soviet scientists had access to the information, including that related to penicillin.

At this point, the dual-use nature of defensive biological warfare research merged with the development and production of life-saving antibiotics. A declassified Central Intelligence Agency (CIA) document offers a clear assessment of its worries then and is worth quoting: "The contribution and support that Soviet industrial fermentation, as exemplified by the antibiotics industry, might conceivably make to a BW program encompasses through principal areas: equipment and instrumentation, the possibility of plant conversion from antibiotics to agent production, and trained scientific and technical personnel."[18]

Around this time the newly formed CIA started its surveillance of antibiotic production in Communist countries. On one level, agents were keeping an eye on antibiotics production since they were considered militarily significant technologies at the time. Moreover, given that they did not know where Soviet BW plants were located, it provided an opportunity to assess Soviet BW capabilities, albeit indirectly. American intelligence agencies had their work cut out for them. They had a dearth of agents well placed within the Soviet pharmaceutical industry and in academia.

Until the CIA was able to infiltrate the Communist scientific community, as the State Security Committee (KGB) already had done with its Western counterparts, analysts relied heavily on making inferences from publicly available resources such as Soviet and Eastern bloc scientific journals and news reports. In the case of biological warfare development, analysts long believed that the technology necessary for producing antibiotics overlapped with creating biological weapons. In particular, they were concerned that growing microorganisms by way of the fermentation process, extracting them from liquid, and freeze-drying into crystalline form could be used. Whether the decision was correct or not, they wouldn't know until decades later.

BY MARCH 1947 THE United Nations Relief and Rehabilitation Administration (UNRRA) limped toward extinction. Its mission remained the same—namely, to provide food, shelter, and health care to civilians hurt by war hostilities and to supply aid for rebuilding devastated countries. Its ability to implement and fulfill those goals was no longer feasible, as the only thing running shorter than their funding was time. For everyone sitting in the Belarusian Mission of the UNRRA in Minsk, it was unfortunate but not unexpected. Present were Theodore Waller, the chief of the UNRRA Mission to Belarus; Konstantin Lastovsky, deputy chief of the UNRRA Supplies Administration; and Professor M. I. Kovalenck, the Belarusian minister of health.[19] It was important that the promised penicillin plant be built in the country, but the administration's imminent demise injected near-fatal uncertainty into the project.

Founded in 1943, the UNRRA consisted of forty-four signatory nations. The brainchild of Franklin Delano Roosevelt, it was founded with the objective of providing the swelling ranks of people displaced by war with a degree of support. Unfortunately, it came into existence toothless and spent its brief stint as a relief agency unable to adequately address the problems it was designed to solve. By 1945 the United Nations (UN) emerged as the dominant international organization and absorbed the UNRRA into its mission. It gradually assumed the responsibilities of the beleaguered administration while delegating its public health responsibilities to the World Health Organization. These duties would also include the construction of penicillin plants.[20]

Ever since the UNRRA's generous offer to supply the parts and blueprints for a penicillin plant to Belarus in 1946, Waller had served as the project's facilitator, updating Kovalenck about the progress being made as well as any setbacks. At first, nothing but good news came out of his mouth, but as months passed, the bad news easily outweighed the good. The original fall 1946 deadline came and went. Even then, though, the receiving countries maintained their optimism and appreciation. Now, months into 1947, they were barely any closer to possessing the promised penicillin plant than in the prior year. Resignation and frustration descended. The Belarusian government could only take solace in the fact that the other countries involved were experiencing the exact same delays.[21]

"I've been anxious to meet with you this week," Waller said. "Because tonight I am going to a UNRRA Conference in Rome. If there are medical problems which are giving your government concern, it may be possible to help reach a solution while I am at the conference."[22]

Kovalenck started off by asking for the easy but still pressing things. The country needed microscopes, X-ray machines, and thermometers. The Germans had confiscated almost all of the scientific equipment, leaving only twenty-five microscopes in the entire country. Without the proper tools, diagnosing sick patients' ailments amounted to a guessing game. They needed the microscopes in order to identify microorganisms; the X-rays were necessary in the diagnosis of tuberculosis and for its treatment. They also needed quinine to fight malaria and asked for penicillin. The supplies they were getting from Russia were insufficient.

Waller noted the minister's requests and then shifted the conversation to the penicillin plants. "Not long ago, I was in Warsaw and Prague," he said. "I talked with the Ministries of Health in both countries about the problems related to the UNRRA supplied penicillin plants. . . . Both countries are concerned about the process of the manufacture of crystalline penicillin with butyl alcohol as a substitute for amyl acetate. Is Belarus going to attempt to produce penicillin with alcohol or does it have a supply of acetate?"

Kovalenck replied that the question was outside his expertise. He was a doctor by training, not a chemist or engineer.

"Will the Ministry of Health be responsible for the operation of this plant?"

"Yes," Kovalenck replied. "The building has already been selected but unfortunately, only two and a half percent of the plant has arrived. I should like to request that you expedite the shipment of the remainder of the plant."

"That's one of the three primary purposes of my trip to Rome. A much higher percentage of the plant has either been shipped or has already arrived in Odessa."

The minister reiterated the paucity of what they possessed.

Waller backed off. He acknowledged that the organization was struggling to provide the parts for a complete plant. "There are some serious problems about certain components of the plant. I am going to Rome primarily for the purpose of trying to solve these problems so that there will be no question about the complete delivery of all components. I have no assurances that certain pieces of equipment essential to the operation of the plant will not have to be procured outside of UNRRA."

Kovalenck raised another very obvious concern. He asked whether a special consultant would be able to assist in setting up the plant and, most important, walk the scientists through the process of producing penicillin. All the blueprints and accompanying directions could not teach them how to coax miracles out of mold. For that, they needed an expert in the field.

"The Administration has been giving the closest attention to the Prime Minister's request for a consultant to assist in the assembling of the plant," Waller said. "We had a man—[Dr. N. L.] Macpherson. However, about a month ago it developed that he, for personal reasons, would not be able to come."

It was crushing news especially because he had drawn up the factory blueprints and specifications. Everything from the basic equipment to the man originally appointed to deliver the technological transfer was missing.

On paper, providing a complete penicillin plant must have seemed a reasonable enough prospect on July 31, 1945, when the Czechoslovakian government put forward the proposal to the UNRRA: "We should like to install a plant out of which we could supply not only the needs of Czechoslovakia but also other countries which are being helped by the UNRRA."[23]

Two months later, the UNRRA Mission in Prague received a telegram from Washington. Herbert Lehman, the head of the organization, agreed to "procure equipment supplies necessary installation [*sic*] institute producing ten billion Oxford units penicillin monthly" for Czechoslovakia. The UNRRA soon decided to extend the offer to four other countries: Italy, Ukraine, Poland, and Belarus. Later Yugoslavia would be given the option of having an old Merck plant disassembled and shipped for reassembly.[24]

Since the United States donated the largest proportion of UNRRA operational funds and its headquarters was located in Washington DC, many assumed it would play the central role in constructing the penicillin plants. Unfortunately, the State Department had other things in mind, especially when it discovered that five out of the six European beneficiaries were Communist countries and to some extent aligned with the Soviet Union. Rather than facilitate, the department sought to obstruct.

The Canadian government stepped in via the Canadian Commercial Corporation and offered to draw up the plans for the plants, procure the equipment needed, and send experts to aid in construction when the time came. Connaught Labs assumed the responsibility of producing the blueprints and specs that would be used to assemble the pieces.[25]

The UNRRA's decision to accept the Czech government's offer and expand it made sense. From a relief standpoint, no other independent organization played a larger role during the waning days of World War II and the early occupation years to deliver the profound benefits of antibiotics to the masses. Having local sources of antibiotics amounted to a humanitarian blessing. In terms of rehabilitation, the penicillin plants and the miracle drugs they produced almost guaranteed that their pharmaceutical industries would be competitive.

On January 11, 1946, the UNRRA held a press conference to announce that it would build penicillin plants in six European countries in need. The administration estimated that the plants would be delivered by the fall of that year.[26] They were too optimistic.

Delays mounted almost immediately. The UNRRA's official history of the penicillin project gives an idea of the problems it confronted:

> Throughout the period of procurement, which was elongated over the time originally planned, various difficulties crept into the overall procurement picture. Amyl acetate was one item extremely hard to locate; recipient countries were advised of this shortage and the suggestion was made that they attempt to locate sources in Europe. . . . Two other large items, the capping machines and cold storage and refrigerating units presented difficulties. Contracts were let on both items but were subsequently cancelled due to contractors' failure to deliver . . . the manufacturers' difficulty in obtaining steel drums and carboys slowed up procurement of some chemicals. . . . Much of the material was not deliverable as previously contracted due to labor problems and raw material shortages.[27]

The biggest obstacle came from the State Department; 10 percent of the parts needed for the construction could only be found in the United States, and without the department's active support, procuring them dragged. Overcoming red tape resulted in considerable delays. And when it came to a specialized centrifuge called a Podbielniak countercurrent extractor, Washington refused to issue the appropriate customs forms for its export.[28] The government deemed it a matter of national security, and since the majority of countries the UNRRA was helping belonged to the Communist bloc, recent embargoes put in place forbade exporting to them.

Thus, the past three months had been as exhausting as it was frustrating for Waller, who had discouraged the Belarusians with varying degrees of success from pursuing the production of crystalline penicillin as it relied on the embargoed extractor. The Americans' stonewalling made the prospect of producing a purer version of penicillin all but impossible. Alternate solutions were needed but in short supply. Everything slowed to a crawl.

ARTURO ROCES LAY ON a hospital bed, wasting away in the Philippines. An acute case of tuberculosis was eating away at his body. Bacteria overwhelmed the five-year-old's defenses. Somehow, the doctors of Santo Tomas Hospital administered a small amount of streptomycin to the boy. It was the last dose available in the entire country. The boy showed signs of improvement, but his relief was temporary. Unable to complete the treatment, doctors watched Roces's condition revert and deteriorate. Unless enough streptomycin could be acquired to complete a full course of treatment, he would certainly die.[29]

On November 23 the Upjohn Company made it available for the boy.[30] On November 28, 1946, a packet containing streptomycin was flown from New York to Manila. From there it was delivered to Santo Tomas Hospital. A month and a half later, Roces was released from the hospital and allowed to go home. The still-experimental antibiotic came through, as advertised, and proved yet again that it would revolutionize the treatment of TB.[31]

Yet, two months after Arturo Roces's release from Santo Tomas hospital, a fourteen-year-old boy in Glasgow died from tubercular meningitis after his family's appeal for streptomycin was rejected by the British Medical Research Council.[32]

Considering that streptomycin had yet to be released to the American public indicates that more was at work in releasing it to the Philippines than just treating an ailing boy. The five-year-old was the son of Joachim Roces, the publisher of one of Asia's first English-language newspapers, the *Manila Times*. The family needed the U.S. Commerce Department's permission for Upjohn Company to send the medication. It was approved on short notice.[33]

Wartime controls on antibiotics was, to a degree, understandable. However, after the war ended, the implementation of constraints continued, and access to streptomycin was tightly controlled. At first, countries or individuals had to petition Washington, which decided the distribution of the antibiotic on a case-by-case basis. Only members of the military had regular access to it. Rationing the latest miracle drug no longer represented a case of national interests; it was about control.

News about streptomycin filled newspapers, yet local doctors and hospitals lacked access to the new drug. Anyone not associated with the military was staring into a store through a glass window. Verdicts were mixed, particularly regarding streptomycin's side effects. On July 4, 1947, the American public finally gained access to Selman Waksman's antibiotic. Headlines announced that the second chapter in the miracle drug story began. That same year, the antibiotic was fully distributed to health care officials in the occupied territories.

When it came to being treated with antibiotics, a firm pecking order existed whether it was in Europe or Japan. Soldiers and other people associated with the military were first in line for penicillin treatment. The civilian population was only treated with the antibiotic under very specific circumstances—syphilis or gonorrhea infections. In U.S.-occupied Germany, the U.S. Public Health and Welfare Section requested shipments of penicillin for the treatment of gonorrhea among German civilians as early as September 1945. Exasperated local doctors struggled to make sense of the fact that administering the medication for non-STD conditions, no matter how dire, was off-limits.[34] Still, the U.S. policy had its good points. It made treatment of STDs popular and prevalent. Self-reporting of infections increased significantly. More and more, Germans enjoyed the benefits of penicillin with increased autonomy. "In January 1946, the German authorities were authorized to supervise most penicillin treatments themselves, and by spring 1946 large quantities of the drug had been made available. By September 1947 supplies had increased to a monthly allocation of 21 billion units of penicillin for the zone: only 2 billion were needed for gonorrhea, 12 billion units were used to treat syphilis, and 7 billion units were available for the treatment of non-venereal diseases."[35]

Meanwhile, the Soviet zone experienced severe shortages of the miracle drug. British and French supplies also lagged. Dispensing penicillin proved to be one of the best arguments for the American way of life. After the military was allotted the lion's share of available medicine, the UNRRA was allowed to purchase whatever remained. The organization then distributed its limited amount to displaced persons or to the health ministries of the countries it assisted. It often competed with the same governments it also served.

The UNRRA's penicillin policies diverged depending on the zone. At first, doctors in the British zone were under strict limitations as to whom they could serve. Only patients suffering from venereal disease could be treated. In addition, only female civilians were allowed to be treated for STDs. Presumably, the troops would not be having sexual encounters with men, but women might pass on their infections, so they needed to be cured. As the men posed no disease problem, they were left to their own devices.[36]

In the American zone, the penicillin that the UNRRA dispensed to local hospitals was to be used only in the cases of non-venereal diseases. In the instructions for the proper way to dispense penicillin, officials voiced their concerns about doctors failing to administer adequate amounts of the antibiotic. "The action of penicillin is bacteriostatic. In order to produce this effect it must reach a minimum concentration in the blood and body fluids of 1/50 Oxford Florey unit per cent. . . . If this is not done so, the infective microorganism may become 'penicillin-resistant.'"[37]

Resistance was indeed becoming a serious problem in countries that used the antibiotic on a regular basis. Resistant bacteria had been induced in laboratory settings since 1940, and, as noted previously, Abraham and Chain published a paper reporting that bacteria exposed to penicillin eventually produced an enzyme they called penicillinase, which resulted in the complete inactivation of the antibiotic.[38] Other studies followed and confirmed that bacteria were able to develop defenses that allowed them to survive.

A 1945 paper titled "Penicillin Resistance of Staphylococcus aureus and Its Clinical Implications" went one step further by showing that resistant bacteria could be found in clinical settings. Maj. Harold Plough took samples from lesions on patients at Lovell General Hospital. He discovered that out of forty distinct strains of *S. aureus*, 40 percent of them showed resistance to penicillin. Most of the patients with resistant bacteria had been treated with penicillin on previous occasions, confirming that exposure to the antibiotic caused resistant colonies to form. When Plough dug deeper, he discovered that formerly susceptible strains developed resistance in as little as forty-eight hours.[39]

More reports of resistant strains in clinical settings surfaced. They were even more concerning as they involved infection *by* resistant strains and not simply their appearance due to active treatment. In 1947 microbiologist Mary Barber published a paper titled "Staphylococcal Infection due to Penicillin-Resistant Strains." She had started monitoring resistant strains of *S. pyogenes* in Hammersmith Hospital in London. Over the course of a year, she had seen infections spreading through the hospital. The first sentences of her paper communicated her apprehension: "The incidence of strains of *Staphylococcus pyogenes* that are grossly resistant to penicillin is clearly increasing rapidly. The rate of increase in this hospital at present is so rapid as to be somewhat alarming."[40]

As the world would soon learn, this was only the beginning.

"YOU'RE LYING, YOU STINKING jackal!"

The lone voice coming from the audience belonged to Iosef Amromovich Rapoport, one of the Soviet Union's leading geneticists. Its target, I. I. Prezent, stood at the front of the lecture hall. The affront echoed through the Soviet Ministry of Agriculture Club lecture hall, interrupting the speaker at the podium and shattering the strained civility between members of the audience. The scientists and politicians attending the August meeting of the LAAAS grasped the audacity and foolishness of the interruption. Even though Prezent was not a scientist, he helped construct the anti-genetics movement in the Soviet Union along with its chief architect, Trofim Lysenko, who was also in attendance. Now, his words were cut short, forced into an ignoble pause by a verbal slap in the face. The gesture was rooted in scientific understanding but drenched in politics. Rapoport knew what he was doing. It was career suicide. He did it anyway. That's how much was at stake. For geneticists in the USSR, it was a matter of literal life and death.[41]

Rapoport had a lot to lose, but his courage came as no surprise to people who knew him and knew of him. In fact, he had proved his mettle during the Great Patriotic War when he volunteered for the Moscow People's Militia, even when his age should have dictated otherwise. Ultimately, Rapoport suffered a gruesome injury, costing him the use of his right eye. He returned to the front when younger men would have gladly gone home, having done their duty. He received a promotion for his bravery.[42]

If he had one shortcoming, however, it was his inability to withhold his criticism when he believed it necessary to speak. He criticized his army superiors, perhaps costing him the title Hero of the Soviet Union. More important, during the second day of the LAAAS conference when the members inspected Lysenko's farm and listened to lectures about the practical uses of creative Darwinism, Rapoport found that his irritation was like an itch, impossible to ignore. So he scratched it. Rather than offering a direct critique, he opted for a stated fact: "The transformation of animals and plants cannot be achieved merely as a result of our wish."[43]

It was a topic the acid-tongued scientist knew something about firsthand. Since his return from the service, Rapoport focused his research on the origin of mutations in organisms. In particular, he produced important work exploring the way chemicals can be used to force mutations to occur in a host's DNA. His work drew on the notions of chromosomes and DNA, and the fact that offspring receive their characteristics directly from their parents. The field was steeped in genetics and put him at odds with most other scientists in the USSR. It certainly put him at odds with Lysenko, Prezent, and the people sitting around him.[44]

Rapoport's exclamation, omitted from official published transcripts, represented one of the last, forceful public declarations against Lysenkoism for decades. It was also futile. The event had been carefully choreographed and its speakers shrewdly selected. Even before Lysenko's opening remarks, the fate of Soviet geneticists had been decided. They were dead men walking. The conference was simply a formality.

During the Great Patriotic War, Trofim Lysenko had bided his time in Siberia, relegated to the margins of Soviet science and planting rows of crops away from the public eye. But as the dust of an uneasy peace settled across the Soviet Union, Lysenko found his influence diminished and his enemies emboldened. The father of creative Darwinism had no intention of relinquishing his hard-earned influence. As one conflict passed, another flared into existence. The war against bourgeois Weismannist-Morganist-Mendelist genetics resumed with a vengeance, only this time, the sides were more evenly matched.

The wartime alliance of the Soviet Union, Great Britain, and the United States served Soviet geneticists well. According to Soviet science historian Nikolai Krementsov, "The scientific community saw its authority greatly expanded during the war. Scientists became state experts and advisers, replacing the party ideologists and functionaries who had occupied these positions since the mid-1930s."[45]

Much of the genetics community's gains took place where it mattered most—in administrative positions and in the political realm. The scientists had learned the hard lesson that while ideological and theoretical fights were one thing, the real impact was made on the administrative level, where decisions on policy were made. The veracity of their scientific research was secondary. For once, they played Lysenko's game and by his rules. If the purge years of the 1930s had taught them anything, it was that controlling how decisions were made outweighed any amount of scientific data, at least in Stalin's Soviet Union.

Anton Zhebrak embodied the new approach perfectly. In 1945 he was appointed to head a section of Agitprop, putting him in the highest levels of government and allowing him to act as the genetics community's voice in the party apparatus. Other geneticists ascended to important positions in higher learning institutions such as Moscow State University and Timiryazev Agricultural Academy.[46]

During this time, Soviet geneticists employed their acceptance and praise from Anglo-American scientists as leverage. After being cut off during the 1930s, communication between international scientists resumed when Hitler invaded Russia in 1941 and was reestablished during the war years. The correspondence list included some of the most important American geneticists such as Joshua Lederberg, Theodosius Dobzhansky, and Hermann J. Muller. They would play central roles in the development of a "second front" from abroad in defending genetics in the Soviet Union.[47]

The détente involved more than transatlantic correspondence. Western academic journals, the fountain of knowledge essential to scientific discovery, became available to Soviet researchers for the first time in nearly a decade, and local Russian-language journals carried regular columns highlighting the latest Western scientific discoveries. In addition, the Soviet Academy of Sciences elected American and British scientists into its ranks. The names include a who's who of early twentieth-century geneticists such as Walter B. Cannon, Henry Dale, J. B. S. Haldane, Gilbert N. Lewis, and Ernest O. Lawrence.[48]

By 1946 the anti-Lysenko geneticists had gained enough ground to try to establish a new genetics center and have Lysenko removed from his membership of the presidium of the Academy of Sciences. They tried, but after a protracted struggle, they failed. The inability to remove Lysenko was a fatal blow for genetics in the Soviet Union. Newly emboldened, Lysenko moved to eliminate his enemies once and for all.

The goodwill between East and West did not last long once the war ended. In the summer of 1947, relations took a serious turn for the worse. Coincidentally or not, Stalin initiated his ideological campaign called *Zhdanovshchina* (era of Zhdanov, Stalin's spokesman on cultural affairs) against Western influence in the Soviet Union during the summer of 1946. Two public decrees in popular magazines announced its arrival. They sought to bring attention to and stifle "the pernicious influence of bourgeois culture" on Soviet society, and they stressed that "servility and slavishness before Western culture" were unacceptable. It was as if the country had stepped into a time machine and returned to the 1930s, which had been plagued with isolationism. While science had escaped immediate peril, its luck ran out in 1947.[49]

According to Krementsov, the so-called Kliueva and Roskin affair harkened the beginning of the end for Soviet genetics' halcyon days. The incident involved two Soviet scientists—Nina Kliueva and her husband, Gregorii Roskin—who collaborated to work on a cure for cancer. During the 1930s, they investigated the effects of live and dead trypanosomes on tumors, having observed that the parasite destroys the cells it infects. After the war, they returned to the project, in part inspired by the work done by the Oxford group, the OSRD, and the researchers in Anglo-American industry.[50]

Initial clinical tests showed promise. Trypanosome displayed little to no toxicity in human beings while causing the dissolution of tumors. After publishing their results, the researchers came to the attention of the State Department, which subsequently sent U.S. ambassador Walter B. Smith to Kliueva's lab. Impressed with what he saw, the ambassador approached the Academy of Medical Sciences with a formal proposal that offered complete U.S. funding and equipment in exchange for access to Kliueva and Roskin's research. Soon after the visit, the scientists published their findings in book form for the public. Everyone from the Politburo down was sufficiently pleased with events thus far. Soviet science had cured cancer after all.[51]

In the autumn of 1946, Kliueva and Roskin received two more American guests—Stuart Mudd, the president of the American-Soviet Medical Society, and Robert Leslie, a founder and business manager of the society. They were eager to advance Americans' access to the lab. As a result, the U.S. surgeon general extended an invitation to Vasilii Parin, the Soviet Academy of Medical Sciences' new academician-secretary, to visit the United States. During Parin's visit, he brought a copy of Kliueva and Roskin's manuscript as a gift. He promised to facilitate a visit by American cancer specialists to the Soviet Union. At that point, everything went belly-up.[52]

On January 28 Andrei Zhdanov interrogated Kliueva in the Kremlin, accusing her of placing the interests of the Soviet Union second to that of United States. As proof, he cited the fact that American scientists possessed a copy of the Kliueva-Roskin manuscript. According to Krementsov, "Zhdanov's 'interrogation' of Kliueva was almost certainly a charade. As he knew, Vyacheslav Molotov had been privy to the decision to share information on KR research."[53]

After further investigation of everyone involved, including Parin but not Molotov, Zhdanov concluded that wrongdoing had, in fact, occurred.[54]

The Kliueva-Roskin affair fueled the resurgence of Lysenkoism and further emboldened him to seize control of Soviet science. It culminated in the LAAAS conference in 1948.[55]

Lysenko opened the meeting with a speech that Stalin had played a major part in finalizing. He immediately set the tone for upcoming remarks by saying, "In the post-Darwin period the overwhelming majority of biologists, instead of further developing Darwinism, did all it could to vulgarize it and to stifle its scientific basis." From there, he went on to reestablish that two types of biology existed in the world—materialistic Soviet Michurinism in the East and a reactionary, metaphysical science embodied in the Weismannist-Morganist-Mendelist genetics espoused in the morally bankrupt West.[56]

One by one scientists marched on stage to declare a final ignoble end to bourgeois science. It was as if the conference was a funeral and the lecture hall a graveyard, and each speaker took his turn to throw dirt on the coffin of fact-based science. The Lysenkoists spewed disdain on what they labeled a Western pseudoscience and spit venom at its practitioners.[57]

Prezent declared, "We are called on here to debate. We will not debate with Morganists, but continue to unmask them as representatives of a detrimental and ideologically foreign and essentially pseudoscientific trend imported from abroad."[58]

By the time Lysenko took the stage to deliver the conference's closing remarks, the fight was over. Genetics had been crushed.

Biology Departments in universities across the Soviet Union reeled as a result of the LAAAS conference and Lysenko's declaration that creative Darwinism was now the de facto version of genetics throughout the Soviet Union and, in all likelihood, throughout the Communist scientific community worldwide. The concept of a single, unified, international science disappeared overnight, only to be replaced by the recycled belief that two opposing sciences existed between the East and West. Scientific nationalism was in ascendancy, and its arrival opened up new opportunities for ambitious colleagues to attack and discredit each other. The purges that followed had more to do with professional advancement than with academic scientific rigor.[59]

Two and a half years of struggle between geneticists and Lysenkoists culminated at the LAAAS conference. Rapoport's voice would be the last stand for almost two decades, and the harm to the life sciences in the USSR would take even longer to heal.

LATER THAT YEAR, NIKOLAI Borodin returned to England in yet another attempt at procuring a penicillin plant. While there, he negotiated with Ernst Chain regarding a role as an adviser in constructing a penicillin plant in the Soviet Union.[60] The futility was starting to take its toll on Communist Party officials. He heard that his superiors in Russia had all been demoted or imprisoned for their failure. His entire department had been liquidated. Stunning changes were sweeping through Soviet science once again. The Klioueva-Roskin affair had a further destructive effect on research as scientists were being arrested. Borodin had survived Stalin's first purge implemented by Lysenko. He wasn't sure he'd survive this round.[61]

On August 27, 1948, Borodin mailed a letter to G. N. Zarubin, the ambassador of the Union of Soviet Socialist Republics in the United Kingdom. The letter opened, "Although I love my Motherland and my people, I, by my own personal and free will, have decided not to return to the USSR. Accordingly, I renounce my citizenship of the Soviet Union."[62]

With that, Nikolai Borodin's defection was complete.

7

Germany was up for grabs. It was also in ruins. At least that's how the four former Allied governments saw it. On one side, France, Great Britain, and the United States tried their best to speak in a single unified voice, while on the other, the Soviet Union expressed the whims of its leader. Each administered a section of Germany and its former capital, Berlin. Each believed Germany's fate would define the direction Europe's recovery would take. Each wanted to ensure that a reconstructed and ascendant Germany posed no threat to the new world order taking shape on the continent and around the globe. Finally, each understood that the deutsche mark lay at the center of whatever solution the group pursued. A prosperous and peaceful Germany was everyone's goal; achieving that was a whole new matter entirely. The Russians and the Americans were keen to speak at each other rather than do the heavy-lifting true compromise demanded. By the summer of 1948, East and West had come to a veritable stalemate.

Black markets and bartering for goods thrived in the absence of a stable currency. So did inflation. According to one report, a case of Lucky Strike cigarettes served as the standard currency and eventually reached the tulip-craze heights of $2,300 per carton.[1] Something as simple as reintroducing the deutsche mark ended up being fraught with potentially calamitous repercussions. It was as if the four powers were maneuvering through a minefield. Everyone had national motivations behind their positions. If the U.S.-led Allies introduced the deutsche mark in their zones and in the process excluded the Soviet Union, the decision would be the death blow to any dream of a united Germany—or Europe, for that matter.

The Americans and the British opted to move forward with a

common currency in both of their zones. It elicited the expected response from the Russians, further driving a wedge between the former Allies. They expressed shock, and Soviet newspapers railed against Western duplicitousness.[2] While Churchill introduced the notion of an iron curtain splitting continental Europe in half and Stalin's actions bringing the Eastern bloc countries to kneel reinforced the idea, the introduction of the deutsche mark transformed the metaphor from an eloquent abstraction into a brutal reality.

On March 15, 1948, Stalin called a meeting with his close advisers: Vyacheslav Molotov, Andrei Zhdanov, Lavrenti Beria, and others. They devised a plan to put pressure on the West. Little by little, the Soviet military would tighten the entry and exit to Berlin, which was situated some hundred miles inside the Russian zone. The objective was to gradually starve the French, British, and American zones.[3] Soon after the meeting, Red Army soldiers began implementing what became known as the Berlin Blockade. The people in Berlin had enough food and supplies for a couple of months, maximum.

The Allies did not expect Stalin's willingness to engage in an overt show of force. In some respects, the blockade forced the hands of countries close to the Soviet Union, and an unintended consequence of the episode resulted in the Benelux countries, Denmark, Norway, and Italy joining the North Atlantic Treaty Organization (NATO).[4] Making matters worse, the nightmare scenario of Russian leaders for hundreds of years was taking shape: the Soviet Union was close to being surrounded by hostile—in this case, capitalist—nations.

On June 28, 1948, the first British C-54 landed in Tempelhof Airport carrying supplies. The next plane touched down five minutes later. Four thousand tons of supplies were delivered to Berlin. That amounted to one plane every three minutes and forty-five seconds, an astonishing feat. Stalin's plan crumbled. On May 12, 1949, the blockade was lifted nearly a year after it started.[5]

The first overt conflict of the Cold War came down to money, on the surface at least. It foreshadowed one of the many battlefields on which the Cold War would be fought—weaponized economics.

WHILE LYSENKO AND HIS followers organized the expulsion of geneticists and evolutionary biologists from Soviet institutions, a different kind of purge was taking place in most of the Western world. Bacteriophage therapy, while never the predominant approach to dealing with infections, began to disappear entirely. But not before some researchers engaged in experiments tantalizingly similar to that conducted over a half century later.

Phage therapy had a considerable track record in North America, though nowhere as entrenched as in France and the Soviet Union. Félix d'Hérelle, of French-Canadian birth, later held a position as a professor of protobiology at Yale University's Medical Center. He held the professorship while also working at the Pasteur Institute.[6]

From the start, Western discourse on bacteriophage therapy suffered from an unfortunate feud between d'Hérelle and Frederick Twort and his many supporters. While it originated in claims of discovery, Twort's having discovered bacteriophages slightly before d'Hérelle, the debate ultimately revolved around the nature of bacteriophages themselves. It was with one of Twort's supporters, a Nobel laureate named Jules Bordet, that the scientific discourse turned personal. D'Hérelle dismissed Bordet's work as "the history of an error," and Bordet led a decades-long assault on everything d'Hérelle touched. In particular, Bordet took every opportunity to discredit d'Hérelle's assertion that bacteriophages were viruses.[7]

Bordet and the scientific community, in general, rejected the viral nature of phages out of hand. Instead, they insisted that bacteriophages were lytic enzymes. The assessment was later further bolstered by another Nobel laureate named John Northrop.

For nearly twenty years, textbooks taught that phages were enzymes. In 1940 the advent of the electron microscope allowed Helmut Ruska, Edgar Pfankuch, and Gustav Kausche to prove that bacteriophages were in fact viruses of varying shapes and sizes, vindicating d'Hérelle. Three years later, Salvador E. Luria, Max Delbrück, and Thomas Anderson went a step further by describing two coliphages in considerable detail. Unfortunately, the waters surrounding phages had been muddied, and attempts at using them for therapeutic purposes suffered as a result.[8] Journal articles continued to question the effectiveness of phage therapy on the grounds of lacking a clear idea of what constitutes a bacteriophage. If something that simple remained a mystery, much more so were the complex workings of phages in the body. *Science* went so far as to suggest that phage therapy's shortcomings arose because "men who had to use it have not understood it well enough to get uniformly good results."[9]

Assessing their efficacy was difficult without standardized methods and materials. This became painfully clear when, in an attempt to clarify the state of bacteriophage therapy, the American Medical Association waded into the scrum. With Morris Fishbein at the helm, the *Journal of the American Medical Association* addressed clinical uses of phages on three separate occasions. Prior to that, the editor penned a pair of editorials questioning the effectiveness of phage products that pharmaceutical companies sold on the market. Always eager to take on causes he viewed as "quackery," Fishbein commissioned a review of existing literature pertaining to phage therapy in 1934 and then 1941.[10] His selection of authors strongly suggested a bias against the notion that phages were viruses and that their therapeutic uses were effective.

The 1934 review, titled "Bacteriophage Therapy: Review of the Principles and Results of the Use of Bacteriophage in the Treatment of Infections," was authored by Stanhope Bayne-Jones and Monroe D. Eaton. At the time, Bayne-Jones had already shifted to more administrative roles than research ones, having served as the president of the Society of American Bacteriologists, New York State Association of Public Health Laboratories, and the American Association of Immunologists. Between 1931 and 1935, Bayne-Jones was a member of the influential Council on Pharmacy and Chemistry of the American Medical Association, and it was in that capacity that he undertook Fishbein's request to review the bacteriophage therapy literature.

From the outset, the paper was an exercise in rhetorical contradiction. Starting from the description of the nature of bacteriophages, it assumed contrary positions to that of d'Hérelle. While admitting that phages may be viruses, it concluded that most likely they were enzymes. When clinical evidence suggested therapy may hold promise, the paper subsequently undercut that position with more evidence of its ineffectiveness. This pattern was repeated throughout the two-part review. Though to be fair, the shoddy standards many researchers held while conducting and reporting their experiments did not help.

Finally, in the second installment, Bayne-Jones and Eaton tipped their hand and verbalized the stance they had been insinuating. It's worth quoting at length.

> It is impossible to read these many reports of the successful bacteriophage treatment of suppurations conditions without feeling that a great many of the authors are extremely uncritical. It is difficult to believe that success in from 95 to 99 per cent of cases has been due to a therapeutic agent that has proved so disappointing in the more critically conducted experiments. . . . Many of the conditions treated are self limiting and, in those which are not, the usual methods of surgical intervention have been practiced. The fact that the patient has recovered has, therefore, little significance.[11]

Seven years later, Albert P. Krueger and E. Jane Scribner continued the critical assault on phage therapy. As noted by Walter Summers, Krueger was a "partisan" in the general bacteriophage debate and a "protégé" of Northrop's, who was partial to Bordet's concept of phages as an autocatalytically activated lyric enzyme.[12]

Krueger and Scribner's review in the *Journal of the American Medical Association* echoed Bayne-Jones and Eaton's even down to the rhetorical strategy of presenting positive phage strategies for the primary purpose of using them as target practice. Successful reports of phage therapy were discredited for faulty experimental design. In instances where that was not the case, Krueger and Scribner attacked studies for focusing on conditions that were self-limiting, implying that the body had simply healed itself. Their paper went so far as to say that sometimes the solution containing the phage elicited the positive reaction and not the phage itself.[13]

The paper's ultimate conclusions kept in line with the previous paper's, stating that the in vitro performance of phages has no bearing on its clinical performance. Once the phage solution enters the body, it "operates on a much less efficient scale and plays a negligible part in the clinical application of phage. There is no substantial evidence that the spontaneous development of phage in the infected host has any bearing on the process of recovery."[14]

Krueger and Scribner then escalated the attack on bacteriophage therapy, breaking from the report seven years earlier. If the conclusions from the Bayne-Jones and Eaton report amounted to gentle diplomatic prodding, Krueger and Scribner did away with all niceties and declared war. According to them, "While it has become almost axiomatic to state that the use of phage is entirely innocuous, we have not found this to be the case. The literature provides numerous accounts of reactions ranging from mild to severe following the injection. . . . Animal experimental work has shown that lysates may contain enough soluble toxin or Reynal's spreading factor to be actually dangerous."[15]

In other words, it was only a matter of time until bacteriophage therapy, not the disease being treated, caused the death of a patient. Coming from the Council on Pharmacy and Chemistry of the American Medical Association, this conclusion represented a virtual prohibition on the clinical use of bacteriophages.

It's worth noting that Krueger and Scribner used the phage therapy review as a platform to once again assert that bacteriophages were enzymes: "The nature of bacteriophage is no longer in question. It is a protein of high molecular weight and appears to be formed from a precursor originating within the bacterium."[16]

They were wrong.

Of course, there were problems with phage therapy. Researchers still lacked an understanding of how it acted in the body. However, the most obvious and public-facing issues were problems of industry. Even from the most reputable companies, the quality of the phage mixtures left much to be desired.

U.S. pharmaceutical companies sold bacteriophage cocktails over the counter. In particular, Eli Lilly maintained a stable of products, a combination of topical gels and liquids. They were marketed as Ento-jel, Staphylo-jel, Strepto-jel, Colo-jel, Ento-lysate, Staphylo-lysate, Strepto-lysate, Colo-lysate, and Neiso-lysate. (The "Colo" products were mixtures of the three specific phage cocktails.) According to Eli Lilly, their products could be used to attack and dissolve bacteria, stimulate phagocytosis, and serve as a more effective biological antiseptic than chemical versions. They could be administered topically, subcutaneously, intramuscularly, intraspinally, intraperitoneally, and intravenously.[17]

Preparation of bacteriophage solutions was also described: "The usual method of preparation is to add a small amount of lytic material to a broth suspension of young, actively growing susceptible broth culture, and the incubate until clearing occurs. The cleared culture is filtered, and when the sterility is assured, Merthiolate, 1:5000, is added. The filtrate is now ready for use."[18]

Production of therapeutic solutions had a lot of room for improvement, even under the best circumstances, and efficacy suffered as a result. Making matters worse, commercially sold products from less reputable companies were sometimes devoid of any phage whatsoever.[19]

In stark contrast to the ambiguity and complexities of phage therapy, the literature, research, understanding, and clinical applications associated with sulfa drugs was clear. Their advantages and shortcomings were well defined. Chemically, they were simple compared with phages. Prior to the appearance of penicillin, sulfa drugs helped clear the way for chemotherapeutic approaches to bacterial infections. When penicillin became available to the public, it reshaped the therapeutic landscape for good. It's said that one thing businesses can't stand is uncertainty. For pharmaceutical companies, injecting viruses into patients and hoping for the best defined uncertainty. It's little wonder they embraced the "sure thing." Penicillin was effective and safe, and it helped win the war.

ERNST CHAIN'S RELATIONSHIP WITH Howard Florey never recovered after their falling out over the latter's trip to the United States. Although Chain remained at the Dunn School until 1948, his tenure was fraught with tension. He never was able to shake the notion that as a continental Jew, a healthy dose of anti-Semitism limited his opportunities and recognition for his achievements in the penicillin project. As a result, outside of the laboratory he tended to keep to himself, preferring to spend his leisure time playing the piano as opposed to joining collegial Oxford actives with his colleagues. His suspicions were not without merit.[20]

When the war ended, Chain saw an advantage in Britain's position as a leader in an antibiotics industry still in its infancy. The Americans had vindicated his earlier instincts regarding protecting their discovery of penicillin when Andrew Moyer patented the process derived at the Northern Regional Research Laboratory with Norman Heatley's assistance. Adding insult to injury, the patent was filed in Great Britain, since working for the government excluded him from applying in the States. Chain proposed to the Medical Research Council that an antibiotic committee be set up to coordinate and fund British research, much the same way Vannevar Bush's Office of Scientific Research and Development did for penicillin. It was the only way to compete with the Americans, who already enjoyed a decent head start and more available resources. The council members rejected the idea "due to a mixture of their antipathy to Chain over his advocating patents for penicillin research and also due to the lack of a tradition in Britain for cooperation in research between universities, government, and private industry." Undeterred, Chain took his proposition to Whitehall, only to meet with rejection yet again.[21]

Chain moved on from Oxford soon afterward; in fact, he quit England altogether. Britain's loss was the world's gain as the Istituto Superiore di Sanità in Rome offered him a position as the director of its new Biochemistry Department. There he set up a modern pilot penicillin plant that was used to produce the antibiotic and, at the same time, to train budding chemical engineers in the basic technique used to produce penicillin. He was also able to pursue his own research in the labs under his direction that spanned an entire floor at the institute.[22]

Liberated from the cloistered confines of Oxford, Chain was free to increase his collaborations with non-British labs that had similar interests. More important, he was able to help countries across Europe acquire the technology and know-how to produce antibiotics. He was a true internationalist at a time when a new internationalism was taking shape, first with the UNRRA, then with the United Nations, and later with the World Health Organization (WHO). He acted as a special consultant to the UNRRA's penicillin plant program and then as the chairman of the antibiotics committee for the WHO. Under both of those organizations, Chain had the biggest impact on sharing antibiotics, in particular with countries such as Czechoslovakia and Yugoslavia, which were already covered in the

UNRRA's mission. Very often, Chain became an advocate for those countries in the world forum. He also authored a detailed pamphlet that outlined step-by-step the production of penicillin and how the equipment should be set up in a plant. He distributed it to any country that was interested, regardless of politics. The benefits of penicillin were above borders and political affiliation. It was something to be shared by humanity.[23]

In 1948 just before resigning from Oxford, the Soviet Union reached out to Chain and asked for his help in setting up a state-of-the-art penicillin fermentation plant. As you'd expect, he agreed to do what he could. To move the process along, three scientists—V. I. Zeifman, G. A. Cherniavskii, and N. M. Borodin—traveled to England to learn what they could at the Dunn School. In addition to mentoring the Soviet scientists, Chain also wrote a detailed hundred-page manual documenting the technology involved in penicillin production. The document was funded by the Technopromimport, an industrial trade association controlled by the Soviet Ministry of Foreign Trade. It even included sensitive information Chain had acquired while consulting for the Swedish pharmaceutical company Astra and the British company Beecham.[24]

For a nation that conceived of and helped create the UNRRA, the United States gave every signal that it was hell-bent on undermining it. In the case of distributing food and clothing to countries such as Poland and Yugoslavia, the politicized reality of an overwhelmingly U.S.-funded organization providing aid to Communist countries complicated efforts. (Even though Poland hadn't yet fully become Communist, the country was snugly sitting under Stalin's thumb.) Congressional lawmakers, who controlled the government purse, took offense to the notion that American taxpayers' money was being used against their interests. The realization that the UNRRA would not adjust its mission to accommodate American politicians played a major role in their seeking an alternative strategy more in their control. It was a major contributing factor in the birth of the European Recovery Program, better known as the Marshall Plan.[25]

The same tensions played out in the very public struggle over the Podbielniak countercurrent extractor, which played an important role in the most up-to-date penicillin production methods. The extraction process—that is, taking the actual penicillin out of the fermentation liquid—was every bit as critical as finding the right mold, the right substrate, and the right fermentation method. Having a high-yielding strain of mold was useless if most of the active ingredients washed away with the waste liquid. In fact, one of the drawbacks of the Heatley-Chain method was that the majority of penicillin disappeared, partly because of the extraction method they employed, and the product they did get was littered with impurities that destabilized it. (Penicillin's early iconic yellow color came from harmful impurities.) In fairness to Heatley and Chain, though, it would have been impossible to have such a large piece of machinery inside a lab setting, let alone during wartime.[26]

The Podbielniak countercurrent extractor set itself apart from other methods due its ability to minimize the decomposition of penicillin. It was also sensitive and nimble enough to deal with the constant changes in the nature of fermentation liquids from batch to batch. "Each broth was radically different. Culture strain and potency information was withheld. Deforming oils were different and sometimes conveyed troublesome slimy and emulsifying characteristics to the broth." On top of that, sometimes corn steep liquor, by now the fermentation standard, was not used, and a yeast raw material base was substituted.[27]

Besides resulting in purer extractions, the Podbielniak extractor allowed for the separation of the different penicillins that were found in the broth. For example, it could be set to extract only penicillin G. This allowed manufacturers to manipulate the concentrations of penicillin in the products they took to market. To top it all off, using the countercurrent extractor significantly lowered the price of producing penicillin and not only made the process feasible but also profitable.[28]

The differences between extraction techniques went from 100 to 400 Oxford units per milliliter in 1945 with solvent-based methods to upward of 5,000 Oxford units per milliliter using the countercurrent extractor. (To be fair, the potency between the two isn't even comparable.) While the technology and actual extractor had been around since the 1930s, the penicillin separation technique was new. As a result, the application of the extractor to fermentation broth was patented in the United States in 1946.[29] For all intents and purposes, the Podbielniak extractor belonged to America, and the government guarded it closely. If anyone outside the United States wanted one, that individual would need to obtain an export license.

Then came Ernst Chain.

In early 1948, after visiting Czechoslovakia and inspecting the (nonoperational) penicillin plant donated by the UNRRA, Chain informed the scientists that the machinery and setup had been practically obsolete when they received it in 1946. Perhaps trying to right a wrong, he took responsibility for procuring a Podbielniak countercurrent extractor for the Czech government under the auspices of the newly formed WHO. According to Slawomir Łotysz, "On April 26, the day after he met Herbert Kaiser of Podbielniak Inc., the sole producer of the extractors, Chain assured Dr. Bruno Schober from the Ministry of Health in Prague that 'the supply of the machines for Czechoslovakia will not meet with any difficulty.'" He couldn't have been more mistaken if he'd said penicillin grew on trees. A year later, not a single screw from an extractor had been exported.[30]

So why the snowballing on the part of the State Department? In today's parlance, it was a matter of national security. At this point, only a handful of countries possessed the capability to produce antibiotics on a large scale. The Podbielniak extractor got caught in a larger battle being waged by the United States and the Soviet Union, one that featured the former trying to deny the latter access to antibiotics. Without the countercurrent extractor, producers were at a significant disadvantage when it came to producing crystalline penicillin, which was purer and more potent than the so-called amorphous yellow penicillin earlier methods produced. U.S. control of the extractor gave the Americans an easy and effective way to control global penicillin production. It was a risky strategy. Even the *New York Times* later commented that "the United States will have a hard time convincing the world that shutting off supplies of medicine is an essential security measure."[31]

Anglo-American fears extended beyond the realm of medicine. In addition to submerged fermentation vats, officials from both countries believed that the Podbielniak extractor belonged to the dual-use technology George W. Merck warned about in his report on biological weapons. According to a confidential document that listed industrial machinery under embargo, the extractor was "effectively controlled by the U.S." That meant "such control of the item so identified would limit the war potential of the Sino-Soviet bloc through the ability of the U.S. to significantly deprive (quantitatively or qualitatively) the bloc of materials, equipment, services or technology."[32]

In the end, the State Department rebuffed the numerous attempts at obtaining an extractor. The requests only served to reinforce the suspicion that the UNRRA was being used to aid Communist countries at the expense of American taxpayers. U.S. lawmakers viewed the attempts by the UNRRA and, later, by the WHO to procure extractors as a backdoor attempt at stealing industrial secrets.

The countries that needed the countercurrent extractor had very few options at their disposal. In the end, the best they could do was to continue pressuring the State Department publicly.

The policy was set. Washington was willing to completely deprive anyone associated with a Communist government of antibiotics from the machinery necessary to produce it to the crystalline salts. It didn't matter that most citizens lacked any choice. Victory mattered. Making a point mattered. Being right mattered. In the realpolitik of the Cold War, compassion had no place. The suffering would be indiscriminate and complete.

TO REDUCE ERNST CHAIN'S immediate post-Oxford years to jetting between Eastern bloc countries and physically patching up the holes in Communist science that prevented them from making antibiotic inroads would be a disservice. Far ahead of his time—nothing new for him—Chain understood that antibiotics' success transcended politics because it was in everyone's interest to have access to the best medication possible. He and Edward Abraham were among the first to document the effects substandard penicillin produced in bacteria. As doctors and patients would learn years later, resistance didn't recognize borders, nor did it care for politics.

Chain contributed much more for the field of antibiotics through the work he did at the Instituto Superiore di Sanità in Rome. He was recruited by its director Domenico Marotta, who was determined to reverse the scientific atrophy that occurred during World War II as result of the country's relative isolation from Western science. Chain enjoyed Marotta's confidence and, as a result, was given a wide berth in terms of research. During a time when Italy's priorities lay in rebuilding the country and feeding its population, the building of Chain's world-class, state-of-the-art laboratory reflected a determination to recapture some of the dignity and prosperity of the country's past. The construction of the pilot penicillin plant, the Fabbrica della Penicillina, represented a calculated stab at the future.[33]

Anyone who had listened to Chain's Nobel banquet speech would have been surprised by his activism and desire to preach the benefits of science—namely, penicillin—as opposed to its destructive potential, or the atomic bomb. He warned others against the abuse of scientific discoveries. "Polite opportunism and passive retreat into the ivory towers of abstract thought will not absolve them from it. Scientists now realise what the cost has been of not having resisted with all their power barbarism between 1933–1939 on the plea that this was the job of the politician."[34]

The Instituto Superiore di Sanità grew into one of the most important centers of antibiotic research and development. It trained scientists and chemical engineers interested in commercial penicillin production. So many promising students passed through the institute's doors that Chain's disciples could be found in pharmaceutical companies around the world. Its new Biochemistry Department was the first international center dedicated to antibiotics and attracted researchers far and wide. Among its R&D accomplishments was the development of semisynthetic penicillins during a partnership with the British pharmaceutical company Beecham. The first so-called broad-spectrum antibiotics such as methicillin, ampicillin, and amoxicillin targeted bacteria not affected by penicillin. Unfortunately, people allergic to penicillin reacted to the semisynthetics as well.[35]

Chain's tenure at the institute had its controversies, though. The Beecham partnership may have been fruitful from a development standpoint, but the agreement, and other similar deals, had critics. It highlighted the conflict of interest semiprivate deals carried. Abusing the system that administrators at the institute helped design became a constant temptation. Domenico Marotta was arrested on charges that he benefited from the deal.[36]

The Instituto Superiore di Sanità showed that the United States, the United Kingdom, and Canada were not the only countries capable of assembling top-quality penicillin plants and competing on an international scale. For a few years, the Italian pharmaceutical industry effectively competed on the world's stage for a slice of the lucrative antibiotics market.

In the Netherlands, the Nederlandsche Gist-en Spiritusfabriek (NG&SF) produced its own penicillin during the Nazi occupation with limited access to scientific journals, specifically the Oxford group's *Lancet* paper and subsequent research by other labs on penicillin.[37] This placed the group in a prime position once the war ended. According to the research of Marlene Burns, J. W. Bennett, and Piet W. M. van Dijck on NG&SF's penicillin program, "By 1946, NG&SF was supplying all the penicillin needed by Dutch hospitals; by 1948 it was supplying all the penicillin needed for the country; and by 1949, it began exporting penicillin." NG&SF grew into one of the world's top antibiotics producers.[38]

The situation in Japan exemplified the unique status the country enjoyed under U.S. control. While it can be said that no occupation is a good occupation, the Americans' determination to engineer their former enemy into a close (and non-Communist) ally did come with some advantages. In this case, Japan was on the receiving end of the construction of penicillin and streptomycin plants.

As with other countries battered by the war, Japan suffered from the breakdown of its health care and sanitary infrastructure. As a result, the immediate postwar years saw an explosion of infectious diseases. In particular, separate outbreaks of typhus and tuberculosis threatened the fragile peace. Both events were among the largest in recent history and worried Japanese and occupation officials.[39] In addition, venereal diseases surged during a time when poverty and destitution gripped the country as a result of damage done during the war. Transactional sex, whether it be promiscuity or prostitution, offered women a means to earn money, usually from the American soldiers tasked with running the occupation. From the lowest private to the high-ranking generals, having a local "girlfriend" and a wife at home was common and accepted. Unfortunately, this practice put the men in direct and intimate contact with locals and increased their likelihood of contracting a disease. And that is exactly what happened.

Antibiotics offered an obvious and expedient way to counter the uptick in infected soldiers; however, for the strategy to be effective, the civilian population—a very robust reservoir for disease—needed to be treated as well. Otherwise, the soldiers would simply keep getting reinfected and require more treatment, more funds, and more antibiotic. Public health officials were perfectly aware of the danger that misusing antibiotics presented—namely, resistance. To address the problem of venereal diseases, a robust response needed to be implemented. Rather than importing penicillin from the States, General MacArthur and SCAP public health officials made the radical and forward-looking decision to construct an antibiotic infrastructure in Japan.

As with the UNRRA's efforts, it served multiple purposes. First, it provided a local source of penicillin and streptomycin. This relieved the strain of having to purchase medicine at cost from pharmaceutical companies, ultimately saving money. Maintaining a reliable local supply removed some of the uncertainty at a time when the world seemed to have an insatiable demand for antibiotics. Second, the construction of local plants served a reconstruction purpose. The Japanese pharmaceutical industry, and therefore a sector of the economy, would receive a boost, almost automatically putting it on par with the handful of other countries capable of producing antibiotics. It would be the only country in Asia capable of producing consistently high-quality products.

EVEN BEFORE PENICILLIN BECAME available to the public, the story of its discovery had already transcended science and become a part of popular culture. In particular, Alexander Fleming's carefully crafted version of discovering *Penicillium notatum* from petri dishes left by an open window had been retold in print, in film, and on television. He'd "gone viral" before going viral was a thing. Later, just to make the story complete, he won the Nobel Prize, sharing it with Florey and Chain. Yet in the long run, Fleming's impact on the nascent field of antibiotics was limited. To borrow a term from the sports world, he was "one and done." In the search for the next antibiotic, Selman Waksman served as the prototype, playing the percentages. Laboratories around the world analyzed tens of thousands of soil samples in the hopes of hitting the jackpot. Of course, the likelihood of finding one viable antibiotic was pretty good, regardless of the crudeness of their methods. That was how the next major antibiotic class emerged from the laboratories of Lederle/American Cyanamid in 1948.

The discovery was made in the laboratory of the brilliant biochemist Yellapragada Subbarow. Benjamin Duggar, one of the researchers under his supervision, made the discovery after doing what amounts to laboratory grunt work, much in the way Albert Schatz did for Selman Waksman. After testing thousands of strains of actinomycetes from soil samples collected around the world, Duggar whittled it down to a few strains with promising antibiotic activity. The most active of the bunch came to be known as *Streptomyces aureofaciens* (later it would be renamed as *Actinomycetes aureofaciens*). Because of the gold-colored crystals that resulted from the extraction process, the new antibiotic was called Aureomycin; its chemical name was chlortetracycline. It was the first member of a new class antibiotics called tetracyclines.[40]

While it provided lukewarm results in initial animal testing, it was a revelation when tested in humans. It was the first of the antibiotics to be labeled broad spectrum. Where penicillin mostly worked on gram-positive bacteria and streptomycin worked on gram-negative bacteria, Aureomycin attacked both. Bacteria, such as *Brucella melitensis*, that managed to escape the chemotherapeutic activity of both of the older antibiotics showed susceptibility to Aureomycin. The antibiotic also covered most of the bacteria attacked by its predecessors with less toxicity. As the first broad-spectrum antibiotic, it proved a game changer. More important, Aureomycin was able to rein in the penicillin-resistant staphylococci that were beginning to plague hospitals around the world.[41]

At about the same time Duggar was making his discovery, a parallel discovery was being made at Pfizer by Robert B. Woodward. Like his counterpart at American Cyanamid, he tested thousands of soil samples collected from locations around the world. He would discover the second member of the tetracycline class, Terramycin; its chemical name is oxytetracycline. Its broad-spectrum activity was similar to Aureomycin's, and both tetracyclines would go on to revolutionize and do irreparable harm to antibiotics in the near future.[42] But that's a story for much later.

FOR A BRIEF WINDOW of time, Western researchers followed the logical paths the discovery of penicillin and bacteriophage therapy carved into the medical landscape. At first, researchers investigated whether the chemotherapeutic antibiotics such as sulfonamide and penicillin had any effect on bacteriophages. They were testing whether the antibiotics acted on viruses. Phages were simply models.

Scientists discovered that for the most part, no effect occurred. Tyrothricin and actinomycin A showed no activity against phages. Penicillin demonstrated no activity as well. Penicillin B showed some efficacy for *E. coli* phages. Further testing demonstrated that streptothricin, streptomycin, and clavacin at high levels could inactivate certain phages.[43]

Penicillin's impotence against viruses may have seemed a disappointment, but canny researchers saw an opportunity. If penicillin attacked bacteria one way and bacteriophages employed a whole different strategy, was it possible to join the two into a super dose of antimicrobials?

In one study conducted by none other than Albert P. Krueger, staphylococci were treated with penicillin, bacteriophages, and a combination. Together with his coauthors, he established that while penicillin alone and phages alone showed their expected efficacy, the combination caused the staphylococcal cultures to lyse at a quicker pace and earlier in the process.

In 1948 J. Smiles, F. V. Welch, and W. J. Elford performed a similar experiment at the National Institute for Medical Research in London. Once again, the combination of penicillin and bacteriophage proved quicker and more efficient at clearing bacteria.

From an evolutionary standpoint, the combination had its advantages. Phage-antibiotic synergy (PAS), as it was called, showed promise. A 2016 study into the advantages of combination antimicrobial therapies explains, "The logic of combining phages and antibiotics stems from an evolutionary understanding that two sufficiently different selective pressures are likely to be more effective than either alone." The authors added, "Antibiotics belonging to different classes and having different mechanisms of action exhibited PAS when combined with phages . . . , compared to the few synergistic combinations reported for antibiotic cocktails."[44]

In the end, the line of inquiry came to nothing. A time would come in a few years when the pincer attack of PAS might have made a difference, perhaps even saved a few lives. By then, the sharply divided world would be reflected in laboratories and journals across the globe. The idea of combining antibiotics and bacteriophages would be abandoned for sixty years; then it was resumed in earnest.

8

In August 1949 he stood in front of nearly two hundred thousand of his countrymen, facing them the way kings and popes did. Tiananmen Square stretched out before him; the Forbidden City loomed behind. He was a long way from Yan'an and the caves where members of his Communist government spent their time, waiting for the right moment to relaunch their crusade against the Nationalist Party that controlled the country. He was a long way from the helplessness of having his wife captured and killed. He was a long way from being forced to leave his infant daughter and the rest of his family. The latest epochal moment in the Middle Kingdom's illustrious history belonged to one man—Mao Zedong.

Reading from a sheet of paper, Mao pronounced: "People all over China have been plunged into bitter suffering and tribulation since Chiang Kai-shek's Kuomintang reactionary government betrayed the fatherland, conspired with the imperialists, and launched a counterrevolutionary war. . . . Now the people's liberation war has been fundamentally won and a majority of people has been liberated."[1]

Mao gave little indication of the rout his soldiers had inflicted on the Kuomintang military. After a protracted internecine struggle, cities fell one after another as if a divine force had intervened. Beijing in January. Nanjing in April. Shanghai in May. Changsha in August. Most of September was spent ironing out the administrative details of how the newly reborn country would be run. Now he formally announced the People's Republic of China to the world.

For some time, President Harry Truman had harbored doubts about the Chinese Nationalist leader Chiang Kai-shek. His faith had not only wavered but also withered. When Lt. Gen. A. C. Wedemeyer returned from the Far East with a report requested by the president, Truman's doubts only grew. According to the general, "Corruption [has] caused the loss of confidence in the Government and basic freedoms of the people are jeopardized due to oppression by government police agencies." Truman ordered the report be classified top secret and buried it so that its recommendations could not be referenced. Only the secretaries of state and defense saw it. With each passing day, the prognosis of Chiang's chances diminished, even with a numerical advantage troop wise.[2] By the time the Nationalist forces were driven off the mainland and onto Formosa (now Taiwan), nobody doubted that Washington had backed the wrong horse. It was a costly mistake.

Less than a week before Mao addressed the crowd in Tiananmen Square, the foundations of America's postwar sense of security (and perhaps entitlement) crumbled with President Truman's admission to the American public that the Soviet Union had tested an atomic bomb of its own. The advantage that had given the Americans their swagger and international assertiveness was relegated to the so-called ash bin of history.

Nothing came easily that year. Even when the West won, it lost in the long run. The year started with the crisis in Berlin still unresolved. A steady stream of planes continued to descend into Tempelhof Airport. Lives were being saved, no doubt; yet it didn't take a foreign affairs genius to see the airlift for what it was—a bandage over an ugly gash in need of stitches.

The tug of war between the United States and the Soviet Union showed no sign of relenting. Each time one country appeared to pull closer to scoring a decisive blow, the other responded with something in kind. A coup d'état in Czechoslovakia installed a Communist government and led to the suspected suicide of Jan Masaryk; a contested parliamentary vote in the Republic of Korea (South Korea) saw a staunch anti-Communist named Syngman Rhee elected as president. The deutsche mark was introduced in the British, French, and U.S. zones of Berlin; Stalin responded by blocking all travel into and out of the non-Communist zones. The Berlin Blockade was undone by the Berlin Airlift. To resist Communist expansion in Europe, the United States, the United Kingdom, Canada, France, and seven other nations established the North Atlantic Treaty Organization; four months later, Soviet scientists successfully tested an atomic bomb. Less than a week after President Truman informed the American public about Stalin's bomb, a victorious Mao Zedong stood in Tiananmen Square and announced the founding of the People's Republic of China.

Mao assumed control of a divided and damaged country. Twenty-three years of conflict—the first phase of the civil war (1927–37), the Second Sino-Japanese War (1937–45), and the second phase of the civil war (1945–50)—resulted in widespread poverty and disease. The savagery of the Japanese alone would have been enough to leave a weakened collective, but the brutality China's sons and daughters inflicted on each other left them compromised. Between 2 million to 3.5 million people died.

The survivors inhabited a country hobbled by sickness and disease. Shortages complicated efforts to provide health care. After the Japanese left the country, Deputy Roy Hendrickson of the United Nations Relief and Rehabilitation Administration described the situation on the ground after completing a tour of the country. "Everywhere throughout China we witnessed a shortage of coal accompanied by lack of important building materials, such as lumber and bricks, and lack of medical supplies, hospitals, doctors, and clothing. The food situation is already getting acute in some districts and there will be progressive deterioration of hot food situation unless help can be made available as soon as possible."[3]

Local hospitals were saddled with shortages that created a dangerous environment. An American doctor named Ernest Lippa spent a few months in 1949 deep in Communist Chinese territory. He reported on the state of health care. "As a result of the careless and unsanitary operating-room procedures, it was impossible to perform aseptic surgery and nine out of ten cases became infected. Some of the patients died, others remained maimed for life because an infected joint would stiffen and some required protracted hospitalization. If the patient was a Communist Party member, penicillin and sulfa drugs were used lavishly. A peasant got such drugs only as long as he could pay an exorbitant price."[4]

Conditions in China were identical to the postwar conditions in Greece, Poland, and Yugoslavia except on a much larger scale. Even with the full cooperation of the Kuomintang and the People's Liberation Army, the UNRRA found conditions challenging. In particular, getting supplies from the coast inland proved a hurdle.

Outbreaks occurred on a regular basis. Cities, countryside—it didn't matter. They flashed and moved with amorphous crowds of people. Refugees from other parts of China. Soldiers returning home. Hankow. Shanghai. Kwantung. Changsha. They carried their infections, depositing a trail of germs in their wake and spreading misery without relief. Anthrax. Japanese encephalitis. Trichinosis. Brucellosis. Glanders. Rabies. Typhus. Typhoid. Plague. Syphilis. Gonorrhea. Sometimes, simply staying alive was the battle.

SINCE THE END OF the war, the Truman administration tried to hinder exports to the Soviet bloc. The First and Second Decontrol Acts allowed the government to control local scarce commodities. After experiencing a degree of success, the administration established an interagency committee to formalize the classification of exported materials according to a three-tier system, depending on their war-making potential. It would soon learn that manipulating American exports was easy enough. Controlling the trade of its allies was an entirely different story.[5]

As fate would have it, Congress was in the process of legislating a bartering chip (or sledgehammer, depending on one's point of view). Officially known as the European Recovery Program, it would be better known as the Marshall Plan and provide $12 billion of aid in the form of grants, which Western European countries could use to rebuild their shattered economies. A body called the Economic Cooperation Administration was created by the Economic Cooperation Act to administer the Marshall Plan.[6]

Before final passage through Congress, an amendment was added that "barred any country receiving US aid if it exported any product to a non-participating European country which might contain a US-supplied commodity that would ordinarily be refused a US export license."[7] An ad hoc subcommittee composed a list of possible exports to be restricted. It consisted of four classes, with class 1 being all military goods and equipment that could be used to manufacture weapons. The next class, 1A, was composed of semi-military items; class 2, indirect military significance such as trains and mining equipment. Class 3 was composed of textiles, clothing, or office equipment, and class 4 included everything else. American officials would strategically alter the list's contents and categorization to their advantage.[8]

The Podibielniak countercurrent extractor fell under class 1A, while antibiotics fell under class 2.[9] This system provided the framework for withholding both items from countries the United States deemed hostile.

The American officials' European counterparts would propose lists of their own that usually omitted exports essential to their economies, much to Washington's frustration. Even Great Britain, arguably its closest ally, refused to unconditionally limit its trade with the Soviet Union.[10]

After Chiang's defeat, the State Department recommended placing a trade embargo on China, one designed to prevent it from becoming "an adjunct of Soviet power."[11] Once again, U.S. desires ran contrary to those of its treaty-bound NATO allies, which had their own vision of what should and should not make it to Chinese shores. In Washington's eyes, this situation would not do. In particular, the United States demanded that London curtail all goods contained on Washington's versions of the class 1 and class 1A lists. At some point or another, most European trade passed through Hong Kong, then a colony of the British Empire, and the British made money off all of it . The British were concerned that if they abandoned that trade, it would simply be picked up by another European country and be lost permanently. Eventually, they'd learn that their fears were well-founded.[12]

The other NATO countries, while wary, did not view the People's Republic of China as much of a threat as the Truman administration did, particularly when it came to trade. Even members of the U.S. government were split by the embargo. For starters much of the exports to China consisted of basic items such as oil and steel. Companies from Texas to Trieste were reluctant to stop selling their commodities.

They belonged to a new list, class 1B, denoting goods that would be controlled by limiting the amount exported, as opposed to forbidding complete exportation. U.S. oil companies had less choice on the matter and simply had to watch as their British competitors took over contracts they were forced to abandon. Secretary of State Dean Acheson asked Secretary of Defense Louis Johnson to moderate the ban. Even U.S. plans for the revival of German and Japanese industries ran into problems with embargoes of their own making.[13]

The Joint Chiefs of Staff stressed that the constant inflow of Soviet aircraft, munitions, and fuel represented significant threats to the already-foundering position of the United States in Asia. If there was any doubt as to how they viewed recent events, they clarified it by declaring that "the United States and the USSR are now, to all interest and purposes, engaged in war—except for armed conflict."[14]

On the Soviet side, the establishment of the Council for Mutual Economic Assistance was designed to counter the creeping Western European threat by serving as an economic counterweight. Moscow hoped that it would prevent the countries within its sphere of influence from defecting to the Marshall Plan.

IN GERMANY, THE AMERICANS had something to prove. Literally. At an early stage in the Cold War, they realized that bullets would not decide the next conflict. The Marshall Plan and, later, the Point Four Program proved that. The next war would be one of ideas and perception. They needed to market the American way of life as one of high ideals, hard-won success, and historic bounty. In other words, the United States needed to show and prove to the people of the world that democratic capitalism was capable of putting food in their stomachs, roofs over their heads, and clothes on their backs. The American way was the path to opportunity and prosperity.

Food represented a visceral symbol of the affluence the Americans hoped to communicate. It also represented one of the basic necessities the war had made scarce in occupied territories. Making matters worse, the problems were not solely logistical in nature but also administrative. "Concurrently, in cascading sequence, wartime destruction and dislocation wrecked the transportation and communication systems, creating critical breaks in not only the traditional food distribution systems from the ground to storage and then on to the market, but also in the ability to administer and communicate regarding food production across the region."[15]

But since 1948, the overall food situation in the British- and U.S.-occupied zones had improved, thanks to increased grain imports. This resulted in larger rations and a variety of foodstuffs becoming available. In no way did this mean that all of the occupation's problems had been solved, but definite strides had been made.[16]

With the starvation problem ebbing into the past, the time had come for the occupation forces to do some selling. Calmer waters allowed planners in the Soviet and U.S. zones to begin indoctrinating Germans to the central ideas that defined their countries. It boiled down to capitalism versus Communism and democracy versus authoritarianism. The legendary CBS newsman Edward R. Murrow understood immediately what was taking place. There was a "psychological war between the U.S. and USSR for possession of the German mind."[17] Unlike the blunt hammer approach employed by the Communists (capitalists bad, Communists good; Stalin is a genius, Truman is a joke), the Americans walked along an indirect path to their ultimate goal. Rather than issuing direct denunciations of Communism, U.S. news outlets published controlled critiques of elements of the Soviets' ideology. "The program will be positive in nature, and not merely destructive and tendentious with regard to communism. It will show how true democracy guarantees the rights of the individual and how a true democracy requires government by the people as opposed to government for the people by a small ruling clique."[18]

Once the kinks lay exposed, officers at the U.S. Information Control Department assembled pieces for print and radio broadcast that extolled related American virtues absent in the Communist model. It was done on purpose and at the behest of Gen. Lucius D. Clay. Department officers were presented with the challenge of promoting the benefits of the American way of life. Disparaging the enemy's ideology was off-limits. Officers had to keep the messages positive and stay away from the negative. Keep away from the obvious; embrace the subtle. It was very much about manipulating the German subconscious.[19]

One way the Americans achieved their goal was by establishing

"Little Americas" across the country that were filled with products, people, and culture imported from the United States. Many of the people coming to settle in the occupied zone were partners of officers, a sharp reversal of previous directives that forbade spouses from joining active duty soldiers. Little Americas put the nuclear family—devoted and prosperous—on display for the world to see. It also dramatically decreased fraternization between soldiers and German women and, by extension, the transmission of sexually transmitted diseases. Moreover, it had the knock-on effect of reducing the number of illegitimate children born. Some estimates indicated that occupation soldiers fathered more than thirty thousand German American children. The situation had gotten to the point that Germans often quipped, "In the next war, just send the uniforms, you left the Army here."[20]

Penicillin played a significant role in communicating the superiority of the West's way of life and standard of living, especially that of the United States. While it's doubtful many of the displaced persons or German citizens knew the story of how penicillin came about, how the British discovered it, and how the Americans mass produced it, they naturally understood one invaluable, indisputable thing: only one of the four zones possessed a consistent supply of antibiotics, and it was administered by the United States.

As noted previously, penicillin in the U.S. zone, as in the British zone, at first was reserved exclusively for treating syphilis and gonorrhea, much to the disappointment of German health officials. By January 1946 supplies of the antibiotic had increased to the point that the stringent rules began to loosen, and German doctors were authorized to administer penicillin treatments themselves. The supply of penicillin continued to increase through 1947. By that September, "supplies had increased to a monthly allocation of 21 billion units of penicillin for the zone: 2 billion were needed for gonorrhea, 12 billion units were used to treat syphilis, and 7 billion units were available for the treatment of non-venereal diseases."[21]

On the Soviet side, two companies supplied the majority of the penicillin and streptomycin—Pharmazeutische Werke Madaus and Jenapharm. At the time, U.S. intelligence reported that the USSR possessed seven plants, each of which produced penicillin in wildly varying amounts. The output of the two UNRRA plants in Kiev and Minsk hovered around 15,000 Oxford units per month. Factory No. 40 and Factory No. 7, both in Moscow, produced 20,000 and 15,000 units of penicillin, respectively. A plant in Sverdolovsk produced a meager 5,000 million units while a plant located in the Pharmakon Factory in Riga contributed 10,000 million units to the cause. A new plant being constructed in Dzaudzhikau (now Vladikavkaz) promised to double the total amount of penicillin in the Soviet Union. Stalin had personally approved the establishment with the understanding that it would add 80,000 million units per month.[22] Even he grasped the urgency of the situation.

Unfortunately, he might not have been cognizant of the challenges facing the antibiotic industry in the Soviet Union and its satellites.

THE LENIN ALL-UNION ACADEMY of Agricultural Science conference in 1948 tore a fresh, life-threatening gash along the neck of genetics in the Soviet Union. What followed for weeks, months, and years afterward can only be described as the gradual bleeding out of the life sciences. The dark campaign against Russia's geneticists was only just beginning.

The process started a few days after the LAAAS conference at a meeting of the Academy of Sciences. Its members passed a resolution supporting "without qualification the decisions reached at the LAAAS session, and decreed the abolition of a number of laboratories pronounced hotbeds of reactionary Morganism (the laboratories of cytogenetics, botanical cytology phenogenesis, and others)."[23]

Capitulation from the scientific community moved at a breathtaking rate. Resistance collapsed. One after another, frightened voices recanted. The scientists confessed their ignorance. Ivan Michurin was right. Lysenko was right. Creative Darwinism was right, while their own life's work was misguided.

Nikolai Kaftanov, the minister of higher education, called a meeting of the country's university staffs. The meeting's objective was to devise a plan to eradicate "reactionary Morganism" and the misguided theory's principal adherents from the halls of higher learning. The Academy of Medical Sciences followed suit. The rhetoric deviated from policy to polemics. It grew into a race toward the extreme. Denunciations of living geneticists. Vilification of dead scientists. According to Zhores Medvedev, a Russian scientist who lived through the purge, "Kaftanov's speech was reproduced as a pamphlet in an edition of 110,000. This document was saturated with demagoguery and slander."[24]

Kaftanov was not done. During the following days, he issued detailed orders that were sent to universities all over the Soviet Union. The communiqués indicated that any faculty members who opposed Michurinism must be expelled from their institutions. There were names. Shmal'gauzen. Zavadovsky. Sabinin. Alikhanyan. The list went on.[25]

And still it wasn't done. A two-month-long search was implemented to root out any remaining Morganist elements. Like a pestilence, they had to be eradicated. To ensure Michurinism assumed its rightful place at the zenith of Soviet science, all genetics courses that espoused Morganism-Mendelism were abolished, their textbooks destroyed, and all non-Michurinist research projects eliminated. This went for all fields, not just agricultural sciences: veterinary medicine, dentistry, medicine, biology, microbiology, psychiatry, anatomy, and even geology. Not a single Morganist-Mendelist was spared.[26]

All over the country geneticists either bowed to Lysenko or suffered ostracization. The purge was as widespread as it was indiscriminate. Any hint, any mention of genes or chromosomes, regardless of how long in the past, meant being vulnerable to attack. Stature meant nothing. Research meant even less. After all, when all was said and done, Lysenko had fudged most of his experiments, and Prezent never performed a single one. Genetics was being wiped away in bold but misguided strokes.

Even influential scientists such as Leon Orbeli, who worked with Ivan Pavlov, succumbed to the incessant harassment by the Michurinist attack dogs. He had proven to be a man of principle during his tenure as the academician-secretary of the Department of Biology of the Academy of Sciences. Rather than turn a blind eye to pseudoscience, he offered a very public and passionate defense of modern genetics. His career paid the price. Lysenko made a point of going after him. By 1950 the man had been stripped of every single position.[27]

Even Georgyi Gause fell afoul of the sweeping Morganist-Mendelist witch hunt. Two years after being awarded the Stalin Prize in Science and Engineering, he came under attack for his groundbreaking work in population genetics, research that earned him acclaim and immortality in college textbooks the world over. According to *Pravda*, he was attacked "for years of spreading Mendelian views with the connivance of the institute's director, P. G. Sergiev." What's more, Gause's attackers accused him of hindering important antibiotic work by ignoring Michurin's teachings.[28]

The accusations leveled against Gause highlighted the threat and subsequent damage Lysenkoism played in the development and production of antibiotics in the Soviet sphere. Nobody was off-limits, or so it seemed.

EASTERN BLOC COUNTRIES LINED up to denounce the United States for its unapologetic cruelty. For years, they'd been made to wait as equipment for their penicillin plants trickled in one box at a time. Even by January 1949, the factories still lacked essential equipment. A few months earlier, the delegations from Poland, Belarus, Czechoslovakia, Yugoslavia, and Ukraine shared their experiences at the Conference of War Devastated European Countries. They took turns recounting the same basic story. The U.S. Customs Service was actively obstructing shipments by refusing to issue export licenses even though, for example, the Podbielniak countercurrent extractor was technically a medical supply.[29]

The Americans stood firm, and the standoff continued.

The World Health Organization, which had taken over for the UNRRA, invited the countries to a "Penicillin Plant Conference" in February 1949. Polish, Czechoslovakian, and Yugoslavian experts submitted field reports describing their incomplete plants rapidly reaching obsolescence. After some debate, a plan of action evolved. Poland's and Czechoslovakia's factories were much closer to completion, so they would be supplied with Sharples centrifuge extractors. They were good enough to produce amorphous penicillin, and for the time being, the factories would have to make due. Yugoslavia's operation had suffered the greatest delays, so transitioning toward a Podbielniak countercurrent extractor process plant was more realistic. Unfortunately, the WHO still hadn't solved how it would obtain export licenses from the United States.[30]

When the executive board of the WHO met again on February 21, 1949, things grew even testier than in previous sessions. Poland, Czechoslovakia, and Yugoslavia accused the United States of hindering their national programs aimed at eliminating venereal diseases, something the WHO had pushed them to address for years. Now that they were in a position to make progress, thanks to modern medicine, they were being denied the tools to accomplish the task.[31]

In particular, Poland took aggressive steps toward addressing the STD crisis. Its campaign, called Operation W, called for the widespread use of penicillin, with ten-day courses of antibiotic for each patient. People identified as carriers also would be forced to divulge a list of past and present sexual partners to the government. Refusing to cooperate could result in the Polish militia forcibly bringing people to the hospital. WHO officials applauded the campaign. As a result, they lent their support to the three countries' efforts at procuring countercurrent extractors. They were so enthusiastic that they inquired whether a non-U.S. company would be willing to manufacture Podbielniak countercurrent extractors for them. Nobody, however, volunteered to publicly engage in a blatant breach of international patent law.[32]

Officials at the WHO vowed to begin steps toward procuring extractors for all of the countries. The U.S. representative objected to taking such an action, claiming that such activities were "not appropriate" to the organization. Plus, the representative added, there was no proof that the U.S. Customs Service had refused export licenses.[33]

Perhaps out of desperation or anger, the delegates from the Eastern European nations threatened to leave the organization if the World Health Organization could not provide them with the plants they had been promised. They vowed to follow in the footsteps of Russia, Belarus, and Ukraine, all of which had pulled out of the WHO already.[34]

The optics of the situation were terrible for the United States, so the following day, it marched out its own expert, Dr. Justin F. Wait, who disputed the organization's charges. He argued that the demands of the Eastern bloc countries and the WHO amounted to red herrings. They did not need the Podbielniak countercurrent extractor since there were other centrifuges on the market capable of doing the job. He was right. Before Western companies used the Podbielniak countercurrent extractor, they had used other centrifuges. However, his argument was disingenuous. He failed to mention that when penicillin manufacturers transitioned to the Podbielniak extractor, they were able to cut down on costs, increase their efficiency (thus, further reducing costs), and extract a much purer, crystalline form of penicillin that had become the world's standard. It increased the viability of producing the antibiotic. The methods Wait was suggesting the Communist countries use were essentially obsolete.[35]

Officially, the withholding of the Podbielniak extractor and lifesaving antibiotics fell under two mechanisms—the Export Control Act of 1949 and the Mutual Defense Assistance Act of the same year. In 1951 the Mutual Defense Assistance Act was supplemented by the Battle Act, which banned assistance to countries doing business with the Soviet Union. It was an attempt to plug the holes in the leaky embargo put in place years earlier. The Export Control Act was actually an extension of the legislation the Roosevelt administration had put in place in 1940 that was designed to avoid wartime (though technically prewar) scarcities of critical commodities and to limit exports to Imperial Japan. When hostilities ended, the act was supposed to expire, but events in Europe and Asia compelled the Truman administration to extend it. The administration's hunch was more than vindicated in the years to come.[36]

The rationale behind the Export Control Act was summed up by Averell Harriman: "Mutual security can best be advanced by increasing the total strength (military, economic, and political) of the free nations relative to that of the Soviet bloc. . . . In other words, trade with the Soviet bloc becomes a security problem when such trade contributes more to the strength of the Soviet bloc than it does to the free nations."[37]

Harriman went on to clarify that the objective of the embargo was not the complete cessation of trade with Communist countries, pointing out that it "would not serve our present economic defense objectives." He stressed that embargoes needed to be well defined and specific. The Export Control Act did not cut off all trade with the Soviet bloc, only the export of select industrial goods and raw materials that would strengthen the Communist countries' ability to wage war. Luxury items weren't subject to any controls. Neither were shipments of grain, crops, and livestock.[38]

Behind the scenes, the Americans' stance was much less unified than it appeared. According to Mauro Capocci, in late 1949, the Podbielniak company expressed its desire to be taken off the embargo list, as it wanted the opportunity to sell on the international market. "A colloquium took place in late December1949, with Podbielniak trying to convince British authorities, with the help of American representatives, to lift the embargo. Yet, the UK Foreign Office resisted, and with the backing of the Ministry of Defence insisted that the technology would improve Soviet defensive capacity and that it may be of 'extreme importance from the point of view of bacteriological warfare.'"[39]

British officials also took issue with the contradictory position private U.S. companies took with regard to official policy. They felt that the Americans' behavior was inconsistent, with the U.S. Department of Defense wanting one thing and the Department of Commerce another.[40]

No doubt, Washington also agreed with the British Ministry of Defence's stance regarding biological warfare. As has already been discussed, BW was a major concern of policy makers and scientists in the United States. There is one additional point that may have worried Washington and Whitehall: countercurrent extractors—particularly newer, more technologically advanced machines—were integral to the development of nuclear weapons. Besides their use in extracting antibiotics from the spent solution they grew in, countercurrent extractors were essential for reprocessing spent nuclear fuel.

AUREOMYCIN CHANGED THE ANTIBIOTIC playing field for pharmaceutical companies as well as medical professionals. In an industry still coming to grips with the curative powers of penicillin, it showed the way forward. It gave them a new product and, more important, provided them with a strategy to build on. The narrow focus of penicillin was good, but the broader spectrum of Aureomycin was much better. It made the doctor's job infinitely easier.

Rather than having to pinpoint exactly which pathogen was causing an illness—something not always possible during emergency situations—a broad-spectrum drug that killed a wide swath of microbes was the safest bet. It bought the responsible physician time to pinpoint the source of an illness without the pressure of a patient's condition worsening. Unfortunately, not everyone proved responsible; instead, broad-spectrum drugs gave them a shortcut.

Aureomycin also showed pharmaceutical companies the financial incentive to develop their own proprietary drugs, since it was the first major patent-protected antibiotic to hit the market. Penicillin and streptomycin were in the public domain and fair game for anyone to attempt to produce them. The hurdle for entry into the antibiotics business was low as a result. Aureomycin made it higher, and that meant less competition. Only the really well-funded companies could hope to compete.

After the introduction of the broad-spectrum antibiotics Aureomycin and Terramycin, pharmaceutical companies around the world raced to join the parade. Empty patches of soil appeared around the world like some bizarre environmental hiccup. Selman Waksman's method of casting a wide net and hoping for the best—essentially trawling for antibiotics—remained the preferred method of discovery. Not only was the ghost of Waksman's methods haunting laboratories, so was the bacteria that provided him with streptomycin. In 1947 David Gottlieb discovered and isolated chloramphenicol from *Streptomyces venezuelae*. Yet again, it represented a whole new antibiotic class that came to be called amphenicols.[41]

Gottlieb's isolation of chloramphenicol was important but not significant. The truly groundbreaking event in the history of chloramphenicol and antibiotics in general took place in 1949. A team of researchers at Parke-Davis Research Labs was able to decipher the chemical structure of the molecule and completely synthesize the antibiotic.[42]

Ever since the early 1940s, the synthesis of antibiotics—in that case, penicillin—had been the holy grail of research in the field. The Office of Scientific Research and Development expended huge sums of money in a parallel program to synthesize penicillin from scratch. Its researchers failed and recognized that for the time being, the beta-lactam ring that gave penicillin its magic also made it impossible to synthesize. Chloramphenicol did not have an unstable beta-lactam ring, making it much easier to synthesize. Ultimately, it lived up to the hype chemists had projected on the hypothetical penicillin. Synthesizing chloramphenicol was quicker and cheaper than extracting it from a fermentation process.[43]

One more discovery occurred in 1949. Abelardo Aguilar, a researcher for Eli Lilly working in Iloilo, Philippines, wandered through his backyard and dug up random patches of dirt. One of those samples ended up yielding yet another new class of antibiotics called macrolides. The compound, called Ilotycin but better known by its chemical name, erythromycin, had a spectrum of effectiveness that allowed it to become the drug of choice for people allergic to penicillin and other beta-lactams.[44]

Unfortunately, chloramphenicol and erythromycin proved to be too toxic for extended use and were prescribed only when other antibiotics failed. In the case of erythromycin, subsequent macrolides would have less unwanted side effects.

THE PEOPLE'S REPUBLIC OF China needed help. Badly. Almost twenty years of conflict had left the country hobbled and divided. It had a dearth of professionals but an abundance of capable citizens. The reconstruction of the country demanded more than just workers' slogans and honorable pledges. It needed money. More than that, it needed professionals.

Even before the civil war officially ended, the Chinese Communist Party had engaged the Soviet Union for guidance and assistance. In February 1949 a delegation headed by Liu Shaoqi secretly visited Moscow to meet Anastas Mikoyan. Eventually, Mao would declare his policy of "leaning to the side of the Soviet Union." In December the chairman personally went to Moscow to negotiate a treaty with the Soviet Union. His objectives were clear: he needed military and material support. On February 14, 1950, Prime Minister Zhou Enlai signed the Treaty of Amity, Alliance, and Mutual Aid between the Soviet Union and China in Moscow. He also signed the Convention on Soviet Union's Granting a Loan to the People's Republic of China of 30 Years' Duration. In addition to trade agreements, the

Soviet Union mobilized its considerable manpower and resources to jump-start Chairman Mao's first five-year plan. The Russians also pledged to send an army of technological and scientific consultants to China. Just like that, the USSR became the largest trading partner of the nascent People's Republic.[45]

The Soviet Union sent thousands of scientists and engineers to China. They served primarily as technical advisers, teaching the Chinese more than working with them. Moreover, tens of thousands of Chinese engineers and scientists studied in the Soviet Union, learning to read and speak Russian while also familiarizing themselves with Soviet approaches to their fields. Students learned from Russian textbooks.[46]

Chinese universities underwent drastic reorganizing, swapping out the U.S. model for a Soviet version. This meant less general education and more technical training. Scientists were required to learn to speak Russian and read Cyrillic. When a survey of the Chinese Academy of Sciences was taken in 1954, 93.2 percent of all the staff were learning Russian, 73.5 percent could read scientific literature in Cyrillic, and 26.8 percent were able to translate Russian papers into Chinese.[47]

When the civil war ended, thousands of scientists and students returned to China after studying or working at universities in America and Europe. While the government remained wary of them, they could not turn their backs on the knowledge and skills the returnees brought with them. They also acted as a balance to the Soviet Union's influence. However, the scientists who had trained abroad found themselves in a situation eerily mirroring that of their peers in the Soviet Union.[48]

Soviet scientific advisers imported Trofim Lysenko's theories of creative Darwinism, causing a Chinese version of Lysenkoism to take hold. The scientists educated abroad and indoctrinated in modern genetics had no choice but to admit that genes did not exist.

BY 1949 SOVIET AND American scientists had retrenched into their labs and, at the urging of their governments, only shared research that did not fall under the category of "state secrets." As a result of the Klіueva-Roskin cure-for-cancer affair, the USSR Supreme

Soviet passed a law that formalized punishment for citizens found divulging state secrets. People found guilty would be confined in a "reformatory labor camp for a term of eight to twenty years." The Council of Ministers determined what fell under the category of "state secrets."[49]

According to Nikolai Krementsov, "The 'patriotic' campaign radically curtailed the international activities of the Soviet scientific community."[50] Soviet journals that were translated into English were discontinued immediately. The Academy of Sciences went a step further and ordered the academy's journals to stop translating abstracts and table of contents into foreign languages. Soon the party ordered all medical and technical journals to follow the Academy of Sciences' lead. From that point forward, whatever correspondence remained between Soviet and Western scientists fell into uneasy silence.

9

On June 25, 1950, a scourge ripped the Korean Peninsula from the inside out. It infected men's minds. An inchoate madness settled. Communist gunfire rolled down from northern hills, accompanied by the crush of Soviet-made T-34 tanks. The forward thrust of the invading forces tore through straw-roofed hamlets, destroying everything unfortunate enough to lie in their path. The heralds of Kim Il Sung's ambition had arrived.

The Korean People's Army of the Democratic People's Republic of Korea (DPRK) was rampant, their South Korean counterparts were in retreat, and the U.S. military was unable to establish even a rudimentary toehold. Disheartening losses followed in quick succession. Osan. Seoul. Chonan. Taejon. General MacArthur's mighty Eighth Army backpedaled from the thirty-eighth parallel to a thumbnail portion of the southeast called Pusan. Meanwhile, a mass of humanity tracked its every step.[1]

The swift southward march of the Korean People's Army while beating back the South Koreans displaced thousands of people, transforming citizens into refugees. Each dirt-scraped face was a an unfortunate reminder that refused to go away, though both sides wished the refugees would. At first, the combatants pushed them to the side. When that didn't work, they just killed them. Few questioned the logic, much less morality, of such brutal acts. Nothing mattered more than obeying orders. Without them, the house of sand that wars were built on would crumble. And this was war.

It would be a long time until things made sense again.

Since the dropping of the atomic bomb, significantly new weapons hadn't been developed. Most countries spent the intervening five years shedding the remnants of being on a war footing and demobilizing troops. Thus, the weapons of World War II were used in Korea, though how and which weapons were employed differed. For example, the use of napalm in incendiary bombs became the norm, whereas during the previous war they had been used specifically on fire-bombing missions.

The Korean conflict was the first war with antibiotics available from start to finish. The treatment of casualties, however, underwent important structural changes. In particular, the introduction of mobile army surgical hospital (MASH) units and the use of helicopters to transport critically injured casualties revolutionized care. The relative proximity between the battlefield and a supporting MASH unit radically decreased the time for treatment whether it was the administration of antibiotics to thoracic surgery. The first-time use of helicopters as evacuation vehicles also brought the front still closer to the hospital.[2] In terms of antibiotics, from surgeons to battlefield medics, everyone's increased familiarity with them meant that the life-saving drugs were administered not only correctly but also much sooner, usually within the first two to three hours of injury. Studies during World Wars I and II established that the least amount of infections occurred in wounds addressed within six hours of being injured. In Korea standard treatment before evacuation from the battlefield MASH unit to Tokyo consisted of surgical debridement and the administration of penicillin with streptomycin.[3]

Yet even with the shortened trip to full medical care, microbiological reports at the time indicated that the injured patients arriving at the MASH units already suffered from contaminated wounds. The nature of the infections depended on the season. Staphylococci and streptococci were prevalent in the winter months; fecal bacteria and clostridium predominated during summer months. Reported infectious complications included abscess, meningitis, encephalitis, anaerobic infections, uncomplicated fungal infections, and superficial wound infections. The highest mortality rate was in the meningitis group, where six of eight people died. Overall, however, infections continued decreasing when compared to the two world wars.[4]

Resistant bacteria were becoming prevalent in wounded soldiers. Samples collected in Tokyo reflected an astonishing rate of resistance. Forty-eight of fifty-eight samples demonstrated resistance to penicillin; forty-nine of fifty-eight samples were resistant to streptomycin. Of the fifty-eight samples, seven displayed resistance to penicillin, streptomycin, tetracyclines, and chloramphenicol—in other words, to just about every antibiotic on the market at the time. It was believed that the use of combined penicillin-streptomycin prophylaxis led to the high incidence of resistant strains.[5]

The potential for epidemic diseases threatened to burst into the open as well. On the one hand, soldiers tended to have varying degrees of prophylaxis in place through vaccination programs, careful hygiene (when possible), and access to health care in the event that they fell sick. American, British, Australian, United Nations, Korean, and Chinese troops usually represented low risks of transmitting disease. The civilian populations in North and South Korea, on the other hand, carried diseases unseen and presented medical teams on both sides with challenges.[6]

Brig. Gen. Crawford Sams, who served as MacArthur's chief of the Public Health and Welfare Section in occupied Japan and later during the Korean War, recalled his first trip to Pusan before tanks and troops crisscrossed the peninsula. "During the repatriation of Koreans in 1945 and 1946, two cases of cholera unfortunately got ashore at Pusan from a group returning by ship from China. Within a few weeks, cholera followed the rail line, literally, and reached Seoul. Some 17,000 cases occurred with over 11,000 deaths. Smallpox, typhoid, diphtheria, and typhus—the wildfire diseases associated with devastation and mass movement of people—were prevalent in Korea as well as Japan."[7]

It was a stark reminder that there was more to conducting a successful military campaign than bullets and bombs.

EVEN AS THE EARLY days of the Korean War raged and South Korean soldiers and American GIs learned how to fight while "advancing in another direction," the U.S. embargo of Communist countries—in particular, China—struggled for effectiveness. Unilateral embargoes on goods that can be obtained elsewhere are tantamount to self-harm, but the Americans did it anyway.

Three days after the outbreak of war, the United States imposed a complete embargo on all exports to North Korea. A month later, all export licenses for exports to China were revoked. Government officials felt as if the Europeans and other UN members failed to provide sufficient support for the war and the embargo. The British continued to sell petroleum to China, claiming that they were legally bound to honor contracts made prior to the declaration of war. The Dutch were in a similar position, only in terms of kerosene.[8]

Congress suspected that the country's Western European allies were knowingly serving as backdoor sources for smuggled goods into China. It had grown so out of control that Republican senators proposed legislation to stop all U.S. economic and financial aid to those allies. After the war, U.S. intelligence discovered that during nine months in 1951, almost two thousand Western ships had docked in Chinese ports. As one commentator put it, "It was now accepted in U.S. government circles that the Europeans did not share the same enthusiasm as did the United States for halting trade with China."[9] From that point, the United States discarded the conceit that its actions were meant to serve the collective; now, the national interest trumped everything. The government also kept close covert tabs on its allies' shipments sent to Communist countries.[10]

For their part, elected officials in Europe found it increasingly difficult to justify to their citizens' economic self-denial and the stifling of potential growth that Washington dictated. Moreover, centuries-old trading links between Western countries such as Britain with Russia proved too strong to break. Basic goods such as eggs, wheat, pork, and cheese were paid for by shipping machinery, tools, and engines eastward. Moreover, long-standing contracts could not be legally abandoned without cause, whether American politicians fully grasped the depths and complexities of European trade. Either way, the Americans threatened to withdraw their support for the European Recovery Program at any time.[11]

The flow of antibiotics between East and West was spotty, particularly during the 1951–52 years of the Korean War. According to the Department of Commerce, the United States shipped a total of $697,000 worth of antibiotics to the People's Republic of China in 1950, most likely during the first half of the year. Meanwhile, Hong Kong received a whopping $11,678,000 worth of product, not altogether surprising considering it was still a British colony. Macau also imported a paltry $13,000 worth of Soviet antibiotics.[12]

The following year U.S. exports fell off the proverbial cliff. A lump sum of zero dollars' worth of antibiotics reached China, most likely for the obvious reason that their soldiers sent General MacArthur into retirement. However, the supplies of antibiotics entering the port of Hong Kong also shriveled to $19,000, reflecting how American officials viewed the British administration's unwillingness to curtail trade with China. Just to complete the picture, Macau's level of trade remained about the same. During the following year (1952), the tourniquet continued to tighten, and even Hong Kong's imports hovered around $3,000. Compare that with the nearly $12 million sent the previous year, and it might as well have been a zero. The following year saw more of the same.[13]

America's NATO allies were only consistent in their inconsistency. While most of them refrained from furnishing China in 1952, they clearly believed supplying members of the Soviet bloc at their own discretion. Their better judgment told them that antibiotics should not be deprived from any nation due to politics. Every NATO member nation exported to at least one Warsaw Pact country.[14]

Exports to China painted a very interesting picture. During 1952 only four countries were on record as having shipped antibiotics to China. The group consisted of Switzerland (technically a neutral country), France (hell-bent on thumbing its nose at Washington), the United Kingdom (famous for the "special relationship"), and Hong Kong (technically, a British colony). Excluding the first two, whose actions can be considered true to form, that the United Kingdom and her colony conducted the overwhelming majority of antibiotic trade with their staunch ally's enemy must have raised eyebrows. In tallying their pharmaceutical exports, the British made no distinction between antibiotics and other drugs. So their total exports to the world came in at an impressive $88,625,000. Exports to China totaled $241,000. Not so bad. But the real significant numbers come from the tiny colony of Hong Kong, which somehow managed to export $12,064,000 worth of antibiotics to China. Considering how difficult production was and how limited raw materials must have been (and still is) in Hong Kong, clearly the $12 million of antibiotics from Hong Kong were originally part of the $88 million the United Kingdom exported to the "world." That made the British the largest supplier of illicit antibiotics to Communist China. In the eyes of U.S. officials who still maintained an embargo on China, that was $12 million worth of smuggled goods. Surely that must have been some sort of record.[15]

The following year, the antibiotics trade was a little like standing in a long, slow-moving line at the grocery, and as a cashier opened another, people raced toward the opportunity. Trade figures indicate that's exactly what happened with other penicillin-producing nations. What only a year before was four countries exporting to China ballooned to twelve. Even countries new to penicillin production such as Japan traded with China. Once again, Hong Kong led the way with its $14.27 million dwarfing the second-highest supplier, the United Kingdom ($543,000). The United States was on its own when it came to keeping antibiotics out of Communist China's hands.[16]

The figures offer another insight. As of 1953 most Soviet bloc countries were still net importers of antibiotics. In other words, their native industries hadn't quite figured out how to consistently produce antibiotics—in particular, penicillin, streptomycin, and Aureomycin.

WHENEVER THE SUBJECT OF antibiotics in popular culture arises, the first reference cited most often is Carol Reed's film adaptation of Graham Greene's screenplay *The Third Man* (1949). Set in postwar Vienna, it tells the story of the search for a man named Harry Lime, whose mysterious disappearance attracts the attention of his friend Holly Martins and Major Calloway of the British Army Police. As it turns out, among Lime's many crimes, smuggling a new drug, penicillin, is his most lucrative. The product's size and value make it perfect for smuggling and selling on the black market. Set in a city divided between victorious World War II participants, multinational hustlers, apathetic citizens, and law enforcement converse in a lingua franca drenched in ambiguity and doublespeak.

According to one account of the screenplay's genesis, the story line revolves around the Eastern European correspondent for the

Times of London named Peter Smolka. Elizabeth Montagu—one of the film's producers and the sister of Lord Montagu of Beaulieu—had introduced Greene to the reporter. According to Montagu, she believed the meeting could prove mutually advantageous, as Smolka knew the seedy side of Vienna well and could provide information Greene wanted. In turn, Graham Greene could help Smolka publish a few short stories he had written.

"Graham went to have tea with him and Smolker [*sic*] gave him the stories," she said in a 1999 interview with the *Guardian*.[17]

Greene found the inspiration for *The Third Man* from one of the stories he heard about an antibiotic scam and the black markets in Vienna. The scam artists stole penicillin from hospitals, watered down the solutions, and sold the diluted antibiotics to unsuspecting Austrian doctors. The ineffective medicine often caused their patients to die. The scam with tragic consequences became a central theme in the movie.[18]

And so it was in real life.

The relative scarcity of antibiotics, their undeniable effectiveness, and the mythology that was developing around them made them natural products for the black market. Their small size made smuggling them all the more convenient. From Europe to Asia, racketeers exploited both the public's clamoring for the new "miracle drug" and the shortages, many of which resulted from U.S.-led embargoes, that seemed to plague every country except the Anglo-American nations. The artificial restriction of supply had the not-surprising side effect of inflating the prices of antibiotics above market value on the black market. In one instance, a sample of a dozen five-milliliter vials sold for as much as $15,000.[19]

Payment often took different forms particular to the region. In occupied Germany, the brutal devaluation of Nazi government currency meant that something else needed to assume the mantle of a currency with intrinsic value. It wasn't gold or silver or even the American dollar that rose to the status of semilegal tender. No, the most valuable commodity in occupied Germany—in all zones—was American cigarettes.

Occupied Germany was one massive black market in the days prior to the reintroduction of the deutsche mark in West Germany and the ostmark in East Germany. One GI recalled, "Our first introduction [to black marketing] came in a subtle way, like a civilian approaching us and asking if we wanted to sell a pack of cigarettes. Just to put things in perspective, cigarettes were the most desirable commodity in Europe at the time. They had become a medium of exchange and in many cases, people would rather be paid in American cigarettes than in money from any country."[20]

Anecdotal evidence suggests that the prices for antibiotics usually exceeded what regular citizens could offer. One East German mother lamented not being able to "purchase" antibiotics for her ailing son. "Dear nephew, I pray you, save my Frantz! I send the prescriptions that may give him back his life. If communists we could apply and perhaps get the drugs after a long wait. Not being of the party or useful to it, we have no hope in that directions. The black market offers no hope either. I have tried to barter dried mushrooms from the woods, goose feathers, and cabbages from my garden. They laugh at me. So high are prices that only other black marketeers and big political can be rich enough to buy."[21]

Smuggled antibiotics meant for East Germany and Soviet bloc countries tended to flow through Tangiers and Switzerland when not sent directly from non-Communist sources. During the immediate postwar years, Republican Spain also served as a major avenue for shipments of penicillin. Its proximity to Algiers and Morocco worked in its favor, as did the blind eye Generalissimo Francisco Franco turned to smuggling. When the tiny bottles of penicillin finally made it to the black market, they were sold from local bars as they were the places most likely to have refrigeration.

In the Far East, Hong Kong, Tianjin, and Macau dominated trade "clandestine or otherwise," although Chinese ports started accepting more commerce on their own. Hong Kong's status as an open port had long encouraged entrepreneurial souls to ply their trades there, and black markets proliferated after World War II. In 1954 the *Wall Street Journal* noted that in Hong Kong, a "capitalist oasis, on rim of China's red desert, a free market blooms." Besides the obvious tensions between it and the Communist behemoth on its western border (while also pointing out the idiosyncratic nature of the city whose tallest building belonged to the Bank of China), the writer highlighted the smuggling nexus everyone knew it to be. According to the article, "Anything and everything can be bought. Even the trade in human beings into and out of Red China can be easily financed at well known prices. It's true there is a strict control on the Hong Kong-China border, and the railroad that used to go from Kowloon to Canton now ends at the frontier. But this only increases the prices for smuggling."[22]

The technical term for Hong Kong's trade role is a "transshipment and warehousing gateway" between China, Southeast Asia, and the rest of the world. While archaeological evidence indicates that rural villages have populated areas in the New Territories since the eleventh century, the island of Hong Kong was populated mostly by Chinese pirates. Its geography, particularly the hundreds of small islands scattered around the mouth of the Pearl River delta, made it the ideal haven for pirates, smugglers, and anyone else looking for a place to hide. Narcotics in the form of opium and later heroin played a major role in the development of the island. Later, illicit tobacco and cigarettes from China grew into a booming trade. Gold, of course, was always welcome.[23]

During the early Cold War years, the British colony played a singular and, for the Americans, disconcerting role in the dissemination of antibiotics to China. Because the nature of Hong Kong's primary industry was as an export-import economy, the difference between legitimate and illicit was often as thin as thread. Major shipments of drugs, medical equipment, and consumer goods passed through Kowloon Bay, only to be repackaged and sold to mainland merchants who ferried it through Shenzhen. Quality varied, particularly when sourced from factories outside the Anglo-American alliance. Nonetheless, the porousness of Hong Kong's border with mainland China wreaked havoc on Washington's dreams of cutting off antibiotics and other materials deemed to serve "strategic" roles in Communism's ability to wage war or, in the case of the Korean conflict, supply the DPRK military with goods.

In 1950 antibiotics consisted of $14.6 million worth of trade. As mentioned earlier, that figure remained consistent for at least the next two years.[24] Hong Kong imported $85.9 million worth of foodstuffs from China and exported medicines and chemicals worth $63.7 million. Antibiotics played such a major role in trade that when Chinese demand dipped, the overall export numbers to the mainland dropped.[25]

Prices for antibiotics, obtained legally but resold on the black market, were jaw-dropping. According to a CIA report, "Despite US efforts to impose restrictions, there has been a brisk trade in antibiotics from the West to the East. Because a small quantity of antibiotics sells for a high price (penicillin is $300.00 per pound, as compared with ammonium nitrate at $0.035 a pound or soda ash at 2 cents a pound), the drugs are adaptable to smuggling."[26] Prices for completely unregulated medicine could mean even more unscrupulous gouging.

In a classic *Casablanca*-style wink and a nod, the destination of antibiotics was the worst-kept secret. The analyst indicates that "many instances of smuggling have been reported, and the quantities involved are believed to be large—particularly the quantities which go to the Chinese Communists."

Even the *Wall Street Journal* pointed out the obvious but added a twist. "The U.S. would also like to see Hong Kong exports to Red China impeded. All the same, some commodities—medical supplies, antibiotics and the like—move even with American approval. And undoubtedly this trade is of great importance to the Chinese Communists."[27]

The smuggling of antibiotics worked because there was an obvious market and maybe even a need for it, as was the case during embargoes. The problem, in terms of antibiotic resistance, was a question of stewardship. There weren't many ways of ensuring quality control. The smuggled antibiotic could have lost its potency due to any number of factors: expiration, improper storage during transport, and dilution of the product as in *The Third Man*. Even when the medication is in pristine condition, problems of stewardship still arise. Under doctors' supervision, patients often fail to complete the course. A person purchasing antibiotics in the black market was unlikely to take the proper dosage. These factors, in turn, make the prospect of resistance arising very likely, if not certain.

10

Stalin no longer played the primary role in shaping the Soviet economy, particularly with the final five-year plan of his time in power. Whether it was because he chose to focus his limited energies on more important matters, such as devising his last fabricated plot to persecute Russian Jews, or because he came to view five-year plans as ineffective, his subordinates handled that for him, devising and writing up policy for him to edit and approve. The Politburo debated and shaped the document. It was one of an increasing number of avenues where aspiring successors could jockey for position.[1]

The Politburo called for an increase in the production of antibiotics in the fifth five-year plan (1951–55). By the end of the cycle, antibiotics were to amount to 30 percent of the total production of drugs in the Soviet Union. According to its calculations, that would turn a net importer of antibiotics into a self-sufficient country.[2]

By this time, the pharmaceutical industries in the Soviet Union and its Eastern bloc satellites produced enough antibiotics to decrease Western imports to a bare minimum. In 1953 intelligence sources estimated that 19,700 billion units of penicillin were produced by the Soviet Union's European satellites.[3] Due to a combination of limited supplies and equipment, as well as a paucity of technical know-how, most of the penicillin coming out of Eastern Europe was still of the yellow, amorphous type first produced in the United States and the United Kingdom in the early 1940s. Countless reports indicate that the injection of this penicillin was accompanied by significant pain. The discomfort resulted from the impurities that give amorphous penicillin its yellow color.

Soviet antibiotic plants ran into multiple issues. During a session of the Academy of Medical Sciences, Academician-Secretary A. I. Nesterov reported on the various antibiotics being studied in the Soviet Union, including Zinaida Ermol'eva's work on ekmolin. Nesterov also singled out the research done by V. L. Troitskiy and Kh. Planel'yes, who "applied the advanced materialistic teaching of Michurin" on the problem of antibiotic resistance and proved that antibiotics caused physical changes in the bacteria, which were subsequently passed on to its offspring. This was in opposition to the Western notion that genes for resistance are coded into the bacteria's DNA and positively selected for over time. Purely in terms of the development of antibiotic resistance, time would show that both arguments held merit; however, the understandings of the underlying mechanisms differed. The Michurinist scientists observed a phenomenon but lacked the tools to address it. You could even say they didn't even have a toolbox at this point. The so-called traditional geneticists, with their notions of heritability and genes, had the fundamentals that would allow them to confront epigenetic changes head-on sixty-some-odd years later.

Nesterov's report also voiced some frustration with the "inadequate extent of work aiming at the development of new antibiotics and at the creation of new antibiotic preparations, which are urgently needed." He went on to explain: "One of the principal causes of this lag is the shortage of installations and apparatus for the production of new antibiotic preparations on a semi-industrial scale. One must also recognize that there is very limited amount of investigations on the mechanism of the action of antibiotics within the animal organism."[4]

Western embargoes were obviously having some effect on the ability of Soviet science to develop and produce antibiotics. Anecdotal accounts indicated that the penicillin produced in the Soviet Union was substandard, most likely amorphous penicillin. A 1950 analysis of samples of Soviet penicillin acquired in Germany showed that it consisted primarily of penicillin K, the least effective form of the drug. This could explain its substandard performance especially when coupled with the presence of impurities.

The exact findings from laboratory analysis follow:

1. The sample is identified as amorphous sodium penicillin.
2. It contains 14.2% penicillin G and 44.3% penicillin K.
3. Its potency is 833 units per milligram.
4. Its pH in aqueous solution is 5.3.
5. It is sterile.
6. It is free from pyrogens.
7. It passes the (U.S. Food and Drug Administration) safety test.
8. Its potency on a vial basis is 212,000 units per vial.[5]

For context, in 1945, U.S. manufacturers were producing penicillin with a purity between 800 and 1,000 units per milligram, and while the sample would pass the FDA safety test, it would ultimately be rejected due to the high levels of penicillin K. The maximum level allowable was 30 percent.

To make up for shortcomings in its pharmaceutical industry, the Soviet Union imported the difference from Warsaw Pact countries. This often came at the exporting country's expense. A closer look at Jenapharm in East Germany is instructive.

Since the cessation of hostilities, Jenapharm played a key role in the Soviet bloc. By the time Russian troops swept into Berlin, a modest amount of penicillin was already being produced there, albeit by the inefficient surface fermentation method. Still, for an institution that had been isolated from Western scientific literature, it proved the technical abilities of the scientists. Jenapharm quickly transitioned to deep fermentation once given the opportunity. Not only were the scientists able to produce significant quantities, the penicillin's quality was often on par with that of Western antibiotics. In the years that followed, it would be one of two Soviet Bloc factories capable of producing streptomycin and Chloromycetin, with the other being the Roztoky factory in Czechoslovakia.[6]

By Soviet standards, Jenapharm's output was impressive. In 1951 it produced penicillin ointments, powders, and calcium salts, as well as Jenacain penicillin, made up of novocaine and penicillin. The factory was also able to manufacture limited quantities of streptomycin and, later, Aureomycin. Western embargoes hindered production of the latter.[7]

Still, supplementary supply was necessary. With the Soviet Union siphoning the cream of what penicillin plants were producing, smaller countries were often left with shortages as a result. Take, for example, East Germany. In the first half of 1952, Jenapharm produced 165 billion units of penicillin; however, during that same time frame, it exported 290 billion units to the People's Republic of China and the Democratic People's Republic of Korea. By September 300 billion units made its way to North Korea alone. With the remaining factories in East Germany—Pharmazeutische Werke Madaus, Schering, VEB Arzneimittelwerk, and Biopharm (Langenhennersdorf)—producing roughly 330 billion units combined, it's easy to see how a domestic shortage could occur.[8] The similarly successful Roztoky plant in Czechoslovakia was also exploited by the Soviet Union.

According to contemporary CIA documents, the production of antibiotics varied across the Soviet-sphere of influence. Like the Soviet Union, countries such as Poland, Bulgaria, and Hungary produced primarily amorphous penicillin.[9]

Again, Western embargoes played a significant role in hampering the production of antibiotics. In addition to the aforementioned discussion in the Academy of Sciences conference, reports indicate that Hans Knöll encountered problems producing Aureomycin at Jenapharm because it was "on the embargo list, [and] supplies come in very irregularly." In Poland the Western "embargo . . . had an adverse effect and . . . caused delays in building up industry in Iron Curtain countries." Penicillin and streptomycin were at the top of the list when it came to shortages in pharmaceuticals.[10]

A CIA report speculated, "There is some evidence that the European Satellites shipped most of their own production of antibiotics to the USSR, which may indicate that imports from the West were necessary to provide for internal requirements."[11]

While undoubtedly scientists in Communist countries still faced a learning curve and a trade embargo that could make procuring even the most basic supplies such as Erlenmeyer flasks difficult, it's hard to believe that those reasons accounted for the quantities of substandard antibiotics coming out of most Soviet bloc plants.

Communist scientists and industrial engineers were fully capable of matching their capitalist counterparts. The October 4, 1957, launch of Sputnik 1 and the April 12, 1951, launch of Vostok 1 carrying Yuri Gagarin proved that much. The vast trove of CIA files documenting the Soviet antibiotics industry offers a possible explanation for its problems—the industry itself.

Given the complexities and fragility of the penicillin production process, it was tailor made for sabotage. CIA documents from the 1950s indicate that officers paid close attention to each and every antibiotic plant in the Soviet Union and its satellites. If the factory appeared vulnerable to subversion, the reporting CIA officer noted it. "The Jenapharm plant's greatest problem with its penicillin production lies in the sterilization of the boilers. There is also a great danger of injecting unsterilized air during the manufacturing process. Sabotage acts are therefore comparatively easy to carry out and are difficult to uncover, and they result in lasting damages, because unsterilized boilers have to be laid up for many months."[12]

In addition to maps of the factory grounds, many reports also contained rough floor plans. Detailed biographies of the plant's workers were often included. The traits the reporting officer chose to highlight suggest that he or she may have been looking for candidates to pull an inside job of sabotage. Take, for example, another report regarding Jenapharm: "Jehnert (fnu), an assistant for the past four years to L. Fischer, head of the foreign trade section at Carl Zeiss, Jena, was transferred several months ago to Carl Zeiss's brand in Göttingen, where he is at present technical director. REDACTED. Jehnert is an anti-Soviet."[13]

An East German newspaper article published on September 7, 1953, corroborates the theory that the CIA was actively involved in manipulating production plants. The author, Horst Willim, the chairman of the Central Committee of IG Chemie, gets straight to the point in his opening speculation: "For years, the espionage organizations sponsored by the US, by West German firms, and by the Eastern Bureau of the SPD (West German Social Democratic Party) have been engaged in establishing a network of agents in the plants and cities of the GDR [German Democratic Republic]."[14]

A portion of the Communist bloc's penicillin production problems very likely resulted from sabotage by foreign powers. One successful act of sabotage would have knock-on effects physically (contamination of machinery) and mentally (questioning production techniques that would have been sound under normal circumstances). The constant setbacks and adjustments could have stunted the employees' development as technicians. These issues would have had negative effects in terms of resistance because documents indicate that the USSR and its satellites struggled with penicillin production well into the late 1950s at least. The impure, low-potency, high–penicillin K antibiotics would have spurred the development of resistant bacteria.

BY THE EARLY 1950S, the Lysenkoist purge of Morganism-Mendelism wound down to a steady baseline. Geneticists who had held their ground openly were demoted and stripped of their titles. Other geneticists altered their work so that it fell safely within the parameters of Michurinism. Presumably, they hadn't surrendered their dedication to the scientific method, not yet at least. News of groundbreaking discoveries taking place in Soviet laboratories filtered into the popular press in Communist countries and a handful of Western outlets with an internationalist bent. For Michurinist scientists, the midpoint of the twentieth century became the halcyon days of creative Darwinist experimentation.

During the 1950s in Georgia, the Eliava Institute remained a bastion of bacteriophage research. Like Ermol'eva and Elford and Krueger, the research teams in Tbilisi investigated the complementary interactions between bacteriophages and antibiotics, especially penicillin and gramicidin S. Their findings fell in line with the other studies and showed that under certain circumstances, the combination displayed greater efficacy than using either alone.

According to Dmitriy Myelnikov, Soviet scientists did not share the view that antibiotics alone was a magic bullet. "While greatly appreciated by Soviet scientists, physicians and medical authorities, antibiotics were not necessarily magic bullets, but rather parts of a broader arsenal. By contrast, in the United States, between 1945 and

1955, the focus on broad-spectrum antibiotics and antibiotic mixes, driven by pharmaceutical companies, obscured other interventions, and concerns over resistance only emerged later."[15]

A brisk business in phage therapy was also happening in other parts of Europe as well. In Germany the pharmaceutical firm Behringwerke had been involved in the production of phages since the late 1930s. Meanwhile, in France, basic and clinical research into therapeutic uses of bacteriophages were still taking place at the Pasteur Institute, where Félix d'Hérelle had begun research decades earlier. And in 1954 the strategy of using viruses to attack bacteria found a permanent home in the Ludwik Hirszfeld Institute of Immunology and Experimental Therapy in Wroclaw, Poland. There, some of the most important and widely cited work would also be published in English during the late 1970s and 1980s, and play a major role in the rediscovery and revival of bacteriophage therapy in the English-speaking West.

Between 1950 and 1960, European researchers studied the effects of bacteriophages on a wide spectrum of conditions including using adapted phages to treat respiratory diseases, diphtheria, gastric enteritis, staphylococcal infections, dysentery, and cholera. They were just a few of the subject areas where clinical research had been conducted. Most presciently, a handful of phage scientists started exploring how the tiny viruses could be used against the antibiotic-resistant bacteria that were beginning to appear in clinical settings.

WHEN CONSIDERING ANTIBIOTIC RESISTANCE during the antibiotic era, the first significant threat to appear was a strain of *Staphylococcus aureus* that emerged in Australia in 1949. It struck hospital maternity wards primarily, and its contagiousness and virulence led to the first antibiotic-resistant bacteria outbreak to be recognized as epidemic. In time, it would come to be known as the "hospital strain."[16]

At the time, the primary method for categorizing bacterial strains involved bacteriophages. Scientists took well-defined groups—group I, group II, and group III—of phages and observed which bacteria were susceptible to certain groups. Each phage group contained phages that allowed for a degree of specificity. In the case of the 1949

Australian strains, the epidemic strain of penicillin-resistant bacteria tended to be susceptible to group III phages.[17]

While it would be a long time until a true sense of alarm took hold among scientists and health care providers, anyone monitoring the scientific journals of the period would notice patches of resistance taking shape. They shared a common point of origin—maternity wards in hospitals. Bacteriologist Mary Barber first called attention to the phenomenon in England, and a similar situation arose in Australia. It was only a matter of time until the scourge of antibiotic-resistant *Staphylococcus* surfaced in the United States and beyond.

Meanwhile, U.S. drug makers enjoyed the pharmaceutical version of Beatlemania. Everyone wanted some for their ailments. Antibiotic cough gels (Candettes) were just the beginning of the latest elixir. Drug makers put it in toothpaste. They put it in facial creams. They put it in mouthwash. They even put it in deodorant. (Is it any wonder resistance arose?) The industry was more than happy to oblige the public's appetite for the new wonder drugs.

By 1950 a clear structure for the antibiotic industry emerged. It was broken into three primary categories: producers who also sold consumer products, business-to-business producers who only sold to other companies that repackaged the antibiotics, and companies that did not produce antibiotics but resold to consumers under their brand.

The twelve primary production companies would become stalwarts in the antibiotics business for decades. Their output represented the vast majority of antibiotic production. While almost all of them sold some form of penicillin and streptomycin, their bread and butter was in the drugs they discovered on their own and then controlled the patents.

While the sale of penicillin and streptomycin remained brisk for the pharmaceutical companies, there was too much competition for selling essentially the same thing. Each company developed its own antibiotic. Some companies made penicillin derivatives that were just different enough to be patentable. The strategy worked for the most part not only because penicillin continued to have the name recognition but also because for all the resistance that had emerged from the cracks and shadows, it was still a very effective drug.

The real money lay in the newly developed broad-spectrum antibiotics. They represented the latest and the greatest as far as healing was concerned. Parke-Davis sold chloramphenicol. Lederle had Aureomycin (chlortetracycline). Pfizer peddled Terramycin (oxytetracycline). Everyone rejoiced because broad-spectrum antibiotics were godsends for medical professionals. Only later would anyone realize the damage they actually did.

A change in the relationship between doctor and patient also resulted from the dawning of the antibiotic age. Patients became consumers, and doctors often became glorified drug dealers, middlemen between the pharmaceutical company and the user. Often patients demanded antibiotics regardless of whether they had bacterial infections. Eager to avoid unnecessary conflict and equally unnecessarily long days, doctors obliged.

In the United States, advertisements targeting antibiotics to physicians and the public played a central role in building the symbolism and mythology around the drugs and shaped public perception. During World War II, campaigns for penicillin often featured soldiers on the battlefield who were frequently injured, always in danger, and threatened by the unseen enemy just off the page. In *Penicillin: Triumph and Tragedy*, Robert Bud points out a particularly powerful advertisement in *Life* magazine for Schenley Laboratories. In it, a U.S. Army medic kneels over a badly injured soldier on the battlefield. He holds out the wounded young soldier's arm, injecting something into it. On the top right-hand corner of the ad is a close-up picture of bacteria taken through a microscope lens. It allows the viewer to draw the connection between enemies—the gun-toting Axis soldier and the subcellular microorganism. Emblazoned across the top of the advertisement are the words, "Thanks to Penicillin. . . . He will come home!"[18]

Beneath the Norman Rockwell–style sentimentality, the advertising and the images it featured had an undercurrent of a society under siege. While the injured soldiers and the Nazi bad guys were replaced by tomorrow's sickness and plagues of uncertainty, the underlying message was the same: illnesses threatened the republic, and only our enemies—no one need mention their names—stood to gain.

The combative rhetoric didn't change much either. An advertisement for Neo-aqua-drin, antibiotic throat lozenges produced by McKesson & Robbins, shows the close-up of a couple standing in a snowstorm. The man clutches the woman, his head protected by a fedora and hers by a scarf. They are looking at something out of the frame (and behind the reader) and witnessing something terrible. Just behind them, two men, neither fully visible and wearing bemused smirks, are looking at the same thing. What amuses the pair of men (comrades?) elicits consternation and concern from the couple. The man frowns and clutches a newspaper or magazine, tying the fictional event into something current, something in the news. The woman's mouth is open and her brows furrowed. And if there were any questions about the threat, she clutches at the neck of her jacket, holding whatever is in her hand close to her chest. It's a defensive reaction. An impulse. A reflex. If it were a film, the next frames would show shock beginning to dawn. We know the story. We've seen the movie.

Above the image, the advertisement exhorts the reader, "Fight Germs . . . Soothes Throat Fast!" How the accompanying image relates to a sore throat is anybody's guess. However, if the words read, "Fight Commies . . . They're coming fast!" the ad would have made much more sense. But this was America in the 1950s, after the airlift, after the Russian bomb, after Communist troops invaded South Korea, and after the Viet Minh took the fight to the French in Vietnam. Certain things were understood.

The images changed, but the dog whistle continued. The advertising had its intended effect. People wanted their antibiotics. Demanded them. And the doctors, a great many of them, obliged. It was happy days for everyone associated with the pharmaceutical industry.

How long the halcyon days would last, nobody knew. They probably weren't very concerned either. Antibiotic manufacturers had one more significant ace in the hole, and they wouldn't wait long to play it.

IT'S A COMMON BELIEF that when a nation needs an economic stimulus, lawmakers always carry a get-out-of-jail free card: they wage war. Afterward, industries convert wartime manufacturing into peacetime prosperity. Meanwhile, U.S. pharmaceutical companies clearly benefited from the wars raging half the world away in Korea and Indochina.

The money earned as a result of the U.S. government's purchase of antibiotics allowed companies such as Abbott Labs, Merck, Eli Lilly, Upjohn, and Monsanto to consider expansion both domestically and internationally. At home, these companies enjoyed a privileged status near the top of the light industries sector. As in World War II, the government granted them certificates of necessity that expedited their procurement of rationed machinery. This allowed them to increase their manufacturing output, which, in turn, led to higher profits. Revenue from antibiotics spiked in 1951 to over $300 million, the best numbers for most of the following decade. Significantly, the total quantity of antibiotics produced increased steadily, indicating that the prices manufacturers could demand had begun to decrease.[19] Nonetheless, sentiment remained positive in the pharmaceutical industry, a notion reinforced by the brisk expansion abroad.

During the first half of the 1950s, U.S. antibiotic companies built fifty-two plants on foreign soil; however, thirty-seven of the facilities were processing and packaging plants that relied on supplies from the United States. Eventually, more vertically integrated plants were built overseas, though the focus on packaging remained consistent.[20] U.S. pharmaceutical companies also benefited from agreements with international companies to provide technological assistance to their manufacturing arms.

The United States and United Kingdom no longer enjoyed absolute advantages in the antibiotics field, particularly in basic research at the university level and in corporate R&D. The template was public knowledge by now: Look for mold, whether it be in humid cupboards or waste bins at food markets. Dig up buckets of soil from anywhere and everywhere, sometimes the more exotic the better. Even toxic sewage could not be discounted. When that was done, grind it out on the lab bench, isolating and growing bacteria on beds of agar in petri dishes. If testing shows that certain bacteria are susceptible to it, test it more. If not, move on to the next batch. In the end, there were always actinomycetes to fall back on.[21]

Researchers, including those in Florey's Dunn School laboratory, continued studying different strains of *Penicillium* while also shifting their focus to the mold *Aspergillus*. As early as 1943, Flora J. Philpot reported a penicillin-like substance from *Aspergillus giganteus* that was effective against *Staphylococcus*. Later it was called claviformin, though it was identical to another antibiotic called Patulin that had recently been discovered by J. H. Birkenshaw. Antibiotic hunters such as Selman Waksman also turned to *Aspergillus fumigatus*, which produced an active compound they called fumigacin. Before streptomycin became available to the public, researchers at the University of Stockholm reported that an unidentified strain of *Aspergillus* inhibited the growth of *Streptomyces griseus*. Meanwhile, Waksman and Boyd Woodruff continued to mine the actinomycetes bacteria for all they were worth, this time isolating an antibacterial compound they called actinomycin.[22]

Researchers also focused on kojic acid, a common byproduct of mold metabolism, but unfortunately it only displayed antibiotic properties in highly concentrated forms. (In the twenty-first century, kojic acid was given a second life as a mass-market skin-whitening substance.)[23] Potential antibiotics were also reported from Chinese water chestnut extracts, bacteria called *Lenzites thermophila* (Thermophillin), and even *E. coli*.[24]

One of the most significant discoveries, particularly from a twenty-first century antibiotic-resistance perspective, was made by Japanese scientists in the once-shattered institutions of occupied Japan. A team of researchers working at the Kobayashi Bacteriological Laboratory had utilized the labor-intensive method of large-scale screening of soil samples to provide leads. Koyama Yasuo and Kurosawa Akio discovered a new compound that was particularly effective against dysentery and whooping cough, which had been untreatable to that point.[25]

Similar to the U.S. Office of Scientific Research and Development's private-public model, Japanese scientists in academia and industry collaborated to bring the new antibiotic on the market. Specifically, Lion Pharmaceutical, Tohoku University, and Tohoku Pharmaceutical University developed what was called colistin but later came to be known as Colomycin. Clinical trials were conducted by Keio

University, Tokyo University, and Teishin Hospital. Finally, Snow Brand Milk Products assumed the responsibility of scaling up from its lab production to mass production.[26]

Colistin marked a significant milestone in the history of Japan's once globally competitive pharmaceutical industry. Until that point, all antibiotics were either imported or grown domestically with the Americans' guidance. This drug was Japan's own. Soon, the modest-scale antibiotic outfits joined forces with the country's larger, traditional pharmaceutical manufacturers in the so-called keiretsu, a vertically integrated and immensely powerful alliance. Sankyo was one example. The company originally manufactured anthelmintics, DDT, and BHC (benzene hexachloride) and changed directions in the 1950s to focus on antibiotics with the help of licenses from Parke-Davis, Løvens Kemiske, Sandoz, and E. R. Squibb. Shionogi, another pharmaceutical firm, also teamed up with Eli Lilly.[27]

Between 1950 and 1960, five of twenty-two antibiotics on the Japanese market had been discovered and produced by domestic operations: colistin (Lion Kinyaku, 1951), sarkomycin (Meiji Seika, 1954), kitasamycin (Toyo Jozo, 1956), kanamycin (Meiji Seika, 1958), and mitomycin (Kyowa Hakko, 1959). The government played vital roles in funding R&D efforts through both the Ministry of Health and Ministry of Education. This, in turn, spurred pharmaceutical firms to be more aggressive with R&D. What else drove them? Increasing cases of antibiotic resistance in the country.[28]

THE REALITIES OF BIOLOGICAL warfare during the Cold War emerged in a surreal war of words that was never fully resolved. In 1952 the Communist triumvirate of the People's Republic of China, the Democratic People's Republic of Korea, and the USSR took years of Washington's argument about biological warfare and flipped it on its head, the way Marx and Engels did to Hegel. On February 22 DPRK foreign minister Pak Hon-Yong stood in front of the United Nations Secretariat in New York City and accused the United States, and by extension the UN itself, of using bacteriological warfare against the Korean people. The expected media scrum followed. Over the following months, American experts volleyed rebuttals to their Communist counterparts. Sensing that they had the advantage, North

Korea, China, and the Soviet Union laid on layers of accusations and evidence supporting their view.[29]

Stealing a page directly from the Americans' World War II playbook, the Chinese and North Koreans disseminated two films that allegedly documented the aftermath of BW attacks. The footage transported their audiences to a surreal, semi-faceless, postapocalyptic world, one birthed through a disease-infested payload and inhabited by innocent peasants who were victimized, militarized, and weaponized against their will. Their outward appearances betrayed nothing but their poverty. But according to officials, the villagers knew something. They felt the American planes approaching at night. They saw them overhead. They braced for the bombs, liquid fire raining down from blackened clouds. But nothing happened. Not that night. Everyone agreed it made no sense. In the morning, these peasants, angels of the proletariat, woke up and wandered to their fields. They found insects, mostly dead, spread over the white snow like sprinkles on ice cream. Broken bombs stuck out from the ground, pointing to their direction of origin—the sky.[30]

The Communists mobilized an army of phantasm-like figures, wearing rudimentary white biohazard suits from head to toe. They resembled stormtroopers from *Star Wars* as they marched out in their rigid formation one by one, single file, on concrete streets, over dirt roads, and finally in the countryside. Sheets of smoke blanketed the ground as the area was fumigated. Wearing no protection at all, not even gloves, peasants helped collect specimens of the insects dropped from the clouds.

Tests later confirmed that dead rats had been weaponized to transmit anthrax and fleas, the plague. As the films showed weak and broken bodies wasting away on hospital beds, their glassy eyes focused on some distant spot on the wall, we see the attack succeeded. Our eyes tell us as much. And when we hear captured American pilots confessing to dropping bacterial bombs on the population, we feel the joint rumblings of shame and anger.

How could anyone do this, let alone the Americans with their love of freedom, liberty, and equal rights for all? Turns out, they probably didn't. Citing documentary evidence, recent scholarship indicates that the reported attacks were part of a complex propaganda campaign against the United States. The uncertainty it created for the Americans and the Communists inadvertently revealed their continued concerns about the possibility of unconventional warfare.

Documentary evidence indicates that the first steps in the propaganda campaign started in Beijing. According to the account of Chinese People's Volunteer Army field commander Peng Dehuai, he alerted the army to the biological attack on January 29. As a result, he organized anti-epidemiological units and ordered them to neutralize the attack, which he recognized immediately as one using biological weapons. A little over a week later, Peng convened a meeting to address epidemic control.[31]

On February 18 in Beijing, Chief of Staff Nie Rongzhen of the People's Liberation Army informed the Communist Party's Central Committee that UN forces had released insects infected with various pathogens to spread disease among the North Korean civilian population.[32] The following day, Mao Zedong instructed Premier Zhou Enlai to formulate countermeasures. Zhou ordered the lab testing of the insects, the dispatching of anti-epidemiological units and vaccine to the front, a protest statement by DPRK foreign minister Pak Hon-yong, a supporting statement from the Chinese foreign minister, and an appeal by the Chinese People's Committee for World Peace to the World Peace Council opposing the use of biological weapons.[33]

On February 21 Mao informed Joseph Stalin that between January 28 to February 17, U.S. and UN forces had dropped bacteriological agents from airplanes on parts of North Korea. According to Mao, they also fired artillery shells filled with biological agents. Chinese scientists concluded from canvassing the countryside and monitoring the symptoms presenting among the sick that the United States had employed biological weapons. They claimed that their analyses proved that some of the insects carried *Yersinia pestis*, the pathogen responsible for the bubonic plague.[34]

The next day DPRK foreign minister Pak protested U.S. BW abuse to the UN Secretariat. Two days later, the Soviet Politburo considered China's request that the USSR join the campaign against the United States. It was approved, and *Pravda* published Pak's statement, in essence rubber-stamping it with the government's endorsement.[35]

On March 3 China's military command in Manchuria reported to the central army's general staff headquarters that bags full of infected rodents had been dropped. Acting on Mao's instructions, Zhou cabled Lu Dingyi, chief of propaganda of the party's Central Committee, that the Chinese Central Military Commission's Epidemic Prevention Office should direct anti-bacteriological warfare propaganda toward the West. A day earlier, North Korea initiated its own propaganda campaign.[36]

The Communist propaganda machine churned for the remainder of the war. A Western fact-finding mission led by the British biochemist and Sinologist Joseph Needham visited sites where the BW attack supposedly occurred. While the commission was in North Korean, the DPRK government marched out captured U.S. Air Force pilots who admitted to taking part in the BW attack, though there was always the question of coercion.

The Americans denied the allegations, of course. Unfortunately, the Merck report's admission that the United States had an active BW program and the public debate that followed allowed for reasonable doubt. Declassified government documents reveal a degree of confusion in Washington and uncertainty regarding how to address the accusations. The cycle of accusations and denials dragged on well past the cease-fire in Korea. The accusations stuck just enough to linger.

11

While the image of the United States received a schoolyard misinformation beating that would have done J. Edgar Hoover proud, Washington was still winning the overall propaganda war against the Communists. It wasn't even close, to be fair. The country's image still enjoyed some of the shine from World War II, thanks in no small part to two massive and groundbreaking foreign aid programs.

World War II had left economies around the world devastated, and for four years starting in 1948, the European Recovery Program distributed mostly U.S. goods, services, and attitudes to countries across Europe. It wasn't benevolence or charitable largesse. The Marshall Plan, as it came to be known, boiled down to shrewd, calculating geopolitical bribery. It was, arguably, good policy from a political, economic, and propaganda standpoint. By 1952 it was winding down, officially at least.

Americans' concerns about the opportunistic spread of Communism led to the Marshall Plan and the Point Four Program (1949). But if we pull back a bit, it's not a leap to say that the Marshall Plan belonged on the same continuum as the much-maligned United Nations Relief and Rehabilitation Administration and, going back still further, the League of Nations. It was the love child of Wilsonian internationalism and late–New Deal corporatism, and its siblings were the United Nations and its various apparatuses, the World Health Organization, and the Point Four Program. For some, the European Recovery Program heralded the age of foreign aid.

The genesis of the program stemmed from a meeting between Secretary of State George C. Marshall and Joseph Stalin in Moscow in April 1947. The visit left the former questioning Stalin's dedication to ensuring Europe's economic recovery. He was now convinced that Stalin preferred the opposite, a fragile, even shattered Europe. The resultant disenchantment guaranteed conditions favorable to the adoption of Communism. Every empty cupboard, shoeless child, or prospectless job search exposed the inadequacy of the capitalist experiment. Every man with something another man wanted and, in his eyes, deserved revealed the inherent injustice of the so-called free market. Those conditions highlighted the Communist alternative, still an unproven abstraction but brimming with ideals and punchy slogans about workers and utopias.[1]

During the planning stages, Secretary of State Marshall and George Kennan insisted that the Marshall Plan not be framed as opposing any country or ideology, yet the ardent anti-Communist DNA of Winston Churchill's "Iron Curtain" speech, Kennan's Long Telegram, and Truman's NSC-68 and its theory of containment all course through its veins. Its primary mission lay in stemming the tide of Communism by providing monetary, economic, and technical support.[2]

On June 5, 1947, Marshall announced the European Recovery Program during a commencement speech at Harvard University. The venue had been chosen with care. "It is logical that the United States should do whatever it is able to do to assist in the return of normal economic health in the world.... Our policy is directed not against any country or doctrine but against hunger, poverty, desperation, and chaos. Its purpose should be the revival of a working economy in the world so as to permit the emergence of political and social conditions in which free institutions can exist."[3]

Marshall promised the full cooperation of the United States for any nation that desired assistance. He also warned that anyone considering interfering with the aid would suffer the full brunt of the United States' displeasure.

The secretary of state urged European countries to get together and reach an agreement as to the continent's needs. They had to make the first move because "it would be neither fitting nor efficacious for this Government to undertake to draw up unilaterally a program designed to place Europe on its feet economically. This is the business of the Europeans. The initiative, I think, must come from Europe."[4]

European interest was swift. First the French. The British followed soon after. They led the rest of Europe: Austria, Belgium, Denmark, Greece, Iceland, Ireland, Italy, Luxembourg, the Netherlands, Norway, Portugal, Sweden, Switzerland, Turkey. Officially, every European country, east and west, received invitations to take part. Other countries such as Czechoslovakia and Poland were eager to join. The administration openly debated whether the aid package should be extended to the Soviet Union. Ultimately, it was.[5]

At first, Moscow considered Washington's offer. The Russians held numerous meetings in Paris. It was becoming increasingly obvious that the Soviets held significant reservations regarding the U.S. offer of aid. Among other things, Vyacheslav Molotov communicated that Stalin wanted assurance that there would be no conditions involved in the aid package. He did not like what he heard.[6]

In reality, American policy makers were playing a high stakes game and would have been left exposed had the Soviets called their bluff. It never happened. Instead, the Soviet delegation rejected the plan outright and immediately ended negotiations, leaving Paris soon afterward. They saw the Marshall Plan as a threat and ordered Eastern bloc countries to reject it.

Eastern bloc countries had considered participating in the European Recovery Program. Their economies were no less battered than those of the Western countries. Indeed, some were even worse off than the Western countries. Over the course of the past decade, cities in countries such as Poland, Hungary, and Czechoslovakia had fallen to the Nazis, were overrun once more during the German retreat, and then victimized by the Red Army in pursuit of the enemy. These countries needed help and viewed the Marshall Plan as an opportunity. Czechoslovakian foreign minister Jan Masaryk showed interest as did other Eastern European heads of state.[7]

Stalin summoned Czechoslovakia's Communist prime minister (Eduard Beneš, the country's president, was a liberal) and a Czech delegation to Moscow. Stalin voiced his displeasure and ordered them to reject the Americans' offer. When the delegation returned to Prague, they immediately announced the reversal of their position. Distraught, Foreign Minister Masaryk declared, "I went to Moscow as a foreign minister of an independent sovereign state. I returned as a Soviet slave." Later Masaryk would die after falling out of his apartment window. Some called it a suicide, while others were convinced he was murdered. In the aftermath of Masaryk's mysterious death, a commentator made the wry observation: "Jan Masaryk was a very tidy man. He was such a tidy man that when he jumped, he shut the window after himself."[8]

Until this point, the Soviet Union had implicitly tolerated Eastern bloc pluralism. The countries may have been caught in the Soviet Union's orbit, but each still had a distinct, national voice. Some historians argue that the formation of the Cominform (Information Bureau of the Communist and Workers' Parties) marked the end of that brief moment. In retrospect, Cominform participation was doomed from the start. What's more, Stalin displayed more than a little bit of foresight, as it would have been impossible to square the circle of Americanization and Communism.

Western European countries, meanwhile, formed the Western Union, a consortium led by France and the United Kingdom.[9]

Similar to the UNRRA program that preceded it, the Marshall Plan provided direct access to antibiotics by financing the purchase of nearly $9 million worth of streptomycin for countries participating in the European Recovery Program and by building a streptomycin plant at Vitry-sur-Seine near Paris. Merck provided the equipment and technical instruction, and the proposed plant was projected to employ up to 120 workers. The estimated costs included $200,000 worth of equipment shipped from the United States and another $800,000 worth of equipment and materials furnished by French suppliers. During the planning stages, it was projected that the plant would supply 60 percent of total French streptomycin needs and earn between $2.4 million and $3.5 million per year. As an added bonus for U.S. antibiotic makers, the French plant would relieve some of the heavy demands placed on them. (Another streptomycin plant was also built at La Plaine Saint-Denis.)[10]

At about the same time, the Truman administration developed and proposed the Point Four Program, essentially a Marshall Plan for the developing world. The fundamental difference between the two programs lay in the role that technical assistance played over economic aid. During Point Four's first year of existence, Congress allotted the program a paltry $35 million. For comparison, Congress provided Italy and France with $500 million in emergency funds for the first three months of 1948.[11]

Washington viewed the technological transfer of its great knowledge and experience as an invaluable contribution to Point Four's recipient countries. It supplemented their know-how by facilitating private investment from U.S. companies and from local governments, as the U.S. Congress was loath to throw any more funds at a foreign aid scheme that it viewed as a sinkhole for taxpayer money.

"The central premise of Point Four was that U.S. technical expertise—identified as its superior knowledge and vast wealth of information—would be the guiding force behind national development." The program used American technical expertise and a philosophy of "self-help" through mixed public and private investment to promote economic growth. It also intended to create an open and extensive capitalist trading bloc that would foster political stability, democratization, and strategic allegiance with the United States.[12]

Self-help was a critical component. So was private investment. "The Act for International Development, which authorized Point Four, called for coordination among private companies, philanthropic foundations, and supranational organizations to finance international development. The act required U.S. officials and government agencies to identify potential private companies to invest in Point Four countries."[13]

Thus, most of the investment costs such as capital, heavy machinery, and labor would be provided by the receiving company or private foreign investors. In other words, the recipient nations would jointly finance and administer the programs. The goal was for each nation to assume all of the costs in the future and assimilate the programs into the local government structure.

Edward Mason, a distinguished Harvard professor with links to the State Department, offered a succinct summation of Point Four's qualities. He remarked, "It seems to me that this program, particularly after the recent events in Korea and China, has to be essentially viewed as part of the American security program. . . . Will [Point Four] influence the willingness of the people in the underdeveloped areas to throw in their lot with the US? Will it influence them to cut their ties or lessen their ties with the Soviet Union or will it not?"[14]

Truman, upon signing the Act for International Development in 1950, claimed that "Communist propaganda holds that the free nations are incapable of providing a decent standard of living for the millions of people in the underdeveloped areas of the earth. The Point Four program will be one of our principal ways of demonstrating the complete falsity of that charge."[15]

In the 1952 presidential election, the Democratic Party's platform listed the Point Four Program, alongside NATO's and the United States' involvement in Korea, as a key to resisting "Communist aggression" and to "mobilizing the strength of the free world."[16] It represented the "quiet war," which would prove no less important than any other aspect of the Cold War, and fell in line with the State Department's task of promoting the U.S. system to neutral nations.

Technical assistance programs were meant to provide as much assistance to developing countries as possible without actually exchanging monetary aid. Yet, while teaching the hungry man how to fish, the structure of the program—with its emphasis on techniques, technologies, and products used in the United States—undoubtedly served the interests of U.S. companies and, by extension, the U.S. economy.

By 1952 the Marshall Plan was approaching its end point. The monetary aspects of the program were winding down; however, the technical assistance program continued. This responsibility was assumed by the Organization for European Economic Cooperation, which had administered the U.S. and Canadian aid.

Overall, the Marshall Plan contributed to Western Europe's postwar survival. It represented a considerable public relations victory for the United States and pulled Europe deeper into its orbit. Right or wrong, the belief that it single-handedly saved Europe from economic collapse and the grips of Communism emerged. During World War II, the United States had displayed its military prowess; after the Marshall Plan, it led in technical and productive prowess.

ON CHRISTMAS DAY 1948, Providence and Nature gave American Cyanamid animal nutritionist Thomas Jukes a present that completed the revolution Benjamin Duggar started with the discovery of Aureomycin.[17] As told by Maryn McKenna in her book *Big Chicken*, Jukes began investigating the effects of antibiotics on chickens' growth after Merck researcher Edward Rickes stumbled upon the same phenomenon: liquid by-products of streptomycin production had caused chickens to grow faster and larger. At the time, they did not know what caused the increase but speculated that it must have been either vitamin B12 or a mysterious compound called animal protein factor, which scientists had been ineffectively trying to isolate. Jukes's hunch mirrored Rickes's, and he wondered whether the spent mash by-product of Aureomycin production from *Streptomyces aureofaciens* possessed similar elements.[18]

For the experiment, Jukes raised chicks from the moment they hatched and controlled the food they ate. The experimental diets (basal diets) consisted of variable amounts of soy meal, corn meal, alfalfa meal, and bone meal and vitamins. A preparation containing vitamin B12 was prepared for comparison with the spent fermentation mash. In addition, supplements consisting of liver extracts were prepared, since they were commonly used animal protein supplements added to vegetable feed.[19]

Jukes weighed the birds. The control group weighed just 110 grams. Scrawny. The group that received vitamins seemed healthy and weighed between 179 and 203 grams. Average. The birds that had liver extract weighed the most, 216 grams.

Jukes moved on to the pen holding the chicks fed the Aureomycin fermentation mash. "He had dosed them at four different levels, so much mash per kilo of feed. He weighed the four groups, averaged the weights within each of them, recorded the numbers, and looked. And then looked again. The birds that had gotten the highest dose of Aureomycin were the heaviest in the room. They weighed 277 grams."[20]

Jukes and American Cyanamid had something. That much was clear. However, just what that something was nobody had a clue, or at least that's what they let on. Either way, it didn't stop them from filing a patent covering the mixture of spent Aureomycin mash with various types of feed in September 1949. The mixture, known as Aurofac, came to dominate the chicken feed market. The following year, it represented American Cyanamid's primary antibiotic product. By the mid-1950s, the company had added tetracycline to its lineup while dropping penicillin completely. In terms of chlortetracycline, only 15 percent of total production was sold for medicinal use. The remainder went to the agricultural market as an animal feed supplement. By this time, the price of Aureomycin had decreased considerably.

Thanks to farmers' adoption of Aurofac, American Cyanamid led the field in its total share of the antibiotics market (26.6), with Pfizer (11.7) coming in second and Eli Lilly and Merck (11.0) sharing third place. By 1956 Cyanamid produced the most antibiotics by far, almost a half of a million pounds. One third of that was produced for the purpose of including in animal feed.[21]

In 1950 Pfizer joined the broad-spectrum antibiotic race with the introduction of oxytetracycline, or Terramycin. The antibiotic spawned a slew of products: intravenous crystalline Terramycin hydrochloride, Terramycin ophthalmic solution, Terramycin ophthalmic ointment, Terramycin topical ointment, Terramycin troches. The company called it "the most dramatic Pfizer discovery to date."[22]

Once again Pfizer utilized the one tried and true method of finding new antibiotic substances and conducted a systematic study of solid samples sent from around the world. According to the company's 1950 "Annual Report," it entailed a global effort. "Travelers, missionaries, airline pilots, and our sales agents in all sections of the world, each month, sent thousands of earth samples to our biochemical laboratories." Eventually, Pfizer researchers isolated a compound derived from *Streptomyces rimosus*. It was the second broad-spectrum antibiotic to be developed and marketed. It not only showed efficacy against roughly fifty strains of bacteria but also proved to be an effective antibiotic growth promoter and allowed the second-biggest antibiotic company to make a charge for the titleholder's spot.[23]

That antibiotics played a major role in the development of what's come to be known as factory farms is no secret. Yet sometimes, their role can be overstated, and they become the primary culprit in the evolution of benign but inefficient family farms to toxic but ultra-productive industrial operations. That transformation took at least a half century after World War II or longer if you start counting from the earliest examples of artificial incubators.

The integrated broiler industry had its modern roots in the burgeoning field of poultry science that emerged at the turn of the twentieth century. The shift from traditional animal husbandry entailed the integration of scientific fields such as bacteriology and biochemistry, as well as organizational systematizations that quantified egg and meat production. As chickens were studied, information about their genetics grew with the nascent field. For various reasons, they proved to be versatile laboratory animals. The more scientists learned about chickens the easier the birds became to manipulate.[24]

Intensive confinement, once described as "a kind of biological time-space compression," allowed producers to maximize the efficiency of the chickens' growing process. A number of problems, however, needed to be solved. The first hurdle stemmed from the fact that chickens raised according to this method saw little, if any, sunlight, resulting in a nutritional deficiency known as leg weakness. Thus, the chickens could only be confined for limited durations. To solve this problem, researchers at the University of Wisconsin discovered that adding a source of vitamin D to a chicken's diet prevented the condition. So from that point forward, cod liver oil was added to chicken feed as a supplement. That simple solution allowed for the strict confinement of chickens.[25]

Controlling the conditions in the warehouse was the next step in the development of factory farms. Effective solutions to this problem would not be possible until steady and reliable supplies of electricity became available outside of big cities. In the United States, this took place gradually, starting with the enactment of the New Deal's Tennessee Valley Authority in 1933 and the Rural Electrification Act of 1936. Providing energy to chicken farms in the south was particularly important because even though the area was naturally feed deficient, it would grow into the country's primary source of broiler chickens.[26]

Electricity enabled farmers to use "thermostatically regulated incubators substituted for the brooding hen, allowing large numbers of newly hatched chicks to be produced on demand." By 1934 state-of-the-art hatcheries were already producing more than a million chicks per year.[27]

Advances in genetics allowed for improved poultry breeding techniques and accelerated productivity. According to William Boyd, "Stimulated by the rediscovery of Gregor Mendel's work, European and American researchers used chickens extensively in early studies of heredity. William Bateson, considered by some the founder of modern genetics and a major force in the spread of Mendelism during the first decade of the twentieth century, started conducting experiments with poultry in 1898."[28] Together with the Royal Society, Bateson published the first paper on poultry inheritance.

In the United States, researchers applied the new knowledge about poultry inheritance to breed chickens and select for specific traits that increased the economic value of the birds. Livestock groups such as the American Breeders Association embraced Mendel's work with its predictive aspects and reaped the benefits. Unfortunately, not all of the traits breeders desired were simple enough to boil down to basic, sharply defined Mendelian factors. The continuous variation of traits such as size and color indicated that much more complex elements were at work. Chicken breeders and scientists looked outside their field and found key answers in the genetics of fruit flies and the seminal work of Thomas Hunt Morgan. They discovered certain aspects of a phenotype, the external traits produced by an organism's genes, were controlled by multiple genes that were not necessarily located close to each other on the chromosome (multiple-factor inheritance). This discovery explained their difficulties but failed to offer paths to rectify them. It wasn't until the advent of population genetics in the 1930s that scientific knowledge allowed poultry breeders to develop a means to select traits, to predict their expression, and to make proper judgments accordingly.[29]

The development and durability of hybrid corn inspired poultry breeders to search for hybrid vigor (heterosis) among chickens. The "Chicken of Tomorrow" contests between 1948 and 1951 played an important role in the development of broiler chickens. The objective of the competitions "had the explicit aim of stimulating interest in the breeding of broad-breasted, 'meat-type' chickens. They were wildly successful, so much so that by the early 1950s two-thirds of American commercial broilers descended from Chicken of Tomorrow prizewinners."[30]

Antibiotics, with their disease-busting and growth-enhancing capabilities, were simply a single cog in the modern broiler chicken machine, albeit an essential one. The ramifications of the widespread adoption of growth promoters by the U.S. agricultural industry during the early 1950s would damage the antibiotic landscape.

WHEN THE U.S. GOVERNMENT, industries, and universities banded together during the early 1940s to scale up production of penicillin, they met the challenge head-on and surpassed expectations. If there was ever any doubt regarding the capabilities of Americans' ingenuity, it was unconditionally put to rest. When new antibiotics were needed, they threw the might of the country's size at it and emerged with drugs such as streptomycin, bacitracin, chloramphenicol, Aureomycin, Terramycin, and tetracycline. Using skills honed while producing penicillin, pharmaceutical companies such as Merck, Pfizer, Lederle, Eli Lilly, and Bristol-Myers went on production binges. Their enthusiasm became their undoing because undersupply shot past the equilibrium point and into oversupply. It was a disaster for prices.

When the U.S. government first priced penicillin in 1943, 1 million units of penicillin went for $200. It was a high price for an impure, underdeveloped product. Over time, as the product was refined and improved, and the production process was honed in efficiency, its price began to fall. It seemed counterintuitive since the penicillin produced a few years after first coming to market was so much better. But in the end, the market defined the drug's cost, and with twenty-four companies involved in the penicillin game one way or another, too much was in circulation. The lack of a penicillin patent had a lot to do with the oversupply.[31]

The same went for streptomycin and dihydrostreptomycin. As their production processes improved and better yields became the norm, prices fell accordingly until the antibiotics found their price on the market. That the same process and equipment, with minor variations, were used to produce penicillin and streptomycin (Aureomycin and Terramycin as well) served to keep costs of production low. Entirely new plants with unique setups and new equipment were unnecessary.[32]

The Communist invasion of South Korea also played an indirect role in depressing the prices of penicillin and streptomycin. The war helped foster increased demand for antibiotics, particularly penicillin. As mentioned previously, those companies willing to expand to supply the military's needs received preferential treatment when it came to procuring raw materials and help in financing expansion. This was fine so long as the war raged on; however, once the battle slowed down a bit to trench warfare and eventually an uneasy cease-fire, those same pharmaceutical companies found themselves producing more antibiotics than they could sell. The domestic market had been saturated before the war, and afterward the situation was no different. Making a profit from penicillin and streptomycin grew increasingly difficult.[33]

Pharmaceutical companies knew what they needed to do and where profits lay. According to Merck, "Profit on products developed by a particular company and identified with it tends to be more stable than on products of general manufacture." In 1951 Pfizer put it more succinctly: "The higher margins of profit on antibiotics (during the past several years the average profit margin on antibiotics has been greater than the average profit margin on all products) has resulted from introduction of several new specialties." And finally, American Cyanamid was blunt when it admitted to a higher margin for profits resulting from new specialties, "the latest and most important of which is Aureomycin."[34]

Companies soon found that having proprietary antibiotics could not shield them from price depreciation. When Lederle released Aureomycin to the public in 1948, it was the sole broad-spectrum antibiotic on the market. The following year, Pfizer introduced Terramycin and Parke-Davis chloramphenicol—both being broad-spectrum antibiotics as well. The markets failed to differentiate between the brands and treated them the same. Rather than having three separate antibiotics on store shelves, the market reacted as if triple the amount of the same drug was being sold. A year after first coming out with Aureomycin, Lederle was forced to cut prices by 20 percent to remain competitive. Pfizer and Parke-Davis also had to lower their prices until a natural price was found. Then to make the same amount of profit, the companies would not only have to sell more antibiotics but also need to produce more, further risking falling prices.[35]

If the companies wanted to survive, they'd have to either manufacture a market for their goods or find a new market already in existence.

THE HISTORIAN ALFRED ECKES argued that the Point Four Program melded "altruism and enlightened self-interest."[36] He could have said much the same for the Marshall Plan as well. Both programs sought to leverage the transfer of technology to the advantage of U.S. industry. Since the primary strategy of the Point Four Program was to use the country's technical expertise in place of monetary grants or loans, the administrators used training sessions and classroom workshops as vehicles to introduce Point Four participants to U.S. goods. At first glance it made sense. Participants were learning American techniques, so why not use U.S. tools and equipment as well? Once the farmers were satisfied and comfortable using them, there was no reason to change. As the saying goes, if it ain't broke, don't fix it.

The Marshall Plan relied on its technical assistance program to handle the transfer of knowledge when the European Recovery Program handed off responsibilities to the Mutual Security Agency and its program. Agriculture was one of the main industries pinpointed for modernization, and an increase in productivity was the goal.

One of the primary and essential means of teaching the "American model" was to send missions to the United States to observe or attend classes at one of the country's land-grant universities. The Point Four Program's technical assistance program functioned in much the same way. Missions from participating countries were sent to the United States to learn modern U.S. methods of agriculture. They attended schools such as Cornell University, Texas A&M, and Pennsylvania State University. In addition, American technicians flew around the world, observing and advising governments and foreign firms on how their existing operations could be tweaked to maximize productivity.

Records from the Point Four Program show just how aggressively antibiotic companies such as Lederle lobbied to be included in its curriculum. Sales representatives had regular access to Point Four officials, meeting on numerous occasions. More important for the pharmaceutical company, the two organizations often collaborated on projects with Lederle Laboratories in Pearl River hosting Point Four employees. As a result, American Cyanamid was perfectly placed to get its products directly distributed.[37]

Using the Philippines as an example is instructive. By the early 1950s, agriculture in the island country continued to struggle and had not returned to pre-1941 levels. Thus, horses, goats, sheep, carabao, and cattle remained in short supply. The cattle industry hovered around 50 percent of prewar levels and showed no sign of increasing. In addition, 60 percent of existing cattle were being used as workstock and not raised as beef herds. The outlook was bleak, in particular because self-imposed import controls prevented bringing cattle in from abroad. Beef for consumption was mostly imported from the United States (35 percent), Brazil (30 percent), and Argentina (30 percent) and in the form of corned beef and sausages.[38]

The dairy industry was limited as well. Domestic milk production supplied a paltry 20 percent of required amounts. The remainder was imported. Making matters worse, local farmers and the government showed little interest in rectifying the situation. The dairy cows' inability to adapt to the conditions in the tropical country did not help the situation much either. For the dairy and beef industries, low returns on investment further stifled any hope of improvement.[39]

The swine and poultry populations represented the two aspects of the Philippines' livestock industry to have shown improvement. By 1952 the number of hogs had returned to prewar levels, while the country's chicken industry had surpassed pre-1941 levels by 40 percent. Egg production increased accordingly. The vast majority of pig, chicken, and egg production were uncoordinated "backyard" affairs, where each household raised its stocks using methods and feeding techniques from previous centuries.[40]

Due to import controls, traditional feed suppliers were locked out of the market. The Philippine Import Control Commission prohibited the importation of carbohydrate feeds. It did so to protect local farmers, to encourage local feed production, and to conserve dollars. Since the Philippine feed industry was just finding that alternative local ingredients such as the ipil-ipil (a river tamarind tree) could also be used as a precursor to a finished product, levels of carbohydrate feed continued to be below average. Protein supplements such as fish and soy meal were in short supply.[41]

American Cyanamid was uniquely positioned to take advantage of the feed situation in the Philippines. Traditional U.S. feed companies could not export their products to the country due to the uneven nature of its import controls. At best, they could sell isolated ingredients, but that only made sense if they produced their own supplies, and that was not always the case. The pharmaceutical company's main profits came not from the feed (Aurofac) itself but from the Aureomycin added as a growth promoter. At the time, there weren't any import controls on antibiotics, much less antibiotic growth promoters. It's doubtful either group of products registered at all in regulators' minds.[42]

The pharmaceutical company pounced.

In a letter dated January 26, 1953, from E. N. Holmgreen, the director of the Food and Agriculture Division of the FDA, to Ray Johnson, the food and agriculture officer of the Mutual Security Mission to the Philippines, the participation of American Cyanamid was discussed. Holmgreen recounts how "three representatives from the company paid a visit to the Food and Agriculture Division to discuss recent developments in animal nutrition with particular regard to the use of antibiotics in livestock feeding." He mentions that the people at American Cyanamid had been helpful in implementing a number of technical assistance projects involving nutrition.[43] Holmgreen then gently pushes American Cyanamid's products by informing Johnson "the Company representatives agreed to make certain current literature on the use of antibiotics in animal feeds available" and that the "documentary materials are transmitted herewith in duplicate." He closes by stating that the letter should not be inferred as a "recommendation of a choice of commercial sources for the materials advertised." He was just going through the motions there.[44]

A letter dated March 10, 1953, from Johnson indicates that the group decided to move forward with the material from American Cyanamid. Two five-pound drums of commercial antibiotic were en route to Manila and would be included in controlled feeding trials being done for the benefit of Filipino farmers and feed mixers. The antibiotic feed mix would also be used on swine.[45]

Johnson also informed Holmgreen of a series of feeding trials with white leghorn chicks that were designed to show the benefits of a commercial B12 and antibiotic feed supplement. He'd send the results.[46]

Documents show that by 1953, the inclusion of antibiotics in animal feed had become commonplace in the Philippines. The report "Poultry Feed Imports" estimated the food requirements for the roughly 3 million purebred chickens and 25 million native birds. The author of the study calculated 200 million pounds of feed would be required for a full year for maximum efficiency, and 2 million pounds of vitamins and antibiotics would be needed to be mixed with fish meal.[47]

Similar processes went on in other countries participating in the Point Four Program. Brazil, Argentina, and Iran are just a few of the countries that received technical assistance from the United States. And whenever given an opening, American Cyanamid pushed to have Aurofac included in a country's feed training program, with the effort essentially being underwritten by the U.S. government.[48]

12

Acquired or inherited? That was the question. Nagging as much as lingering. Even after Oswald Avery's seminal 1944 study and the consensus view that DNA, not protein, was responsible for the transmission of traits, enough scientists still disputed the notion of inheritance to keep geneticists moving forward and trying to settle the issue once and for all or at least shut up the critics. It was a testimony to Western scientists' vigor that they never settled for good enough and continued searching for more definitive answers.

Whether the Lysenkoist controversy played any role or added to the sense of urgency is unknown. However, that the leading voices in modern genetics actively and publicly contested Michurinist demagoguery at least proves it was very much in their minds.

The ultimate rebuttal to Trofim Lysenko and his Michurinist acolytes came from the laboratory of Joshua Lederberg. A pair of experiments, one in 1952 and the other in 1956, addressed the question head-on. The simplicity and elegance of the studies added to the feeling that the question had finally been put to bed.

The groundwork leading to Lederberg's seminal bacterial genetics work had been laid first by Salvador Luria and Max Delbrück and then by Alfred Hershey and Martha Chase. Luria and Delbrück approached the question of whether mutation or adaptation was responsible for the transmission of traits by using *E. coli* and bacteriophage T1, and by adding a twist of population genetics. They inoculated bacteria and placed them into separate tubes. The *E. coli* were allowed to grow for a predetermined time before they were plated into agar containing T1 bacteriophages and observed for signs of resistance. How they grew would tell the researchers whether pre-adaptive or post-adaptive forces were at work. If the population in the petri dishes arose by adaptive evolution, where each cell had an equal probability of developing resistance after exposure, the colonies on the plates should be more or less equal. However, if the resistant colonies arose with every new generation but before exposure to the virus, the number of resistant colonies would fluctuate between extremes. Luria and Delbrück discovered the latter was true. It marked the first significant experiment to indicate that the spontaneous mutation hypothesis was responsible for changes in the generation of bacteria.[1]

In 1952 Hershey and Chase took it one step further. They relied on T2 bacteriophages to demonstrate whether protein or DNA was responsible for carrying genetic information. First, they inserted radioactive isotopes of sulfur (sulfur-35) and phosphorous (phosphorous-32) into the phage's protein sections—mostly its outer casing—and its DNA, contained inside. These isotopes were significant because proteins are partly composed with sulfur but not phosphorus, while DNA contains phosphorus but lacks sulfur. Next, the bacteria were then infected by the phages, which hijacked the genetic machinery, as viruses do. Then Hershey and Chase removed the phages by agitation in a blender. What was left was placed in a centrifuge, and the phage coats were separated from the bacteria. The remaining bacteria were lysed, and the progeny of the older phages were released. The replicated phages carried only the radioactive isotope phosphorus-32, proving that DNA carried the genetic material that was passed onto offspring.[2]

Unfortunately, while Hershey and Chase's experiment proved that DNA was the genetic material, it did not explain how it was passed on. That was where Joshua Lederberg picked up the mantle. He conducted his first experiment and presented the results in a 1952 paper titled "Replica Plating and Indirect Selection of Bacterial Mutants."[3]

Lederberg immediately addressed the issue at heart. "It has been repeatedly questioned . . . whether a selective environment may not only select but also direct adaptive heritable changes." He proceeded to list fourteen papers, including his previous papers, that "adduced in support of preadaptation."[4] The ideal experiment would show the presence of mutants in a population that had not been exposed to the selective agent. Lederberg, along with his biochemist wife Esther, proved up for the challenge.

The experiment's design, conceived by Esther Lederberg, was so deceptively simple that it's almost comical in retrospect. Lederberg used a cylindrical wooden block with a diameter smaller than a petri dish. At one end of the cylinder was a handle, and on the other end she tied on a sterile piece of velvet cloth, which was called a replicator.[5]

Lederberg took the replicator and gently pressed it against a dish containing a solidified nutrient with large colonies of bacteria on it. This dish was the "master" plate. Making sure to keep the orientation of the cylinder the same, the velvet cloth was pressed on a fresh plate that had an antibiotic on it. The colonies were then transferred, but the only ones to survive were those resistant to the bacteria. The key here is that none of the bacteria had been previously exposed to the antibiotic before inoculating the second dish. It proved that the trait for resistance had existed before exposure and was more capable of surviving in the new conditions.[6]

In 1956 Lederberg collaborated with Luigi Luca Cavalli-Sforza to devise another test for indirect selection, this time in liquid cultures. (The replica plate experiment took place on a solid culture, the agar contained on the plate.) It came to be known as the "sib selection" technique, and it accomplished essentially the same thing—the isolation of a resistant strain without exposing it to antibiotics—only in a liquid.[7]

In the experiment, they took a culture of bacteria and isolated resistant bacteria on a nutrient medium containing an antibiotic. Once they had the resistant colony, they diluted the culture with a liquid and then separated equal amounts of the liquid into test tubes, one of which contained only resistant bacteria. They then repeated the process. One tube (the best one) ended up with most of the resistant bacteria (all from preceding "best" tubes), thus proving that the trait was passed down from generation to generation and not acquired.[8]

The replica plate and sib selection experiments, along with the Luria-Delbrück and Hershey-Chase experiments, were starting points of bacterial genetics and seminal moments in modern genetics. The work could also be considered a crucial strike at what remained of the scientific aspects of Lysenko's creative Darwinism. That it continued to thrive in the Soviet Union testified to its political underpinnings. It was now exposed. Denying the conclusions that logically followed the pair of experiments could only be managed by the most ardent followers of Lysenko, people with so-called skin in the game who were motivated by politics, self-interest, and self-preservation.

JOSEPH STALIN DIED AT 9:50 p.m. on March 5, 1953, surrounded by his family, his doctors, and the men who would run the Soviet Union in his wake. While everyone stood in silence, Lavrenti Beria, the former head of the Secret Police, sprang into action, barking out orders to hospital staff. Stalin's daughter later recalled, "The silence of the room where everyone was gathered around the deathbed was shattered by the sound of his loud voice, the ring of triumph unconcealed." Nikita Khrushchev described him as radiant. As Beria readied to leave the hospital, he shouted to his driver, "Khrustalev, my car!" Those words became famous in Russian history and culture.[9]

Stalin's death sent the Communist world into spasms of uncertainty. The instability the dictator's policies had created fostered resentment and pent-up rage that found expression on the streets. East Germany erupted in riots. Upswells of unrest in Bulgaria and Czechoslovakia followed. Unfair and unrealistic production quota increases often served as their spark. The new Kremlin leaders understood what was happening and moved as best they could to quell the demonstrations. They tried to convince with words, and when that failed, they deterred with tanks and guns and bullets.

Khrushchev finally outlasted, outthought, and outmaneuvered the competition. With the support of General Zhukov, the hero who had saved Moscow and Leningrad, he had Beria arrested and executed. And then there was Lysenko, who had lost his patron and political guardian. Would he survive the next phase in Soviet history?

ON JANUARY 17, 1953, the *South China Morning Post* published a brief article detailing a milestone in the annals of modern science and medicine. The Soviet Union was celebrating the centenary of the discovery of penicillin. According to the article, Soviet scientists claimed the world's first antibiotic had been discovered in Russia by a dermatologist named Alexei Polotebnov.[10] It built off of a 1948 *Pravda* article that had announced penicillin was a Russian discovery, citing both Zinaida Ermol'eva's work and that of obscure nineteenth-century mold researchers.[11] Now, simply being able to produce penicillin no longer sufficed; countries believed that to enjoy credit for having the drug, they needed to have introduced it to the world.

Communist scientists came together in 1955 for the Warsaw International Conference on Antibiotics. Participants from Bulgaria, Hungary, China, North Korea, Poland, Romania, Czechoslovakia, and the USSR attended the seven-day gathering. Over thirty presentations updated the attendees about the state of antibiotic development and antibiotic resistance research mostly in the Communist world but also gave passing mentions about Western developments.[12]

Like microbiologists, bacteriologists, and drug developers the world over, Communist researchers struggled to get a grip on the phenomenon of antibiotic resistance. However, unlike their Western counterparts, who were inching closer to acknowledging what would come to be known as the resistome, Soviet bloc scientists moved in the opposite direction, engaging in some a priori discoveries and confirming "directed modification" (the transmission of acquired traits). "Great interest was elicited by a report presented by Professor Malek, Active Member of the Academy of Sciences of the Czechoslovak Republic. Professor Malek's report dealt with the directed modification of organisms producing antibiotics and with methods of modifying the heredity of those organisms. Malek emphasized the great significance of Michurin's teaching as a basis for studying the modifiability of microorganisms."[13]

According to the report, Professor Malek treated bacteria with "strongly acting agents" to "disturb" their heredity. After breeding the altered unnamed bacteria, the resulting subsequent generations were transformed into antibiotic-producing strains.[14]

Other presentations reported similar findings regarding the "modifiability" of actinomycetes to produce streptomycin, Aureomycin, and Terramycin. Other researchers announced the results of bombarding bacteria with ultraviolet radiation. One researcher from

Hungary claimed that by subjecting actinomycetes to a method of "vegetative hybridization," he was able to transform the bacteria into an altogether different species.[15]

Communist scientists relied on the same labor-intensive analysis of soil samples that was pervasive in laboratories around the world. In particular, Georgyi Gause highlighted his newest antibiotic discovery called albomycin.

Some research was redundant. Researchers from China described studies on the effects of adding corn extract and lactose to penicillin fermentation broth. Another Czech study documented the increased rate of weight gain by adding Aureomycin and procaine penicillin to animal feed.

THE 1950S WITNESSED AN uptick not only in antibiotic production around the world but also in its development. Broad-spectrum antibiotics dominated the market. Extracts of soil crisscrossed countries, if not the globe. Laboratories worked diligently, plating samples and hoping to find their literal version of pay dirt. Meanwhile, applied scientists went to work, devising slight variations on already established fermentation techniques with different degrees of success. The combination of local productions of already existent antibiotic classes as well as genuine discoveries created a labyrinth of names that was almost as variable and confusing as pasta nomenclature.

In the Soviet Union, synthomycin was the name for locally produced chloramphenicol. Gause described it as "synthetic racemic chloromycetin prepared according to a method developed by Soviet chemists." Levomycetin was another local name for chloramphenicol (Chloromycetin) in parts of the Soviet Union, particularly in Stalin's home state, Georgia. It differed from synthomycin in that it was optically active and synthesized at the Institute of Biological and Medicinal Chemistry of the Academy of Medical Sciences.[16] Biomycin was the local name for oxytetracycline, which had been "obtained" by the All-Union Scientific Research Institute of Antibiotics.

Albomycin, a Soviet discovery, belonged to the class sideromycin, which was characterized by chemical appendages called siderophores that possessed antibiotic properties. Most of its efficacy was against gram-negative bacteria, in particular *Enterobacteriaceae*. According to Gause, "Albomycin is effective against penicillin-resistant staphylococci and may be used to treat septic diseases caused by them."[17]

Ekmolin was perhaps the most promising antibiotic developed in the Soviet Union during the 1950s. Discovered in 1952 by Zinaida Ermol'eva and other collaborators, the drug was described as an antibiotic preparation from a species of fish. It is active against gram-positive and gram-negative organisms, depending on the media (broth or 1 percent glucose peptone water). It works synergistically with streptomycin, preventing the emergence of resistant microorganisms and acting on streptomycin-resistant strains of *Shigella dysenteriae*. Streptomycin and ekmolin together are called ekmostreptomycin. Ekmolin also works synergistically with penicillin and showed activity against influenza A.[18]

In Japan the discovery of colistin in 1950 represented a significant discovery. It was synthesized from the *Bacillus polymyxa* subspecies *colistinus* and was used therapeutically in Japan and Europe during the 1950s. In the United States, it came in the form of colistimethate sodium in 1959. By the early 1980s, most parts of the world had stopped using colistin due to its high incidence of nephrotoxicity. Since then, the antibiotic's use has been restricted to lung infections due to multidrug-resistant gram-negative bacteria. Most recently, it has replaced carbapenem as the antibiotic of last resort.[19]

Another Japanese antibiotic called kanamycin was discovered in 1957 by Hamao Umezawa. *Streptomyces kanamyceticus* produced the aminoglycoside, and its spectrum of activity included *E. coli*, *Enterobacter aerogenes*, *Klebsiella pneumoniae*, *Acinetobacter*, and a few other bacteria. Like colistin, the drug exhibited a degree of toxicity and was only used for short durations.[20]

One of the most important drug discoveries at the time came from, you guessed it, a soil sample. This one came from a missionary in Borneo who sent a sample to his friend E. C. Kornfield, an organic chemist at Eli Lilly. Kornfield and his team isolated *Streptomyces orientalis* from the sample and discovered that it produced a chemical called compound 05865 that was active against gram-positive bacteria, including penicillin-resistant *Staphylococcus aureus*. After running tests, they established that after over twenty generations of staphylococci, its resistance to penicillin skyrocketed 100,000-fold; however, the yet-to-be-named compound 05865—though nicknamed "Mississippi mud" because of its brown color while impure—experienced a meager 4- to 8-fold increase in resistance. After tweaking the production process to improve the purity of the antibiotic, clinical trials began. Word about the new antibiotic spread quickly, as did the demand for it. Vancomycin, as it came to be called, arrived at a time when health care professionals possessed very few options to treat penicillin-resistant staphylococcal infections. It was a godsend.[21]

GOVERNMENT LEADERS AROUND THE world continued their push to acquire antibiotic plants in their countries. They could no longer be considered luxuries; they were medical necessities and represented a political imperative. Politicians wanted their names and legacies associated with the miracle drugs. In India one of the founding members of the modern state, a man who stood beside Mahatma Gandhi against the British, wanted a penicillin factory. Jawaharlal Nehru was determined to get one.

Not long after gaining independence, the Indian government began to explore different avenues that would allow the country to manufacture pharmaceuticals. In particular, officials were interested in drugs that prevented or treated communicable diseases. Not only that, they were determined to provide their citizens with low-cost, high-quality medicine. They looked to Western Europe and North America for solutions and set up the Committee on the Penicillin Project to negotiate the particulars.[22]

Most collaborations between Western companies and their developing world counterparts involved some degree of technology transfer in exchange for part ownership. For the committee, this was a nonstarter. The goal of building a penicillin production facility was part of a larger initiative to jump-start India's industrial sector. Signing a contract whose terms seemed to move in the opposite direction made little sense. Still, the proposals from pharmaceutical companies used that as a start point.[23] "Glaxo proposed to import pure penicillin in bulk and to use Bombay [now Mumbai] as a base for bottling therapeutic doses of the drug. Pfizer offered the government the option of importing crude penicillin in bulk, to be refined and subsequently formulated in India. Merck offered to collaborate in establishing a manufacturing facility . . . although exact terms under which the transfer of technology would occur were not disclosed."[24] The Rahway pharmaceutical company emerged as the front-runner for obvious reasons.

One other option arose while negotiations with the Western firms continued. The United Nations International Children's Emergency Fund (UNICEF) and the World Health Organization approached the Indian government and offered to build a factory for free. The two organizations envisaged the proposed plant as being one among a network of antibiotic research, training, and production centers around the world. The Indian government would also reimburse the WHO for its investment by supplying penicillin to the organization. Dr. K. C. K. E. Raja, the director general of health services for the Indian government, became the point person for discussions between the three parties.[25]

The technical adviser to the committee, G. Sankaran, traveled to Switzerland to meet with WHO officials. There he met with Dr. N. L. Macpherson, the Canadian scientist who had formerly worked with the UNRRA as an adviser on constructing large-scale penicillin plants. Macpherson stated the WHO's position: the offer to build a plant hinged on the plant's functioning in a noncommercial role. He suggested the Indian government forgo Merck's proposal and assured Sankaran that WHO experts could provide both the technical know-how and hands-on assistance in constructing, setting up, and running the penicillin plant.[26]

Sankaran believed that anyone with valuable information about running a penicillin plant would have learned it in the private sector and, therefore, would be prohibited from sharing such information due to their previous employment. Either way, he believed Indian applied scientists needed exposure to the most advanced techniques, and that meant collaborating with private industry—in this case, Merck. Most of India's industrial leaders believed licensed manufacturing represented the most efficient route to self-sufficiency.[27]

As the Committee on the Penicillin Project investigated options, two camps emerged. The country's industrialists, who were mostly based in Bombay, championed the idea of licensing. It represented the quickest path toward production. Moreover, it carried the least amount of risk, since the technology they would be essentially renting had already been tried and tested. Licensing also addressed one of business' central concerns—uncertainty. The implications of adopting this licensing-driven collaborative model would influence the future of India's industrial sector had it been selected.[28]

Meanwhile, the other side, mostly composed of people in Nehru's camp, believed that the difficult step of acquiring the technical skill and knowledge at the heart of the fermentation process was the best option in the long run. Moreover, Nehru had reservations about whether Merck was the sole source of information regarding the current fermentation methods.[29]

An extended discussion about the nature of patents followed and consumed the committee's energies. When an Indian government representative returned from the United States with Merck's terms, Nehru ordered that no commitments be made until a meeting was held.[30]

Ultimately, the UNICEF-WHO proposal fell more in line with Nehru's position than did Merck's. He held strong reservations about collaborating with large multinational corporations, particularly quickly ascendant pharmaceutical firms. He believed they would use their leverage as essential partners to influence the direction of scientific research in India. Nehru described his concerns: "We have built up a considerable number of laboratories and I have specially laid stress on research and the scientific approach, rather than the commercial approach to scientific problems. The commercial approach can pay dividends in a country like the U.S. where the whole basis of the social structure is commercial and individual profit making."[31] Nehru found Merck's capitalist approach was simply incompatible in his socialist country.

In March 1951 the Indian government consulted with Ernst Chain at the Instituto Superiore di Sanità. The former Oxford man stressed that Indian scientists deserved to have a role in the future of the new field of biochemistry. He advised the government to build a state-of-the-art research facility attached to an antibiotics plant, similar to his setup in Italy. He explained the logic behind his suggestion: "Production of antibiotics will stimulate research problems in all aspects of the field of chemical microbiology, and vice versa, advances in research will be reflected immediately on the production capacity of the plant." He urged the government to create an environment where Indian scientists could ply their trade shielded from commercial secrecy.[32]

Chain also reaffirmed Nehru's hunch that Merck's process was not entirely its own. He argued that the *Lancet* article that described the Chain-Heatley process of fermentation guaranteed that most of the fermentation process was in the public domain.[33]

Nehru also turned to Sir Edward Mellanby, the man responsible for Florey's questionable decision to publish the fermentation work done at Oxford. Mellanby highlighted two points: whether the WHO team could complete the project successfully and whether the technical know-how could be adequately transferred. Mellanby took the matter in his own hands and met personally with Macpherson. He came away satisfied that the WHO project should move forward. The Indian government selected the UNICEF-WHO proposal for building a penicillin plant in December 1953 and was seeded a year later. By mid-1955 the plant was producing penicillin, albeit inconsistently at first.[34]

The completed building included six 30,000-liter fermenters that were producing 890,000 mega units by February 1956. This plant served as the cornerstone of India's most important pharmaceutical firm, Hindustan Antibiotics, and the Committee on the Penicillin Project evolved into the company's management.[35]

BY THE MID-1950S, HOSPITALS around the world realized they were under siege. A strain of *Staphylococcus* had emerged and reached pandemic levels in health care settings. This time, the strain was susceptible to group I phages and not group III as with the original Australian outbreak in 1949. Among group I phages, the strain of *Staphylococcus aureus* showed the most affinity for phages 80 and 81, both of which were closely related. Their spread was fast and vicious, and taken together they constituted the first wave of *Staphylococcus aureus*'s decades-long assault on human beings and their antibiotics.[36]

One of the first outbreaks took place at the Royal Prince Alfred Hospital in Sydney. It was the first instance of a phage type 80 bacteria being isolated in patients. In this case, the outbreak occurred in the maternity ward and was ultimately responsibility for nineteen of twenty-four neonatal staphylococcal infections in Australia. The type 80/81 bacteria displayed an unusual virulence, causing the formation of distinct lesions on the babies that were "distinguishable on clinical grounds from those due to other types." Of all type 80/81 strains, 94 percent were resistant to penicillin.[37]

Similar outbreaks in the United States and the United Kingdom followed the Australian case. Infections tended to follow similar patterns. From 1954 to 1958, U.S. hospitals suffered over five hundred outbreaks of antibiotic-resistant staphylococci.[38] Newborn babies developed open lesions (pyoderma) while in the maternity ward. This normally occurred in association with increased incidence of breast abscesses in nursing mothers and pus-filled lesions (suppurative) among family members. Furuncles, carbuncles, and other abscesses were common. Later, it was determined that the two primary points of infection in newborns were the nose and umbilical cord. The bacteria tended to show resistance to penicillin (due to its prevalence), streptomycin (bacteria developed rapid resistance to it), and chlortetracycline (perhaps due its overuse clinically and agriculturally).[39] According to Mary Barber, hospital strain *Staphylococcus* also showed resistance to chloramphenicol, but once the drug's use was severely limited, it regained its potency.[40]

Up to this point, the most important antibiotics belonged to three and a half classes: the penicillins, aminoglycosides, tetracyclines, and, to a limited degree, chloramphenicols. The remainder consisted of minor drugs such as bacitracin and neomycin that could only be applied topically. While scores of other compounds had been isolated from soil samples, they were mostly too toxic for any practical use.

Why were hospitals so susceptible to antibiotic-resistant bacterial infections? In 1958 researchers Vernon Knight, Arthur White, and Thomas Hemmerly presented a paper at the U.S. National Conference on Hospital-Acquired Staphylococcal Disease. They had studied four separate hospital strains of staphylococci, three of which were susceptible to antibiotics and one that was not. One strain came from a sample dated 1932–48, another strain was obtained in

1953–54, and another in 1954–55. A final strain was obtained in a mental hospital. They tested them for resistance to penicillin and tetracycline.[41]

The bacteria from the first hospital showed considerable resistance to penicillin but not to tetracycline. In the second sample from a hospital, *Staphylococci aureus* resistant to penicillin and tetracyclines skyrocketed. Penicillin resistance more than doubled from just under 40 percent to over 80 percent.[42] Tetracycline resistance soared from none to over 60 percent. The next sample, obtained the following year, showed a similar pattern of resistance. Finally, the strains obtained from the mental health hospital, where heavy antibiotic use was not the norm, showed barely any antibiotic-resistant staphylococci. The findings suggest that resistance followed heavy use of antibiotics in a particular setting—in this case, hospitals.[43]

The abundant use of antibiotics in hospitals drove resistance to evolve. It also incentivized pharmaceutical companies to alter their business models. As we saw with the combination of penicillin and streptomycin into a single drug, utilizing two antibiotics as a means of broadening the spectrum of activity made some logical sense. Early reports suggested a degree of synergism between the two. This cleared the way for pharmaceutical companies to concoct more so-called fixed-dose combination antibiotics. These "new" antibiotics were supported by aggressive advertising campaigns that boasted extravagant claims supported by specious facts. According to Scott Podolsky, "Antibiotic resistance reflected a business opportunity for the pharmaceutical industry, eager to market 'specialty antibiotics' to confront resistant organisms."[44] This business decision ended up having major clinical implications.[45]

At this critical juncture, when resistance to chemotherapeutic antibiotics first began appearing in hospital settings, alternative approaches to fighting bacterial infections may have helped. In particular, the use of bacteriophages against *Staphylococcus aureus* leads to a number of tantalizing what-ifs.

At the time, a small but significant body of research indicated that bacteriophage treatment had shown effectiveness against localized exterior infections such as those caused by staph A. As noted in chapter 7, Eaton and Bayne-Jones in 1934 highlighted the efficiency of phage therapy on staphylococcal infections. Seven years later, even hostile reviewers such as Albert Krueger and Jane Scribner could not ignore that the science at the time supported topical treatments with phage mixes, particularly the cocktails that eventually emerged with broad-spectrum phages such as the staphylococcal bacteriophage Sb-1, phage K family.[46]

Besides being effective against staphylococcal infections, research indicated that both phages and antibiotics could be used in tandem, often with beneficial results. In addition to synergistic activity, phages offered yet another benefit. As one recent reviewer recalled, "Very little development of resistance to this family of phages has been observed, presumably implying that the still unidentified primary receptor is a molecule of significant importance to bacteria. Thus, so far as phages are concerned, MRSA (methicillin-resistant *Staphylococcus aureus*) is simply another strain of *Staphylococcus*."[47]

Unfortunately by this time, the blinding glow of penicillin and subsequent antibiotics prevented Western researchers from considering phage therapy. In addition, the American Medical Association's sustained editorial campaign undercutting the strategy had made its once-marginal uses nonexistent. Finally, any chances of stumbling across contemporary research—namely, Russian-language journals—had been cut off by the Cold War climate that had isolated Soviet-bloc scientists from English-speaking ones.

One more possibility cannot be discounted, but it is slightly trickier to establish: bacteriophage therapy was largely ignored because it was considered "Communist" medicine. References to the idea are difficult to come by, especially since something that partisan and crass would be avoided in scientific journals. Even in the ardently anti-Communist *Journal of the American Medical Association*, Morris Fishbein's editorials veered away from blatant politicization. Yet, the sentiment seems to have existed to some degree and to have been passed down from generations of health care professionals. In a 2000 *New York Times* article on the rediscovery of bacteriophage therapy, Chief of the Biochemical Genetics Laboratory at the National Institutes of Health Carl Merril stated that "there's the psychological obstacle of a new treatment coming from the former Soviet Union. It's unusual, to say the least."[48]

FOR A BRIEF, FLEETING moment in 1954, it appeared as if Lysenko's grip on Soviet biology had received a mortal blow from the country's highest official after none other than Khrushchev spoke out against Lysenko and his followers. To observers, Khrushchev's 1953 appeal for an end to "bootlicking and servility" in the agricultural field signified a desire to overturn the Soviet soil that had sprouted Michurin and Lysenko and the entire creative Darwinist cabal.[49] Along with the sharp attacks against Lysenko's theory of species formation, the time seemed right.

The incident in question began when V. S. Dmitriev presented his dissertation to the Academy of Sciences. Dmitriev was an agronomist who had once been in charge of the agricultural section of the State Planning Commission (Gosplan) in 1948 but was dismissed when Stalin's Great Plan for the Transformation of Nature was abandoned. Like most of his peers, he was a devoted disciple of Michurin. Lysenko had taken Dmitriev under his wing and arranged for him to have a research position at the Academy of Sciences and to enroll in the graduate program. When the time came for Dmitriev to submit his dissertation, he produced a work based on Lysenko's transformation of species. Much to everyone's surprise, the doctoral committee members decided to show their backbones and rejected Dmitriev's work. It was also an implicit rejection of Lysenko and his theory.[50]

Lysenko intervened on Dmitriev's behalf and forced the committee to reconsider the dissertation and to grant his degree. The scientists protested vehemently, and much to everyone's surprise, Khrushchev came down on their side. In a rare public rebuke, the press chided Lysenko for his actions. In truth, the premier's stance had less to do with Lysenko and more to do with his disdain for Dmitriev. By the time the year ended, Khrushchev had all but ordained Lysenko the master of Soviet agriculture and biology.[51]

David Joravsky speculates that Khrushchev's embrace of Lysenko could have been a matter of his relying on him because he was the president of the Lenin Academy and the formally appointed chief of agricultural science. Perhaps it was because Khrushchev had a long history with Lysenko, going back all the way to his time as chief of Ukraine, where he had inherited Lysenko as his agricultural adviser.

Joravsky concludes that the most important thing Lysenko offered Khrushchev was confirmation that the virgin lands of the Soviet Union could produce high reliable yields, when no other agronomist in the country was willing to utter the fiction.[52]

Domestically, Khrushchev pinned his reign to transforming Soviet agriculture from tepid yields and occasional famines to the wheat- and corn-producing machine he'd seen in America. He wanted the healthy cattle and the creamy milk that come with well-fed livestock. It all started with grain. Once that was in hand, the rest would follow. That much of the country's land fell short of the required nutrients to support the intensive farming he imagined was a minor detail the proletarian farmers could and would overcome. With the force of Soviet science behind them, planting and harvesting were mere formalities. At least that's how the narrative went.[53]

DURING THE WANING DAYS of the Chinese Civil War, Soviet scientific advisers introduced Michurinist biology to the country. They found its Communist Party leaders were receptive to the Soviet version of genetics and eager to implement it. They couldn't have wished for more pliant subjects or been more willing mentors. Soviet self-interest trumped any sense of benevolence; much like the U.S.-based Marshall Plan, first and foremost, its assistance was steeped in real-world geopolitics.

The Soviet Union sought to perpetuate an image of goodwill wherein the Russian people shared the secrets of their much-mythologized proletarian agriculture. When it came time to rely on symbols to communicate the modernity and prosperity of Soviet life, they turned to images of science, a Communist version that was distinctly far better than that of the West. According to Nikolai Krementsov, the Soviet Union had created its own geopolitical universe "in which science was an extension of politics and subject to the same Cold War distinctions of 'us' and 'them,' 'ours' and 'theirs.'"[54]

Starting in 1952, Michurinism replaced classical genetics in classrooms, textbooks, and libraries. Luo Tianyu's group relied on the party's "mass science" and "science popularization" campaigns to spread the gospel of creative Darwinism. Major libraries continued to receive Western scientific journals but were forbidden to allow access and permission to read them. For the most part, Morganist-Mendelist geneticists maintained a low profile. They were not asked to recant the way scientists in the Soviet Union were forced to do in public; however, the Communist Party forbade teaching anything but party-approved science. In the end, Michurinism in China, like its Soviet counterpart, proved to be nothing more than pseudoscience.[55]

By 1954 events outside China began eroding the foundations of Michurinist biology in the country. The problems started outside the scientific field. After Stalin's death, a growing rift between the Soviet and Chinese leaderships emerged. Mao disapproved of the direction Khrushchev was taking the USSR and took a dim view of his so-called secret speech to the Politburo. The public denunciation of Stalin's atrocities amounted to a betrayal of the form of Communism still espoused by the Central Committee. The reflexive subordination of the Chinese will to Soviet leadership was shaken for the first time.[56]

At around the same time, news began to filter into China that Soviet classical geneticists were openly deconstructing Trofim Lysenko's theory of speciation. His claim that under certain conditions one species can transform into another left him open to all sorts of attacks, even from some of his supporters who felt the quackery went one step too far. The so-called speciation debates were eventually documented in the December 1954 issue of the Chinese Academy of Sciences' *Science Gazette*. The publication forced the press to acknowledge the debate on a national level and document the opposing evidence that undercut the Michurinist prophet's claims.[57]

In December 1955 the Chinese Academy of Sciences invited Hans Stubbe, the president of the East German Academy of Agricultural Science, to give a series of talks on Lysenko's "vegetative hybridization." During the course of his lectures, he ripped Lysenko's research. He had spent five years trying to reproduce the findings without any luck. He concluded there was no evidence of the phenomenon. Stubbe went one step further, denouncing Lysenko as simply incompetent. The conviction of the East German's declaration was so forceful and certain that it shook the academy. News of his lectures went straight to the Central Committee, which, in turn, informed Mao. The chairman was so concerned that he ordered Minister of

Propaganda Lu Dingyi to investigate Michurinism once and for all and report back to him.[58]

Blow after blow landed unanswered. In 1956 Khrushchev held the All-Soviet Union Conference on the production of hybrid corn seed. The genetically modified corn had been a central factor in the abundant corn production in the United States, where it had been developed during the early twentieth century. For years, Lysenko denounced the use of hybrid techniques that relied on classical genetics that he denied existed. He forbade the use of the corn. Then, in a serious blow to his authority, the Soviet Union lifted the ban on hybrid corn. The Soviets were now able to reap the definite and tangible benefits of increased corn production. Meanwhile, the ban remained in place in China, which continued suffering through lackluster harvests.[59]

All this coincided with the initiation of the Communist Party's Hundred Flowers, Hundred Schools campaign. It was a brief moment of respite for scholars from the Communist Party's oppressive control of the literary and scientific fields. Intellectuals were invited to come forward and speak freely about the restraints on their ability to conduct research.[60]

Biologists came forward in droves. Official Chinese Academy of Sciences journals and newspapers published their accounts of being punished and humiliated for disagreeing with the Michurinist theories in Chinese and Soviet textbooks. In fact, they spoke out against the unquestioned constraints Soviet scientific literature—journals as well as textbooks—put on research. They also cited the stifling effects of their fear of being charged with "undermining confidence in Soviet science."[61]

The Qingdao Genetics Symposium, held in August 1956, was the first opportunity for the unshackled classical geneticists to present their theories in the open. The lectures exposed how far behind their Western counterparts the Chinese geneticists had fallen. It became apparent that denying them access to non-Soviet journals had hampered the development of their field.[62] The conference also addressed the rewriting of textbooks to insert basic concepts such as chromosomes, genes, and the recently discovered deoxyribonucleic acid, better known as DNA. For scientists it represented a significant first step toward their regaining a firm footing, but it by no means leveled the field or undid the damage done over eight misguided years. In fact, the argument could be made that the party's new stance was equally damaging because now Michurinist genetics shared the stage with classical genetics as equals. It took another decade for creative Darwinism to be expelled in its entirety.

Unfortunately, there would be much more pain to suffer. Because the Chinese Communist Party had been so taken aback by the criticisms it had invited, the Central Committee used the campaign to compile a retribution list. Mao then initiated the Anti-Rightist Movement in which many of the intellectuals who spoke out were denounced, imprisoned, and killed.[63]

13

A 1957 advertisement for Pfizer highlighted a number of products in its catalog. Atarax. Biostat. Terramycin Egg Formula. Their newest products from 1956. At the top of the list, in the position of honor, was the company's latest antibiotic creation: "Sigmamycin—Newest extended-range antibiotic effective in virtually every situation calling for an antibiotic—including many infections caused by bacteria resistant to other antibiotics."[1]

Virtually every situation.

Bacteria resistant to other antibiotics.

Hyperbole be damned. But that was how Pfizer described it. The new kid on the block. The future. Only the future looked a whole lot like the past, albeit with a little extra window dressing. Lipstick on a pig, some would call it. In this case, the hog's name was Terramycin, and the lipstick was two antibiotics with limited capabilities named oleandomycin and Sigmamycin. The former consisted of two parts tetracycline to one part macrolide, while the latter consisted of tetracycline and oleandomycin.[2]

Pfizer supported Sigmamycin with an advertising campaigns for the ages. The ad team's efforts fed right into the company's game-changing sales force, which introduced the antibiotic to every doctor alive. A healthy public relations campaign ensured the public was made aware of the details, with one *Los Angeles Times* article titled "One+One=Three," claiming that with Sigmamycin Pfizer had essentially accomplished the impossible and created a combination drug greater than its parts.[3] According to a *Wall Street Journal* article, Sigmamycin was "a new antibiotic drug, expected to be a major weapon in treating germ-caused diseases[, that] has been developed by Chas. Pfizer & Co."[4] Truth be told, they even convinced fictional doctors that the most miraculous of the so-called miracle drugs was Sigmamycin.[5]

In *The Antibiotic Era: Reform, Resistance, and the Pursuit of a Rational Therapeutics*, Scott Podolsky recounts how John Lear, the science editor at *Saturday Review*, published an article about antibiotics. He gave it the title "Taking the Miracle out of the Miracle Drugs." During the course of writing it, Lear spoke with numerous infectious disease experts. One of the things he came away with, and then opened the article with it, was that physicians across the country prescribed antibiotics as easily as aspirin. Lear knew the reason why and proceeded to document the pressure pharmaceutical company salesmen placed on doctors to use their drugs. This was especially true for Pfizer and Sigmamycin.[6]

It got worse. Lear went on to recount a dinner he had with an "eminent research physician." After dinner they visited the unnamed researcher's laboratory. While they were there, the physician opened drawers that were bursting with pharmaceutical advertising brochures. He informed Lear that most of what he saw in them was misleading, if not completely false. He then showed him one of Sigmamycin's most famous advertisements, which proclaimed, "Every day . . . everywhere . . . more and more physicians find Sigmamycin the antibiotic therapy of choice."[7]

The use of "testimonials," or claims made by physicians, researchers, or other medical professionals but without the hard clinical proof to support their claims, had a long and mostly checkered tradition. It stretched back to the traveling elixir salesman peddling Clark Stanley's snake oil liniment from the back of his wagon. Baseless but genuine claims continued to dominate the pharmaceutical industry, even as it gained in size and influence. They also represented a major technique used in the advertising industry to blur lines, particularly with science or health-related issues. (If any proof is needed of their centrality to advertising, it took exactly four minutes and twenty-two seconds [including opening credits] for the pilot episode of *Mad Men*, the critically acclaimed series about the U.S. advertising industry, to reference "testimonials" and "doctors." Only rather than antibiotics, it was referring to cigarettes.)

Lear went on to describe how his source showed him an advertisement for Pfizer's combined fixed-dose antibiotic. It repeated the slogan, "Every day, everywhere, more and more physicians find Sigmamycin the antibiotic therapy of choice." This advertisement featured reproductions of eight business cards of physicians, all of whom presumably prescribed the drug and vouched for its effectiveness.

> The doctor said he had himself conducted some experiments with Sigmamycin, and at one point he had written to the eight doctors to ask the outcome of their use of the drug in clinical tests. As he told me this, he reached into one of the drawers and brought out eight envelopes, all stamped "Return to Writer—Unclaimed." I asked him if I might report his experience, and he said that he couldn't get involved in any kind of exposé. He pointed out, however, that there was nothing to prevent me from writing to the doctors myself.[8]

When Lear tried to reach the doctors, he did as thorough a job as possible in the late 1950s. He wrote them letters—no luck. He sent telegrams, only to be informed that the addresses didn't exist. He even tried the telephone but met with the same degree of failure. Turned out, those doctors really didn't exist.[9]

It didn't take long for the federal government's tentacles to latch onto the story of the eight doctors who weren't. On May 24, 1959, the Federal Trade Commission (FTC) called out Chas. Pfizer and Company, accusing it of mailing deceptive advertising material to doctors across the country. One of the FTC's complaints was aimed at the pharmaceutical company's April 1957 Sigmamycin campaign and the eight phantasmic physicians. When describing the effects of the pharmaceutical industry's advertising campaigns, one writer asks, "How can legitimate education compete with the philosophy of the opium pipe and the carefully contrived distortions driven home by the trip hammer effect of weekly mailings, the regular visits of the detail man, the two page spreads and the ads which appear six times in the same journal, not to mention the added inducements of the free cocktail party and golf outing complete with three golf balls stamped with the name of the doctor and the company in contrasting colors?"[10]

Pfizer denied any wrongdoing. No surprise there. Its explanation for the advertising campaign depicting doctors' business cards and prescriptions for Sigmamycin was straight out of Art 101. The faked cards were meant "to indicate in a symbolic way the various medical fields in which Sigmamycin might be employed."[11]

Eight months later, the FTC made its recommendation in the case against Pfizer. Edward Creel, an official examiner at the FTC, found that the pharmaceutical company's advertising had been deceptive. Not only that, he declared that the Sigmamycin campaign violated the FTC Act, most likely the government agency's charge to "prevent unfair methods of competition, and unfair or deceptive acts or practices in or affecting commerce."[12] Even after the company's intransigence, Creel recommended that the charges against Pfizer be dismissed. He claimed that Pfizer had voluntarily planned to discontinue the campaign even before the FTC started its investigation and that the company was unlikely to repeat the same ads. How terminating a fraudulent campaign exonerated Pfizer from knowingly conducting a fraudulent and criminal campaign is anybody's guess. But when the case was appealed by the FTC's own staff counsel, Edward Creel shot it down again, citing his previous decision.[13]

As Dominique Tobbell's book *Pills Power, and Policy: The Struggle for Drug Reform in Cold War America and Its Consequences* makes clear, the pharmaceutical industry had long enjoyed the favor of Washington DC politicians and the cover Cold War rhetoric provided them. "The industry drew from and reinforced the pervasive anticommunist political culture of the 1950s and early 1960s. . . . In every political arena, 'conservatives used anticommunism not only to dismiss the prospect of reform but to impugn the motives and loyalties of reformers.'" Yet, by the time Creel made his second judgment, Pfizer had bigger problems. The Sigmamycin campaign was now a central part of a Senate antitrust subcommittee's hearing on drug price collusion.[14] Things were about to get decidedly worse for the industry.

HOW MANY SHIPS AROUND the world could boast about having their own dairy system, mass producing tons of milk, and distributing it in personalized cartons emblazoned with the word "hope"?

Probably just one. How many civilian "mercy" ships carried millions of dollars' worth of medicine and whose sole purpose was to provide relief to people in developing countries? Perhaps not many, maybe only one. How many ships were designed to project American ideals to the world, to serve as a symbol of democracy, and to counter the creeping threat of Communism around the world? Only one. It belonged to a nongovernmental organization.

In 1955 then president Dwight Eisenhower suffered a heart attack; during his lengthy convalescence, he met Dr. William B. Walsh, a cardiologist. At some point, he asked Walsh to submit a proposal for a medical project for the People to People program. Walsh proposed an ambitious plan to create a mobile hospital on a converted navy ship. A consortium pooled its resources to fund the conversion of a navy ship.[15] He called it Project HOPE.

On September 22, 1960, while John F. Kennedy and Richard Nixon sprinted down the stretch toward the November presidential election, the SS *Hope* embarked on its maiden voyage, setting sail from San Francisco. Its destination: Indonesia. During its thirteen years of service, the SS *Hope* completed eleven voyages to Indonesia, Vietnam, Peru, Ecuador, Guinea, Nicaragua, Columbia, Sri Lanka, Tunisia, Jamaica, and Brazil. By the time the old ship was heading to the Philadelphia Naval Yard on February 11, 1975, its legend loomed large, with the *New York Times* calling it "a worldwide symbol of United States aid to underdeveloped nations." It was also one of the pharmaceutical industry's great public relations moments.

(Incidentally, four days after the SS *Hope* first set sail, Kennedy and Nixon squared off in the first televised presidential debate in U.S. history. Nixon had previously been sick. Campaigning also had him overworked. He was notoriously clumsy, and a month and a half earlier he had banged his knee against a car door while getting out. The mishap resulted in an injured knee that took a turn for the worse when the ever-present *Staphylococcus aureus* caused septicemia. Recovering from the illness may have played a role in Nixon's famous, sweaty-browed, and beady-eyed appearance at that debate.)

While Washington did not believe that the Soviet Union posed a serious threat in leaping past the United States in the pharmaceutical field, politicians felt less assured when it came to deploying medical personnel. Many pharmaceutical industry executives shared their apprehension. Merck's president at the time, John T. Connor, warned that in 1958 the Soviet Union had more qualified physicians per capita than the United States. Apparently, he worried about the "Soviets plan to 'export' their medical talent to underdeveloped countries in their effort to 'sell Communism.'" Connor would be very vocal about Merck's role in rolling back the so-called creep of Communism.[16]

The United States had its advantages, though. Considerable ones. When it came to lifesaving drugs, nobody questioned that the country held the upper hand. (Probably not even the Soviets, if they were honest and abandoned their we-discovered-penicillin sense of denial.) According to Tobbell, "Beginning as early as 1957, legislators argued in Congress and before industry audiences that drugs—and by extension the drug industry—were going to be critical weapons in the ongoing war against communism. On June 3, 1957, Sen. Hubert Humphrey (D-MN) proclaimed to a meeting of pharmaceutical advertising executives the value of using pharmaceuticals to free people in underdeveloped countries from both disease and the communist threat. As he noted, 'No amount of diplomacy or armament can bring peace where the bodies and minds of men are sick.'"[17]

Whether Humphrey was paying homage to Gen. Lucius Clay's declaration in occupied Berlin that "there's no choice between being a Communist on 1500 calories a day and a believer of democracy on a thousand" is anyone's guess. Nevertheless, the underlying logic of Humphrey's and Clay's statements rang true. People around the world would not choose between competing ideologies on an intellectual level; they would make their decision from a visceral standpoint. A hungry stomach, a debilitating illness—those were things people understood. They would also inherently grasp the significance of the people responsible for alleviating their hardships.

In the same speech, Humphrey implored the industry to take the lead in international health by providing antibiotics and vaccines to developing countries around the world. He also urged the companies to stand as examples of U.S. free markets. Companies such as Pfizer, Upjohn, and Lederle seized the anti-Communism mantle. They also adopted the future presidential candidate's Cold

War rhetoric, particularly during times when their business model was under threat.[18]

The opportunity medical diplomacy presented was not lost on President Eisenhower. In his 1958 State of the Union address, he proposed that people around the world, including in the Soviet Union, engage in "works of peace" rather than pursuing the destructive path the world seemed doomed to repeat. Under the auspices of this new proposal, Eisenhower leveraged the U.S. health care industry to find common ground with the Soviet Union. He proposed the establishment of a medical research exchange between the United States, the USSR, and other nations. In particular, he stressed that the Americans and Russians should attack epidemic diseases in concert rather than individually. With the full force of the pharmaceutical industry at his disposal, Eisenhower's plan had much to offer—in theory at least. The industry's considerable role in funding Project HOPE was part of that and a reaction to the "threat" of the Soviet Union's medical diplomacy.[19] (The reality of Communist medical diplomacy would be skillfully exploited by Fidel Castro, who expelled Fulgencio Batista's government in 1959, further stoking America's growing sense of Communist encirclement.)

The pharmaceutical industry was more than happy to oblige, particularly since the negative inertia that started with Sigmamycin's questionable advertising had snowballed into a crash waiting to happen. Yet, the upcoming hearings run by Sen. Estes Kefauver (D-TN) were impossible to ignore, and industry executives soon found themselves under the spotlight, defending their questionable practices.

As Tobbell systematically points out, pharmaceutical industry experts framed much of their defense in terms of the Cold War. From the outset of the Kefauver hearings, the unmistakable rhetoric of the struggle against Communism informed discussions. It took implicit and explicit forms, including Communist production versus free market capitalism.

Connor recalled how Merck had competed with the Soviet Union in India over the construction of a corticosteroid manufacturing plant. The New Jersey company's proposal eventually won the contract. Connor described the episode in terms of conflict, saying

Merck had won "an initial skirmish with the Soviet Union in India." And while the U.S. industry may have won the battle and was currently building plants all over the country, Connor warned that the Soviet threat was still pressing for an advantage. In particular, he pointed out the Soviets' ability to co-opt and successfully duplicate Western discoveries, the implication being that by relying on industrial espionage, they were able to save considerable funds in R&D. Not willing to leave anything to interpretation, the Merck president spelled out his industry's role in the Cold War, reminding "the subcommittee that the drugs manufactured by American firms served as both important symbols of American capitalism and necessary vehicles of foreign policy."[20]

Dr. Walsh of Project HOPE also appeared as a witness on behalf of the pharmaceutical industry. He proved an eloquent and effective defender. He testified that monetary donations from the pharmaceutical industry were used to transform the U.S. Navy hospital ship USS *Consolation* into the SS *Hope*, complete with an infant ward, water purification system, and the "iron cow," which blended powdered milk and fats into milk. Without their support, Project HOPE would not be able to "carry American medical knowledge and health care" to the rest of the world. He went on to describe how drug firms had donated a million dollars' worth of drugs each year and how his requests for aid had never been refused.[21]

The common argument about innovation driven by the free market was used as justification as well. Republican senators went so far as to argue that undermining the pharmaceutical industry by granting the Food and Drug Administration increased oversight was a direct attack on the American way. The pharmaceutical industry also fell back on the argument that the risks and expenses taken by the companies justified their freedom to price their products how they chose. They also used the issue to argue against weakening patent laws to help drive down prices.[22]

Nothing symbolized American innovation more than penicillin. (Not surprising, the senators conveniently forgot to mention that the antibiotic was a European discovery.) Vannevar Bush took the stand, cementing the argument that the pharmaceutical industry played a central role in the country's defense. He reminded members of the subcommittee that they lived "in hazardous times," when the chance of war breaking out was as great as any. In the event that it did, "it would be far more terrible than any war in history. This time, in addition to hydrogen bombs, with their burns and radiation, we might also meet a still more appalling weapon in the hands of men with no conscience: biological warfare." He stressed that weakening the medical system by crippling the pharmaceutical industry made no sense.[23]

Pharmaceutical industry witnesses included Nobel laureates and the foremost researchers in their fields. On some aspects of the hearings, their points were heard and carried some weight. Meanwhile, reformers on the opposing side found firmer ground when it came to misleading advertising such as Pfizer's Sigmamycin campaigns and to the need for proper proof of efficacy.[24]

While the Kefauver hearings' purpose, on paper at least, was meant to address monopolistic pricing of antibiotics by drug companies, that turned out to be its least significant aspect. The importance of the event proved to be its exposé about advertising and drug efficacy.

TO A CERTAIN EXTENT, fixed-dose combination antibiotics such as Sigmamycin and Panalba were supposed to be responses to rising resistance. At least, that's how Upjohn presented them to physicians who were eager for a cure.

The fact still remained that the combination drugs consisted of antibiotics that were already on the market and already vulnerable to resistant bacteria should the two cross paths. Some studies, in particular those sponsored by the producing pharmaceutical firm, suggested combination antibiotics retarded the development of resistance when they interacted with bacteria. However, when confronted with bacteria resistant to either drug of the combination, research indicated that resistance developed at a faster rate. It suggested that at best, fixed-dose combination drugs could be used during very limited circumstances.

With the limitations of combination antibiotics on full display, pharmaceutical companies still sold them and promised the stars. Unsuspecting consumers bought every word. Somehow, the Kefauver hearings' impact was limited, and companies continued selling and marketing their products. There wasn't a clear medical advantage to many of the new combinations, though there were clear business rewards. They allowed companies to offset losses or low profit margins that accompanied the production of antibiotics in the public domain. Most companies, though, developed different antibiotics or at least tried.

The scientific community's understanding of beta-lactams, their chemistry, and their mechanism of action on bacteria was still in its early stages at this point. In the mid-1950s, Joshua Lederberg did a series of experiments that led to important observations about the action of penicillin. He showed that *E. coli*, the gram-negative rod-shaped bacterium, changed into a ball shape when placed in a hypertonic solution. The altered bacteria, which Lederberg called spheroplasts, had fragile membranes and barely any cell wall, so they burst as a result of the pressure. This led him to deduce that penicillin interfered with the synthesis of the bacterial cell wall.[25]

Advances in the knowledge about the molecular structure of bacterial cell walls in bacteria shed further light on how penicillin attacked bacteria. Eventually, scientists were able to discern that the inhibition of cross-linking peptide chains in the cell wall by beta-lactam antibiotics lead to the death and lysis of the bacteria. Since peptidoglycan synthesis does not occur in human or animal cells, the beta-lactam does not interact with host cells during an infection.[26]

Since World War II, scientists tried and failed to synthesize penicillin from scratch. Their chemistry shortcomings also hindered the development of new antibiotics until scientists in Japan discovered that the nucleus of the penicillin molecule could be produced from *Penicillium chrysogenum* without adding the antibiotic's characteristic side chain. Then the isolation of 6-aminopenicillanic acid (6-APA) in 1957 changed everything. It was like baking a Betty Crocker cake. Buy the mix. Blend and bake the ingredients. The resulting cake—naked and anonymous—was 6-APA. Adding distinct side chains to the molecule was similar to decorating the cake with icing, sprinkles, crushed cookies. The 6-APA discovery, made in England at the pharmaceutical company Beecham, opened the floodgates to antibiotics that could genuinely be called new.[27]

Using 6-APA as a starting block, scientists at Beecham added different variations of side chains onto the molecule. Icing on the cake. After a spell, they discovered an addition, ortho-dimethoxyphenyl group, to the penicillin nucleus. The addition halted beta-lactamase by physically preventing it from attaching to the molecule, therefore rendering it impotent. In other words, it destroyed penicillin-resistant *S. aureus* by the bucket. In 1959 the first semisynthetic penicillin to be introduced clinically was called methicillin.[28]

Soon methicillin, another semisynthetic antibiotic, emerged from Beecham's laboratories. This time it contained an amino group that benzylpenicillin (penicillin G) lacked. It was called ampicillin, and it further spread the beta-lactam's spectrum of activity to include gram-negative bacteria such as *Neisseria meningitidis* and some *Enterobacteriaceae*. It wasn't effective against antibiotic-resistant *Staphylococcus aureus*, however.[29]

At about the same time, another novel antibiotic inched into existence, thanks to a process very similar to the new penicillins. The antibiotic class would come to be known as cephalosporins.

Cephalosporins took longer to develop than most of the contemporary antibiotics. It was first discovered in 1943 by Giuseppe Brotzu, an Italian hygienist at the University of Cagliari. While engaged in a study of typhoid infection, he spent time collecting samples from the sewers running under Cagliari. He found that salmonella was not present in the sewage that flowed into the sea. Rather than stopping there, he broadened his line of inquiry to include the reason why. After numerous attempts to culture salmonella in the lab from his samples, he noticed *taches vierges*, or "virgin patches," which were haloes of inhibition. After cultivating the fungus *Cephalosporium acremonium*, he isolated its active compound and tested it on patients with typhoid fever. He was encouraged by the results. In echoes of Howard Florey's penicillin struggles, Brotzu failed to find funding for his research in Italy. He gave up, disheartened by the mounting rejections, and ended up sending his antibiotic fungus to Florey's lab at the Dunn School.[30]

E. P. Abraham took over the research on *Cephalosporium acremonium*. For years he twisted, tickled, and teased it. Whatever chemical that came out of it only had weak antimicrobial activity; however, he discovered that the fungus produced a second antibiotic in small amounts. The molecule's structure was similar to penicillin's, but the beta-lactam ring was fused to a six-membered ring instead of a five-membered ring. It came to be known as cephalosporin C and was much more potent than whatever Brotzu had found.[31]

As with synthetic penicillin, Abraham learned that a cephalosporin without a side chain could be produced, allowing various new side chains to be attached. It was called 7-aminocephalosporanic acid (7-ACA) and, similar to 6-APA, proved a versatile building block for semisynthetic cephalosporins. Eli Lilly discovered more efficient ways of obtaining 7-ACA than the Oxford lab's, and its methods would become the standard. In 1961 Glaxo laboratories in Britain sold the first clinical cephalosporin, cephaloridine. Three years later, Lilly released its version, cephalothin, in the United States. Both drugs were effective against resistant *S. aureus* and are considered first-generation cephalosporins.[32]

Around this time, a new antibiotic class was discovered called ansamycins. Rifamycin, the primary drug belonging to this group, was discovered by Piero Sensi, Maria Teresa Timbal, and Pinhas Margalith while working at Gruppo Lepetit SPA in Milan, Italy. It proved a significant improvement to streptomycin and offered additional hope for tuberculosis patients because it did not foster the swift appearance of resistance the way Waksman's antibiotic did. Rifamycin would become the first line of defense in treating the disease.[33]

Vancomycin was the first antibiotic to be fast-tracked as a response to increases in antibiotic resistance. When it came out, its slight toxicity made doctors choose the new penicillins, which also appeared at the same time. They considered the latter as safer for their patients. This resulted in a lack of resistance developing against vancomycin at that time.[34]

ON JUNE 2, 1957, in the Kremlin Nikita Khrushchev took questions through an interpreter on the long-running CBS political news show *Face the Nation*. Opposite him American journalists readied unrehearsed questions that would run the gamut from war to economic planning. Stuart Novins was the moderator. Alongside him sat the *New York Herald Tribune*'s B. J. Cutler and CBS reporter Daniel Schorr.

The first question dealt with agriculture.

Schorr asked, "To open with a subject that is close to your heart, agriculture. You recently stated that the Soviet Union expects in the next few years to catch up with the United States in the production of milk, butter, and meat. American experts say this is an unrealistic target especially with regard to livestock, an increase of three times in livestock. How do you plan to do it?"

Khrushchev replied by first referencing Lenin and the working classes, and how they called upon the peasants to transform a backward agricultural sector. True to Communist form, he cited the economic improvements made by the proletarian peasantry since the October Revolution. He stressed that the Soviet Union faced the task of catching up with the advanced capitalist countries in terms of production per capita. It entailed matching production in milk and meat. As far as milk and butter were concerned, he claimed his country would catch up with the United States as far as production per capita in the next year, 1958. Meat production was more difficult. By 1960 or 1961, he insisted, they would be caught up. He was confident Soviet farmers and agronomists would solve the task.

"I've heard experts say that no nation in the world has ever been able to increase its meat supply three and a half times in four years. Do you communists have some way of seeing that every cow gets twins?" asked Cutler.

Pigs would make up a big difference, Khrushchev insisted. Production of pork was set to increase, and the possibilities were tremendous. He believed poultry production would be great as well. The country would rely on these alternative meats to bolster its livestock.

He continued,

> As far as the production of cow meat, I believe that in this five-year period we will still be behind. And at the present time, . . . our hope is for the greater production of bacon. We know the British, for instance, like the bacon very much. And we don't see why the Ukrainians or the Russians should not like bacon too. . . . Up to now, our cattle has been killed at the age of one year usually. Now we want to decrease the number of cattle killed and then increase the number of cattle killed when they . . . are two years old.[35]

Of course, food security was the topic, but it wasn't the issue. Beneath the talk of raising standards of living was its implied counterpart of food shortages coupled with a growing demand due to urbanization threatened social unrest. Wary Soviet leaders had learned their lesson from the crises in East Berlin (1953), Poland (1956), and Hungary (1956). Deteriorating living standards drove people out to the streets, an action that the Soviet army suppressed by force.[36] Khrushchev did not want any more incidents.

By the end of the questions about Khrushchev's agricultural strategy, two facts crystallized on screen. First, the soft-spoken, smiling, shoe-wearing Soviet leader intended to grab his country by the scruff and supplant the United States' position in the world. He saw Soviet glory in the promised land and liked what he saw. Second, for all the quiet bombast and exaltations of the Soviet peasant, Nikita Khrushchev, the man who came out on top when all of his peers jostled for Stalin's vacant crown, hadn't the slightest clue how to achieve his goals. He'd need to rely on the giants of Soviet agriculture. He'd turn to Lysenko.

Early during Khrushchev's tenure, it appeared as if the first secretary's rise to power had dealt a mortal blow to Trofim Lysenko's influence. Raissa Berg, a witness to Lysenko's reign, offered an alternate explanation for their initial mutual wariness: "The clash between Khrushchev and Lysenko started long before Stalin's death and thus before Khrushchev came to power. Thanks to Khrushchev the vernalization affair was abandoned, and the winter-varieties of wheat were returned to the fields. During his first years in power Khrushchev was skeptical about Lysenko's practical recommendations and most of them were not used. Khrushchev himself appears to be the architect of his agriculture policy and his grandiose projects have nothing to do with Lysenkoites."[37]

As mentioned briefly earlier, central to Khrushchev's plans for boosting the Soviet Union's meat production lay the humble cob of corn. He viewed it as the fuel for his livestock trains. While corn was edible as a staple crop, Khrushchev acknowledged that his people lacked experience with the vegetable, and its adoption would take time. However, as a source for animal feed, there were few, if any, hurdles to its adoption. Cattle and swine the world over gorged on corn feed, and they grew large and fat. What's more, it seems Khrushchev may have overestimated corn's durability. While it was much more versatile than wheat, as the first settlers to the Americas discovered, corn was still an ill fit for most of the Soviet Union's climate and virgin lands.

The Soviet leader undoubtedly saw the abundance, first from afar and eventually in person, and wanted it for his country. The peasants might not have loved collectivization, but this must have seemed as close to a sure thing as possible. As Berg put it, "Corn became the engine and symbol of industrial agriculture owing to a self reinforcing process: engineers and agronomists found the crop responsive to industrial technologies and therefore concentrated their efforts on it."[38]

The future lay in the industrialized, intensified, and unhealthily cramped farms spreading among Western nations. They had meat. They had milk. They had butter. Their technology and techniques held the key.

According to Berg, Lysenko's uselessness when dealing with hybridized corn caused the initial rift with the premier. It was no wonder the agronomist struggled to make a difference since he and his disciples had spent the past twenty years denouncing hybridization. In their view, the success of inbreeding corn was nothing but capitalist propaganda disseminated for the capitalists' own gains at the expense of unsophisticated Soviet peasants. As early as 1935, Lysenko had denounced hybrid corn at a Lenin All-Union Academy of Agricultural Science meeting in Odessa.[39]

At the infamous 1948 meeting of the LAAAS, one of Lysenko's henchmen lambasted hybrid corn and assured the Soviet public that it was the result of a Weismannist-Mendelist sham. "The Morganists proposed some complicated technical methods to produce hybrid corn (preliminary self-fertilization and selection of inbred lines), which make it difficult for large-scale use. This apparently serves the interests of the capitalist seed firms, since the methods proposed by the Morganists are inaccessible to ordinary farmers."[40]

Unfortunately, no amount of technology could have compensated for the unmitigated inanity of the so-called virgin lands initiative of 1954 in which Khrushchev declared that previously unused land in Central Asia's Great Steppe would be utilized to expand Soviet grain production. The campaign peaked in 1956 when a record harvest seemed to vindicate Khrushchev. Unfortunately, the soil never recovered because of the single-crop cultivation and the failure to follow anti-erosion techniques. By 1960 the soil was destroyed and literally blowing away. Lysenko could not have done anything to avoid the disaster, though his lack of grounding in agricultural reality certainly could have made things worse.[41]

Lysenko may have been a serial hack when it came to science, but he was an astute politician. He took every opportunity to support his patron's agricultural proposals and maintain his position atop Soviet biology, even if it meant contradicting years' worth of declarations. The Soviet premier, however, had no qualms about discarding any advice from Lysenko that did not fit his plans. Nothing exemplified this more than hybrid corn.

In 1955 Khrushchev single-handedly undercut Lysenkoism when he oversaw the purchase of hybrid corn from Garst & Thomas Hi-Bred Corn Company in the United States. Given that increasing the Soviet Union's meat production was an important part of his domestic plan, he envisioned the livestock industry's growth being driven by corn feed consumption, much as it was in the United States. Therefore, a robust and reliable harvest was at the heart of Khrushchev's plans, and he very much tied his leadership to it. So it was telling that when it came time to act, the Soviet Union purchased tons of corn starter seed from one of the top U.S. producers (using Morganist theory and techniques) of genetically modified hybrid corn. Twenty years of denunciation based on Michurinist science by Lysenko, Prezent, Mikhail Olshansky, and others were rendered moot.[42]

Even though Lysenko and his followers had denounced hybrid corn, assuring the public that it was a Western swindle, Khrushchev publicly and politically continued to support and even promote Lysenko and his expertise in general. He also did not have any problem in having Roswell Garst visit the Soviet Union on numerous occasions to lecture on hybrid corn and assist farmers in implementing the associated techniques. Khrushchev even went so far as to insist on including Garst's farm in his 1959 barnstorming trip through the United States.[43]

Khrushchev continued to borrow from U.S. agricultural practices when it came to livestock. The same year the Soviet Union embraced genetically modified corn, it proudly displayed the use of antibiotics in agriculture, both to treat infections and as growth promoters, at Moscow's Soviet Agricultural Exhibition. According to Claas Kirchhelle, "From the late 1950s onwards, countries throughout the Soviet bloc began constructing factories for antibiotic/B12 supplements. Planners' shift toward AGPs [antibiotic growth promoters] coincided with a new emphasis on increasing living standards and meat consumption as well as freeing agricultural labor via industrialized food production."[44]

During the late 1950s, Eastern bloc countries committed to using AGPs in agriculture. Bulgaria constructed an antibiotic plant in Peshtera dedicated to agricultural use. The product was called Biovit-60 and consisted of biomycin, which was a form of oxytetracycline. Similar plants were constructed in Romania and Czechoslovakia. In East Germany, antibiotics became available for agricultural use from 1959 onward.[45]

MEAT MEANS SOMETHING. IN fact, it means a lot. While the space race undoubtedly symbolized technological superiority, the meat race was no less significant and equally reflected technological prowess. In fact, one can easily argue that it was more significant than putting a man on the moon. People can't eat spaceships or digest lunar soil.

The United States had a long history of using meat and its associated symbology as proof of U.S. exceptionalism. The abundance of meat was associated with the westward expansion of the 1800s and the taming of the frontier, which coincided with the rise of the cowboy. President Herbert Hoover was undoubtedly referencing this tradition when his campaign promised Americans "a chicken in every pot," a tactic that ultimately backfired and that Franklin Roosevelt exploited on the way to his landslide victory.

Pharmaceutical companies played an important role in bolstering the country's claim to carnivorous prosperity. Lederle soon found itself competing with other firms hoping to capitalize on the new and prosperous market agricultural antibiotic use provided. More than any other company, Pfizer posed the biggest and most sustained challenge to Lederle. Ultimately, Pfizer would rise to the top of the antibiotic market, largely thanks to its agricultural division's expanding the use of Terramycin to include a sow's milk replacement called Terralac. But it did not stop there. Pfizer's catalog exploded with antibiotic-based products. Medical brands included Cosa-Terramycin, Cosa-Tetracyn, Cosa-Sigmamycin, Penicillin, Maxipen, Tao, Tao-AC, Taomid, streptomycin, dihydrostreptomycin, polymyxin B sulfate, Urobiotic, bacitracin, neobiotic, Viocin, and Candettes antibiotic troches.[46]

Meanwhile, it had even more agricultural offerings: Terramycin A/D Fortified Crumbles, Terramycin Egg Formula, Terramycin Animal Formula (soluble powder), Terramycin Animal Formula for mastitis, Terramycin A/D Scours Tablets, Terramycin Poultry Formula with Anti-Germ 77, stimplants, Terramycin Liquid Concentrate, Terramycin Turkey Formula, Terramycin feed supplements, penicillin feed supplements, Strepdust, Vigofac, Liquamast, Liquamycin, Penicillin G Procaine, Mastalone, Tetracycline-Vet, Terramycin, Combiotic, Combistrep, and Sterane.[47]

It seemed as if the development of "new" antibiotic products was limited only by pharmaceutical executives' imaginations and their marketing departments. From the moment Merck's sulfaquinoxaline gained approval for use in animal feeds to combat coccidiosis in 1948, the therapeutic use of antimicrobials proliferated in the entire food supply line and not just as growth promoters. They were used as prophylaxis in fish farms and to prevent mastitis in dairy cows. By the mid-1950s, they even moved out of the livestock arena and out to the perfectly linear farming rows teeming with crops. Employees sprayed solutions made of streptomycin on crops to prevent common bacterial infections such as American fire blight.[48]

Across the globe, the agricultural use of antibiotics continued to grow. Common antibiotics were accessible once rationing ended, and they became available without prescription in countries such as West Germany (1951), Great Britain (1953), the Netherlands (1954), and France (1955). Each country relied on different drugs.

The Netherlands used tetracycline; the United Kingdom, tylosin. France employed a multitude of antibiotics such as erythromycin, oleandomycin, spiramycin, neomycin, and framycetin. West Germany used bacitracin, oleandomycin, taomycin, and flavomycin. The adoption of AGP technology and how deeply it penetrated European agriculture differed, however. Very often, it depended on the degree to which a country took up the Americans' use of intensive confined housing systems. In 1958 nearly 50 percent of British pigs were fed antibiotics. By 1966 80 percent of feeds in West Germany contained antibiotics.[49]

The AGP trend spread to Asia as well. Japan had become largely self-sufficient in making antibiotics by 1950 and began licensing growth promoters three years later. The island nation engaged in intensive farming, and its farmers embraced antibiotics and made extensive use of them. They used a streptogramin compound called blasticidin S, which they isolated locally on crops to fight rice blast disease. By 1974 annual antibiotic usage hovered around fourteen thousand tons.[50]

The possible ways to include antibiotics in the food supply line ballooned. In Northern European countries, the whaling industry relied heavily on the drugs as an on-location meat preservative. Prior to that, bacterial spoilage and long processing times caused the loss of money. After killing their targets, whalers filled their catch with oxygen to prevent the animals from sinking, but this sped up the autolytic process. To combat it, whalers incorporated tetracycline into their exploding spears or injected the preservative into the corpses. It worked. By 1953 Norwegian sailors had adopted Pfizer's Biostat (oxytetracycline) as their medicine of choice.[51]

Pharmaceutical companies saw yet another opportunity to repackage their antibiotics into "new" products. For Lederle, this meant rebranding Aureomycin as Acronize, a drug that preserves the integrity of butchered meat by washing it with antibiotics. The term "acronize" suggested cleanliness, modernity, and safety. Unfortunately, sometimes it made matters worse. Meanwhile, other companies joined in the market of food preservation.[52]

Dissenting voices began to express concern. In 1961 Antonio Santos Ocampo Jr. from Araneta University in the Philippines questioned the rapid increase of antibiotic use in the country. He went out of his way to point the finger at the "Pfizer people" hawking Terramycin Egg Formula and other combination products.[53]

BY 1960 THE ANTIBIOTIC resistance problem showed no signs of abating. It just continued to accelerate. Tuberculosis remained a challenge due in no small part to streptomycin's tendency to foster almost immediate resistance. Treating STDs such as gonorrhea involved using up to forty times as much penicillin to clear an infection. Gram-negative bacteria, never a serious problem before, joined nosocomial staphylococcal infections as hidden threats in hospital wards around the world. Still worse, the insidious staphylococci bacteria made the leap from health care settings to neighborhood playgrounds. Community-acquired *Staphylococcus aureus* illnesses introduced epidemiologists and public health officials to a whole new reality, and it was not a comforting one.[54]

Pharmaceutical companies continued producing antibiotics. They all basically relied on the same strategies that penicillin and chlortetracycline employed, wiping out really large swaths of bacteria. Their efforts amounted to sticking Band-Aids on Band-Aids. What they needed was a new paradigm, such as the bacteriophages that were always under their noses. Clinicians used them in typing bacteria; virologists studied them like fruit flies. Even phage therapy, long since abandoned in most of the West, was still being used in Eastern Europe, the Soviet Union, and France. But during the Cold War, adopting phage therapy, which was branded "Communist" and "foreign," did not get any attention, much less funding. Anyone suggesting the use of Communist cures was looked upon with suspicion. In retrospect, it was a lost opportunity to at least diversify doctors' arsenals against bacteria.[55]

If there was a glimmer of hope, it came from John Sheehan at the Massachusetts Institute of Technology and Beecham Research Laboratories in Britain in 1959. Sheehan discovered a way to produce the nucleus of the penicillin molecule 6-APA without the side chain that made the molecule functionally penicillin. Freed from the constraints of having to completely rely on organisms to provide the finished antibiotic, scientists then added side chains to 6-APA, each time creating a new molecule. Of the resulting class of semisynthetic penicillins, methicillin—the most significant of the early batch—came from Beecham.[56]

Methicillin synthesis involved attaching an ortho-dimethoxyphenyl group to 6-APA. The presence of the new side chain allowed the beta-lactam core to continue to function even in the presence of beta-lactamase-producing bacteria, most notably penicillin-resistant *Staphylococcus aureus*. The process was called side-chain steric hindrance, and it allowed methicillin to display the same effectiveness penicillin had when it was first used clinically.[57]

The introduction of the new semisynthetic penicillin resulted in a drastic reduction in hospital- and community-acquired staphylococcal infections. In particular, the phage type 80/81 *S. aureus* that had victimized newborns and their families for the entire decade all but disappeared.[58] It was a victory and cause for optimism that would become rarer as time went on.

14

Spectral figures combed the Haitian countryside. They were known as the Tonton Macoute, the bogeymen of Haitian folklore who kidnapped, beat, and devoured disobedient children. But these men were real, dressed in their country denim shirts and straw hats, clutching rifles and handguns. They were searching for their former leader, Clément Barbot. The country's president François "Papa Doc" Duvalier ordered his execution. When "voices" informed Duvalier that Barbot had transformed himself into a black dog, he ordered every black dog in the country slaughtered. Had Papa Doc's bloodletting been limited to four-legged canines scavenging the corners of Port-au-Prince, it would probably have gone down as one of those curious incidents in world history.[1]

Graham Greene, who spent much time in Haiti during the dictator's reign, famously portrayed Duvalier's Haiti in *The Comedians*. The author was not far off the mark when he described the leader in his introduction to the novel. "Poor Haiti and the character of Doctor Duvalier's rule are not invented, the latter not even blackened for dramatic effect. Impossible to deepen that night."[2]

Papa Doc governed with impunity. He belonged to the growing list of despots—Mohammad Reza Pahlavi, Ferdinand Marcos, Ngo Dinh Diem, Rafael Trujillo—supported by U.S. coffers for the simple, some say strategic, reason that they proclaimed to be ardent anti-Communists. Beneficiaries of the Cold War.

During the massacre that resulted from the search for Barbot, the international community and his Caribbean neighbors could only watch. When an investigative committee of the Organization of American States descended on Haiti, Duvalier had truckloads of countryside peasants brought to the city, where they paraded their support for Papa Doc. The charade was designed to impress the visiting dignitaries and at the same time mock them. When he spoke, Duvalier did so in Creole and cursed the clueless committee members to their faces.[3]

When Haiti's historic neighbor and tormentor, the United States, expressed its displeasure with Duvalier's strong-arm tactics against his countrymen, the despot reacted the only way he seemed to know how—with defiance. He imposed martial law and a crushing nightly curfew. "The Tonton Macoutes searched everywhere," an American reported after leaving the country. "Everywhere you see people with their arms in the air, being patted under the shoulders as police frisk them for guns."[4]

The haplessness of their efforts culminated in the media circus that arose when rumors about Duvalier's resignation began to percolate among the international media. Papa Doc's position had become untenable. The Haitian consulate in New York even booked escape flights for the Duvalier family. They seemed destined for the streets of Paris. As it turned out, the Duvaliers weren't going anywhere, not for a long time. The prediction was one generation off, as it was François Duvalier's son and successor, Jean-Claude (Baby Doc), who would end up seeking refuge in the French capital.[5]

On November 22, 1963, as his presidential motorcade snaked through Dallas, bullets cut down U.S. president John F. Kennedy. While much of the world mourned, or at least kept quiet, Papa Doc gloated. Duvalier famously proclaimed that he had killed President Kennedy by placing a voodoo curse on him. He went so far as to order an assistant to go to Kennedy's grave and capture air from the gravesite in an attempt to capture his *loa*, an amorphous entity akin to a person's spirit.[6]

Some say Duvalier's presidency was a product of the Cold War, but he rose to power very much on the perceived magic of penicillin's antibacterial powers.

Since gaining its freedom from France in1804 after the only successful slave revolution in history, Haiti had been plagued by poverty and disease. The tropical climate and overwhelming poverty made it an incubator for disease. By the twentieth century, three main culprits plagued the country: malaria, hookworm, and yaws.

Of these, yaws was the most common, most virulent, and most crippling if left untreated, which it usually was. Health care workers estimated that 80 percent of the rural population was infected. The only other country in the Americas with a comparable infection rate was Brazil.[7]

Yaws is caused by the corkscrewed microorganism *Treponema pertenue*. It belongs to the same family of conditions as syphilis, which is caused by *Treponema pallidum*. Unlike syphilis, which is mostly transmitted through sexual contact, yaws is spread by simple skin-to-skin contact. Children in Haiti tended to be prone to contracting the disease and were considered the main reservoirs. They then carried it for the rest of their lives.[8]

Yaws infection follows a similar course to syphilis infection. Victims are easy to spot. Pustules and open sores riddle their skin. Their noses and lips seem to shrivel and fall. In the same way that syphilis merged with leprosy in the public's perception during the early Enlightenment, the general Haitian populace scorned people suffering from yaws, confusing them with lepers. Families rejected them, and towns ostracized them. In the cities, yaws came to signify the afflicted and unclean peasant. It reinforced ingrained notions about the urban-rural divide.

Like syphilis, yaws is susceptible to penicillin. One shot does the trick.

As a country doctor and *noirist* (supporter of black liberation) intellectual, Duvalier understood the physical, emotional, and social destruction yaws inflicted. It did not debilitate. It destroyed. It reduced the productivity of its victims, in this case making the poor poorer still. Its social stigmatization would be echoed decades later when the human immunodeficiency virus ravaged the country, afflicting men and women in their primes.

In 1943 the U.S. Inter-American Affairs Commission turned its attention to combating yaws around the world. It sent Dr. James Dwindle to Haiti to spearhead a countrywide effort to eradicate the disease. He enlisted local doctors and equipped them with the weapon of choice in that particular war. That was when Papa Doc Duvalier first encountered the almost-magical powers of penicillin.[9]

Dwindle interviewed Duvalier. The Haitian doctor's ability to speak English, French, and Creole certainly played a role in Dwindle's hiring him. He assigned Papa Doc to direct the Rural Clinic of Gressier, located fifteen miles outside the capital; it boasted one of the highest rates of yaws infection in the country. Equipped with penicillin, Duvalier tended to shunned, destitute peasants. He injected them and, for the most part, cured them. People came from all over the region, descending from the Montagnes Noires (Black Mountains), crossing the Artibonite Valley, and risking bandits and criminals on dirt roads at night, in the hope of salvation from the spirochete-induced malady. Spurred by the program's success, the Inter-American Affairs Commission decided to expand the program and establish mobile clinics all over Haiti. To facilitate the process, it sent a group of doctors, including Duvalier, to study and train for two semesters at the University of Michigan. A language barrier and a fair dose of racism, which Papa Doc carried with him for the rest of his life, limited their success.[10]

The experience of eradicating yaws from Haiti transformed Duvalier, at least temporarily. Penicillin captured his imagination. He set aside ethnology for clinical field research. The true success of Duvalier's participation in the yaws program took years to play out. It emerged as he sculpted his public image while ascending the ranks of Haitian politics. The humble country doctor's stature grew. He became a great Haitian physician. A point of pride. As his reputation grew, Duvalier made the transition to politics.[11]

The success of the program, which would not have been possible without penicillin, and Duvalier's position as a doctor created a major portion of his myth. Duvalier, the entomologist, understood his people, their beliefs, and the combination of symbols that would make him king. There is a common saying among Haitians: "Haiti is 70 percent Catholic, 30 percent Protestant, and 100 percent voodoo." Duvalier exploited this. He dressed in black suits and wore dark glasses and a top hat, mirroring the deity Baron Samedi, the skeletal guardian of the realm of the dead. He reminded people how peasants had come from all over Haiti so he could cure them. Duvalier was Jesus Christ. Finally, he was also Papa Doc, a nickname bestowed on him during his time as a country doctor while wielding a symbol of modernity—penicillin.

On September 22, 1957, Francois Duvalier won the presidential election in Haiti. He embraced the rough tactics of prior presidents and then infused them with his own blend of noirist values and voodoo traditions. He also strengthened Haiti's bonds with the African continent. He hosted Ethiopia's emperor Haile Selassie I, bestowing on him the Necklace of the Order of Jean-Jacques Dessalines the Great. He also sent Haitian professionals to work in Côte d'Ivoire and the Republic of the Congo.

Ultimately, Duvalier also located Clément Barbot. Harris Lentz III summed up the manhunt best: "Barbot was finally captured and executed, still bipedal, in July 1963."[12]

BACTERIAL DYSENTERY BADGERED JAPAN'S population. On top of atomic scars and a pacifist constitution, it lingered as a reminder of the country's misguided war. Sanitation efforts were well under way toward making Japan one of the cleanest countries in the world, and the housing situation had returned to prewar normalcy. Yet no matter how much they tried to control it, the disease caused by the *Shigella* bacterium refused to yield. Year after year, case upon case, an unrelenting stream of patients filled hospitals and doctors' offices. Its persistence baffled scientists and public health officials.

Researchers tackled the dysentery mystery on a countrywide scale. They pieced together their findings and analyzed the data for any hint. The strain of *Shigella* circulating among the Japanese population had been transformed by an influx of medicine that had accompanied the U.S. occupation. Doctors used a variety of sulfonamides to treat the cases of dysentery. When one stopped working due to resistance, doctors moved on to the next sulfonamide. The strategy worked for a few years. But then it didn't, and the Japanese were left with strains of *Shigella* that were highly resistant to sulfonamides.[13] Kryptonite had turned to coal. Again. In 1949 the incidence of dysentery stopped falling and began rising. Peak incidence occurred in 1952.[14]

Health care professionals in Japan turned to the newer antibiotics to treat the sulfonamide-resistant *Shigella*. They attacked the bacteria with a cocktail of the newest antibiotics: streptomycin, chloramphenicol, and tetracycline. This way bacteria that showed resistance to one or two antibiotics were always attacked by a third. Sulfa drugs were resurrected as still one more weapon. For a while, they enjoyed a degree of success with the hit-it-with-everything approach. Then in 1955, the worst thing imaginable happened.[15]

A Japanese woman came down with a case of dysentery that defied treatment. She had recently returned from Hong Kong. One by one, clinicians ran susceptibility tests on the sample taken from the woman. The *Shigella* that scientists in Japan isolated from the woman was a typical dysentery bacteria; however, unlike others in the past, this particular strain was resistant to four drugs: sulfanilamide, streptomycin, chloramphenicol, and tetracycline. In the years that followed, incidences of this multidrug-resistant *Shigella* increased to epidemic proportions.[16]

Japanese researchers determined that many of the patients who suffered from the multidrug-resistant form of *Shigella* also carried *E. coli*, which shared the same susceptibility profile. They were able to determine that *E. coli* had been responsible for transferring its resistance to *Shigella*. It did so by way of an extra-chromosomal snippet of DNA, or plasmid, that bacteria were able to pass on to other bacteria.[17] (It stands to reason that antibiotic-resistant *E. coli* would emerge in the gut since many antibiotics were administered orally. If the gut is ground zero, where antibiotics and stomach flora meet, the bacteria will try to survive.)

Multidrug-resistant *Shigella* was a harbinger of things to come. The existence of plasmids revolutionized the way scientists viewed antibiotic resistance. Safe to say, it scared them because of the way bacteria could swap and integrate the bits of DNA regardless of whether they belonged to different species. Plasmids also went a long way toward explaining what Soviet scientists had seen when they reported that bacteria "acquired" resistance. What they were witnessing, at least in part, was the transfer of actual DNA, which thus conferred new genetic traits to bacteria.

The staphylococcal problem also continued to fester in hospital wards. The methicillin miracle proved short lived. By 1962, three years after the discovery of the semisynthetic penicillin, the first strains of methicillin-resistant *Staphylococcus aureus* appeared. The bacteria was proving a much nimbler and more adaptable foe than scientists initially thought. A *Scientific American* article about staphylococcal infections cites "attendant difficulties and inadequacies" of antibiotics. The talk about miracle drugs had dissipated like mist on a windy day. The discourse shifted as the days of easy cures were under threat. Even politicians got into the act, with Congress allocating to the National Institutes of Health $1 million for *Staphylococcus aureus* research.[18]

Picking up where they left off with semisynthetic penicillins, drug developers continued shifting their strategies from curing new diseases to reclaiming the real estate lost to resistant bacteria. The revolutionary days in antimicrobial chemotherapy were drawing to a close, giving way to a conservative reactionary approach. The broader the antibiotic coverage the better. It didn't hurt that broad-spectrum antibiotics provided pharmaceutical companies with a degree of cover, allowing them to give the impression that they were still staking new therapeutic ground. By nature, using the buckshot, sawed-off shotgun approach meant that drug developers had a chance of offering something new by killing some previously untreatable bacteria. Still, they continued to rely on a technology and an approach that were quickly becoming obsolete. Closing your eyes, aiming in a general direction, and shooting went only so far.[19]

In fairness, the corporate researchers had little opportunity of breaking out of their proverbial box. They were restrained by the biotechnological tools available at that time and the corporate structure of the companies for which they worked. While pharmaceutical firms bore the responsibility for developing new drugs, their financial structures obligated them to generate returns for their shareholders. With development and testing becoming more expensive and antibiotic prices continuing to fall, it made little sense to take a gamble on a completely novel antibiotic when older approaches still gave results.

For years to come, pharmaceutical companies would engage in a game of whack-a-mole, where they created new and improved versions of the same antibiotic class. The drugs would work for a little while, only for resistance to arise in a couple of years. Scientists would then produce another variant of the same class. Semisynthetic penicillins were the one example, with methicillin being replaced by drugs such as ampicillin and amoxicillin. They were also able to accomplish similar feats with cephalosporins, a feat made possible with the discovery of 7-ACA, a precursor molecule similar to 6-APA with semisynthetic penicillins.[20]

Amid the iterative approach to drug discovery, some new classes of antibiotics were developed, with quinolones being one example. The first member of the group, nalidixic acid, was discovered while attempting to synthesize chloroquine (the malaria drug). It was primarily prescribed for treating urinary tract infections, which had grown harder to address due to resistance. Quinolones' exceptionally broad spectrum made them the third-most prescribed antibiotic for outpatient purposes. To combat resistance to this class, the FDA attempted to curtail its use. Like the cephalosporins, quinolones underwent numerous generations of manipulation by adding different active side chains, most notably ciprofloxacin, a fluoroquinolone.[21]

IN JUNE 1961, PEOPLE in an Indonesian seaside community near Kendal began falling ill with a stomach illness. In the months that followed, it spread to Bandung, on to Kalimantan, and then to East Java in November. When public health officials took stock in February 1962, 4,107 cases had been reported with 897 deaths (21.8 percent fatalities). The culprit? A strain of *Vibrio cholerae* named El Tor. The strain was known to be endemic on the island of Sulawesi and responsible for seasonal outbreaks; however, this time it was different. This time, the bacteria refused to stay put, and thanks to travelers, it transitioned from a local outbreak into an international epidemic.[22]

Epidemiologists worked frantically to piece together its path outside Indonesia. The data suggested that in June and July 1961, the bacteria was brought to Kwantung in China. News broadcasts reported 234 patients coming down with cholera infections. From there, the epidemiologists believed that travelers in August introduced the bacteria into the Hong Kong area, where 13 cases and 6 deaths took place. Macau reported a similar outbreak. The following month, doctors at San Lazaro Hospital diagnosed the first El Tor cholera patient in Manila.[23] The disease swept south from there all the way to Jolo Island south of Mindanao. In five months, 15,000

Filipinos fell ill, and 2,005 died. Other Southeast Asian countries also reported outbreaks during this time.[24]

The emergence of the El Tor epidemic in Indonesia initiated what would come to be known as the seventh cholera pandemic.[25] It continued to spread north to Japan and by 1963 had expanded westward through Bangladesh, India, and Pakistan, displacing the traditional *V. cholerae* responsible for historic outbreaks in South Asia.[26] El Tor's efficiency is believed to have even driven the classical biotype of cholera to extinction.[27]

By the late 1960s, the cholera pandemic provided Soviet and South Asian scientists with an unprecedented opportunity to test the effectiveness of bacteriophage therapy on cholera. In fact, even before the El Tor outbreak, Russian scientists from the All-Union Scientific Anti-plague Research Institute in Rostov-on-Don of the Soviet Ministry of Health were already in Dakha, Pakistan, conducting trials with phages as both cholera treatment and prophylaxis. They were perfectly placed to confront the burgeoning pandemic head-on.[28] Meanwhile, South Asian scientists had a long tradition, dating back to Félix d'Hérelle's visit in 1927, of using bacteriophages as treatments for cholera and plague.[29]

The study done by the Rostov-on-Don team documented the use of bacteriophage therapy in Pakistan and in Kandahar Province, Afghanistan, where the outbreak had seeped across the border. A phage cocktail was administered to patients suffering from serious cases of cholera to mostly positive results. In addition, an emergency dosage of phages was given to 270,000 people in northern Afghanistan as a prophylactic measure; afterward they reported no new cases of cholera.[30] Unfortunately, the resulting paper suffered from the same shortcomings that seemed to undercut past studies—namely, a lack of randomization and control groups.

The work being done during the early El Tor pandemic improved over time. One study done by researchers from the Pakistani Institute of Public Health and the Pakistan-SEATO (Southeast Asia Treaty Organization) Cholera Research Laboratory tested the effectiveness of phage therapy on patients with cholera and compared it with patients treated with the antibiotic tetracycline. This time, a control group was included; its patients were only given an intravenous fluid to keep them hydrated (the most common treatment at the time). Because it was acknowledged that keeping patients hydrated over the course of the disease resulted in high rates of survival, the team made the crucial decision not to focus on the final outcome of treatment but on the differences observed during the course of treatment. They found that high doses of bacteriophage therapy caused the disease to clear more quickly than in the intravenous fluid control group but at a slightly slower pace than in the antibiotic group. Just as important, the study established that administering high doses of bacteriophage was indeed safe.[31]

A subsequent paper documented a 1969 Soviet-led study conducted at the Pakistan-SEATO Cholera Research Laboratory using bacteriophage cocktails prepared at the All-Union Scientific Research Anti-Plague Research Institute. Cholera patients were administered the phage preparation or tetracycline or a placebo. As with the Pakistani study, the researchers reported that the tetracycline-treated group fared the best; however, the Soviet team found that patients given the bacteriophage therapy and the placebo group performed similarly. The lead author of the paper concluded, "Despite its promise of therapeutic efficacy, the bacteriophage did not eliminate Vibrio cholerae from the intestine, and did not significantly affect the course of the disease. From these studies we can concluded that bacteriophage in the doses and concentrations used is of no value as an adjunct to standard intravenous therapy in the treatment of cholera."[32]

Published in the *Bulletin of the World Health Organization*, the collective papers by Soviet and South Asian researchers on their work treating cholera represented the handful of English-language papers available from 1960 to the early 1980s. While their results were generally positive, though questionable, they serve as proof that serious efforts to explore bacteriophage therapy's potential were still being conducted and on a significant scale. What's more, the results were available to any Western researchers willing to consider them.[33]

DURING THE WANING DAYS of *Life* magazine's run, it received a tip that North Vietnamese civilians were being held in a prison on an isolated island that was no more than a speck in the South China

Sea. In 1970 an American delegation consisting of Rep. Augustus Hawkins (D-CA), Rep. William Anderson (D-TN), congressional aide Tom Harkin, translator Don Luce, and Office of Public Safety director Frank Walton of the U.S. Agency for International Development made an official visit to the joint Vietnamese-U.S. prison hidden on the island. Its name was Con Son Island. For American soldiers trapped in the messy and shapeless conflict, it went by another name—Devil's Island.

The presence of Westerners in Vietnam dates to the early seventeenth century when a Jesuit priest established a French mission there. For a while, Western activity was limited to Christian proselytizing and trade. A century later that changed. The French clergy started a long tradition of Western meddling in Vietnam's affairs. Pierre Pigneau de Béhaine, a Catholic priest, solicited the aid of the French military in restoring the deposed king, Nguyen Anh, and retaking the land lost to the Tay Son, a rebel group led by three brothers. Accompanied by the king's seven-year-old son, Pigneau de Béhaine returned to France to solicit aid from King Louis XVI. With the help of French soldiers, the Nguyen Anh family ascended to the throne once again. A century later, however, the entire country was under the French government's thumb as one of its numerous colonies across the globe.[34]

The Japanese swept the French Army out of what was then known as Indochina during the early years of World War II. After the Axis defeat, France attempted to reestablish its influence in the area. Its people were not received with open arms.

The French had used Con Dao Prison since 1861 to incarcerate dangerous criminals, but by the turn of the century, the calf-shaped island's population consisted mostly of political prisoners. In 1954 the French transferred the responsibility for the prison to the South Vietnamese Army, which continued the practice of incarcerating dissidents there. The gradual ceding of power by the French to the Americans saw the prison change hands yet again, and it continued to function until the Communist North Vietnamese liberation of South Vietnam.[35]

The American delegation arrived with a map in hand and a guide in tow. The men started exploring parts of the prison on their own.

As if scripted by a Hollywood screenwriter, the group discovered structures with deep pits in the ground that were covered with metal grills and barbed wire. Inside, North Vietnamese families wasted away in the sweltering heat. These "tiger cages" ran the length of the room like gestation crates for humans.[36]

Con Dao Prison was a terrible place, no doubt. Because of that (or in spite of that), Con Son Island lay at the heart of a well-known and much-believed urban legend among American GIs. While there's no formal title for the tale, a possible name could be "The Revenge of the Black Syph." It struck deeply at the core of the invading soldier's fighting spirit, posing a direct challenge to his courage, virility, and overall manhood.

According to the story that circulated, a devastating form of syphilis existed in Vietnam. It afflicted men unfortunate enough to have caught the disease from any one of the thousands of prostitutes in bars and nightclubs scattered throughout the country. As its name hints, soldiers infected with the black syph discovered their penises covered in sores. As the disease progressed, it necrotized the skin, turning it black and scabrous. It was incurable. It was humiliating. Most of all, it was the end. The U.S. Army viewed soldiers with the disease as burdens and embarrassments back home. Their foreign-borne uncleanliness could not be allowed to make its way to American shores.[37]

The army hid infected individuals away rather than demoralize the people back in the United States. A boat carried them over choppy waters to their destination—Con Son Island. Devil's Island. Black Syph Island. And that was where they'd spend the remainder of their days in syphilitic agony. Their brains would deteriorate as their disease progressed toward the tertiary stage. They died in secrecy officially labeled missing in action by the military.[38]

Anecdotal evidence suggests that a significant number of soldiers encountered some version of this story even after the war. It struck at the heart of the complicated sexual mores that antibiotics made even more complicated by taking the literal sting out of STDs.

Yet, behind the legend may have been a shred of the truth. As with every war, sexually transmitted diseases spiked with the influx of troops, and commanders fought the same nonfraternization battles as their predecessors. The first major strain of antibiotic-resistant gonorrhea appeared during the Vietnam War when American soldiers were on leave in the Philippines for R&R. They tested positive for *Neisseria gonorrhoeae*, which showed resistance to penicillin, spectinomycin, and tetracycline. More cases of resistant gonorrhea emerged, and eventually the Southeast Asian strain crept across the globe. It would become the most prevalent form of multidrug-resistant gonorrhea in the world.[39]

In a 1971 *New York Times* article titled "The Venereal Disease Pandemic," the authors lamented, "The dosage given today is 48 times what doctors prescribed 20 years ago, and a certain number of cases still defy normal treatment. The resistance problem seems to be aggravated by the importation of new and hardier strains from Southeast Asia. Indeed, V.D. [venereal disease] must rank close to heroin addiction on Vietnam's list of exports."[40]

STDs and penile necrosis weren't the only infections making the rounds in Vietnam. There is some debate as to whether *Acinetobacter baumannii* infections became the predominant complication in war wounds during that particular conflict. Some studies indicate that it played a major role in morbidity and mortality. "These organisms were the most frequently recovered gram-negative isolate from war wounds and the second most frequent bacterium causing bloodstream infection in US Marines with extremity wounds during the Vietnam War."[41]

Despite the increased incidence of *A. baumannii*, the number of soldiers that died of wounds continued the downward trajectory that started during World War II. Increased efficiency of rapid casualty evacuation to hospitals contributed to the improvements. (Surgical admissions accounted for 46.3 percent of admissions but 93 percent of deaths. Sepsis was the third leading cause of mortality in surgical patients; that amounted to roughly 12 percent of deaths. Head injury and hemorrhagic shock were numbers 1 and 2.) After the first twenty-four hours, the most common cause of death was sepsis, or roughly 38 percent total. Causes ranged from intestinal injuries, intra-abdominal abscesses, and pneumonia. Burns were a common injury, and among the burned, infections represented the leading cause of death.[42]

Other bacteria were also present. Wounds analyzed during evacuation from Vietnam to base hospitals in Japan showed the presence of *Pseudomonas*, *Staphylococcus*, and *Escherichia coli*. *Klebsiella* was also found.[43]

Penicillin remained the most prescribed antibiotic, at 91.6 percent of all antibiotics administered. Of the 70.2 percent of wounded American soldiers receiving such treatments, 61.5 percent had it administered intramuscularly, 35.3 percent intravenously, 2.2 percent locally, and 31.2 percent orally. Doctors used it to control beta-hemolytic streptococcal infections as well as gas gangrene.[44]

FOR ALL OF TROFIM Lysenko's power and influence, he never really had a firm grip on either. Instead, it was as if he were a currency pegged to the U.S. dollar, deriving his stability, above all other things, from the link between the two. The very nature of the Michurinist biology he espoused and the research in support of its tenets were flimsy. Lysenko tied his fortunes to his primary patrons—first Joseph Stalin, then Nikita Khrushchev. It served him well until it didn't.

In October 1964 Khrushchev visited the Black Sea. By then, he had started spending more time outside the country, seeking respite from the domestic issues that only seemed to get worse. While he was away, his former supporters banded together to bring him down. They summoned him back to Moscow, and one after another denounced him for his failures. It marked the ignominious end to the Soviet Union's second "leader for life."[45]

Trofim Lysenko's fall from power occurred soon afterward.

David Joravsky's book *The Lysenko Affair* summarized the confused and contradictory climate that existed prior to Lysenko's removal from his perch atop the Academy of Sciences.

> The official formula for reconciliation and a united move ahead came to this: The position taken in 1948 was essentially correct; genetics was still banned. There had been mistaken excesses, but now they were happily corrected. Soviet biologists were once again free to learn from the work of foreigners (though the effort to translate work in genetics provoked constant quarrels, and Soviet geneticists were not allowed to travel abroad); cytology was being revived (though it could not be

reconciled with Lysenkoism any more than it could be separated from genetics); and Soviet biochemists were permitted to study nucleic acids (though this study also was inseparable from genetics and incompatible with Lysenkoism).[46]

The amalgam of internal contradictions provided cover for Soviet agriculture to enjoy practical Western advances such as selective weed killers and polyploid sugar beets, both of which were based on concepts Lysenko vigorously denied existed. It allowed Soviet scientists to continue to deny the existence of chromosomes and genes while also allowing them to enjoy the bounty hybrid corn provided. Ultimately, the weight of the contradictions proved too much, and once the supporting beam Khrushchev's patronage provided was pulled out from underneath them, the entire structure Lysenko had constructed over three decades came down, crushing many of the people who stood under it.

15

The era of Trofim Lysenko and his Michurinist destruction of Soviet science may have drawn to a merciful close in 1964, but the debilitating effects of his policy lingered long after his fall. Thanks to him and the politicians and scientists who enabled him, the biological sciences in the Soviet Union lagged behind the level of their Western counterparts. Over thirty years of faulty science and bad habits would take decades to unwind.

The shackles may have come off, but the wounds had yet to heal. Geneticists in the Soviet Union came out of hiding only to discover a scientific wasteland at home and a new era of recombinant biotechnology abroad. During their years in the wilderness, Soviet scientists missed out on actively participating in the major discoveries in genetics that laid the groundwork for the modern biotechnology era. Lysenko's bullheaded insistence that chromosomes, genes, and DNA were bourgeois myths had relegated the scientists to the roles of observers as genetic discoveries changed the very nature of the life sciences. Here is a partial list of what they missed:

1. George Beadle and Edward Tatum demonstrate their one gene, one enzyme hypothesis (1941).
2. William Astbury obtains the first X-ray diffraction pattern of DNA, showing DNA has a regular, periodic structure (1943).
3. Oswald Avery, Colin MacLeod, and Maclyn McCarty determine DNA, not proteins, transform the properties of cells (1944).
4. Barbara McClintock discovers that genes can move around on chromosomes (1944).
5. Alfred Hershey and Martha Chase show that genes are made of DNA (1952).

6. Francis Crick and James Watson describe the double helical structure of DNA (1953).

7. Arthur Kornberg and others isolate DNA polymerase, which later plays a central role in DNA sequencing (1955).

8. Matthew Meselson and Franklin Stahl demonstrate that DNA replicates semiconservatively (1958).

9. Jérôme Lejeune, Marthe Gautier, and Raymond Turpin discover that Down syndrome is caused by trisomy 21, identifying chromosomal abnormalities (1958).

10. Sydney Brenner, François Jacob, and Matthew Meselson ascertain that messenger RNA ferries information from the nucleus to the cytoplasm (1961).

Soviet science discarded Lysenko and his minions just in time to witness Marshall Nirenberg announce that he had cracked the genetic code by showing that four nucleic acids spelled everything out on DNA.

Did the Lysenko era affect the Soviet Union's ability to conduct basic theoretical and applied science research? The answer is yes.

Zhores Medvedev, a witness to the lunacy of creative Darwinism, summarized the state of post-Lysenko Soviet science in his book *The Rise and Fall of T. D. Lysenko*. "It cannot be said that Soviet scientists made no contribution, but theirs was relatively modest because they lacked the technical and methodological conditions for experimentation on the necessary scale. . . . After 1948, the methodological level of biology in our country dropped sharply. This opened the way for a large number of people incapable of real and serious creative work in science."[1]

Had it not been for researchers of drive, dedication, and vision, the damage done by creative Darwinism might have lingered indefinitely. Yuri Ovchinnikov, for one, was determined to return Russian science to its proud tradition.[2]

Ovchinnikov was a star in the reborn field of Soviet science. His ascent in the ranks of Russian institutions echoed that of Lysenko four years earlier, only Ovchinnikov succeeded using actual knowledge. Like Lysenko, he knew how to play the political side of national science. According to Milton Leitenberg and Raymond Zilinskas, "Ovchinnikov was an astute political operative and had friends and supporters in high places."[3]

Ovchinnikov graduated from Moscow State University in 1957 with a degree in chemistry. His first professional lab position came in 1960 when he was awarded a research post at the Institute of Chemistry and Natural Compounds. However, it was his acceptance into the Plenum of the Central Committee of the Communist Party in 1962 that paved the way for his political success. In 1973 he became a member of the Presidium of the Supreme Soviet of the Russian Republic of the Soviet Union.[4]

As a scientist, Ovchinnikov focused on naturally occurring peptides that possessed chemotherapeutic activity. As part of studying the compounds, he often attempted to synthesize them in the laboratory. Together with Mikhail Shemyakin, he worked on dipeptides, chemicals that were the products of the metabolic processes of microorganisms. Examples included actinomycin, valinomycin, and gramicidin C (yet another variation of the original antibiotic). Later he focused on a protein known as bacteriorhodopsin.[5]

Ovchinnikov's greatest contribution to Soviet science came from his role as an administrator rather than as a scientist. During the early 1970s, he understood the precarious position in which Lysenko's influence had left the life sciences in Russia. The Russians had missed the genetic revolution, and if something drastic wasn't done, they were set to suffer a similar fate during the biotechnology revolution. The only problem was how to procure enough funding for researchers to catch up with current trends and conduct new work.[6]

A firm understanding of how the Communist scientific apparatus functioned and where the Communist Party's priorities lay made the difference. It was succinctly summarized in a quote attributed to Ovchinnikov: "At the Central Committee of the Communist Party, if we offer ten drugs nobody would support us. Nobody would give us money for medicine. But offer one weapon and you'll get full support."[7]

Col. Gen. Yefim Ivanovich Smirnov's professional work in biological warfare stretched all the way back to 1939, when Stalin placed Lavrenti Beria as the official head of the Soviet program. For all intents and purposes, Smirnov ran the organization's day-to-day operations. His influence continued to grow until 1954 when he headed the Ministry of Defense's Seventh Directorate of the General Staff (later known as the Fifteenth Directorate). Until 1985 Smirnov was the most important decision maker. If there was any chance of dragging the country's life sciences into the age of biotechnology and recombinant DNA, he had to be on board. One microbiologist called him "the ideologue par excellence of Soviet bioweapons research from the 1950s to the 1980s." Gaining his support was the single critical factor in realizing Ovchinnikov's grand plan.[8]

According to Leitenberg and Zilinkas, no record exists regarding when Ovchinnikov and Smirnov first met or when their collaboration began. However, they speculate that it must have been some time around 1971 when Ovchinnikov was first made aware of the advances in biotechnology Western scientists had achieved, particularly in recombinant DNA and the potential it unleashed. Ovchinnikov pitched his idea and "concluded that the only way to quickly gain support from decision makers for a program that aimed to match Western developments was to play the military card."[9]

Thanks to Ovchinnikov's shrewdness, the Soviet government officially declared biotechnology as a field of importance. Even though the BW program probably wasn't his primary concern, he ensured that researchers developing new weapons used the latest genetic techniques. He was fully aware that for over a decade, military scientists relied on antiquated techniques that had been developed in the West a half century earlier. They relied on exposing pathogens to chemicals or radiation to force mutations in DNA. Potent strains would then be separated from the less potent ones, and the process would be repeated until the pathogens exhibited the characteristics they desired—namely, increased infectivity, virulence, and hardiness. Unfortunately, the scientists probably had limited, if any, knowledge of the microbiology and genetics behind the changes they induced. An element of luck would play a role in their progress.

When Leonid Brezhnev assumed control of the Soviet Union in 1964, he brought a different temperament to the role of general secretary. He also promoted a variation on Khrushchev's "catch up and overtake" strategy that involved matching the United States missile for missile, nuclear warhead for nuclear warhead, and biological bomb for biological bomb.[10]

Ovchinnikov's framing of the establishment of a new BW program that relied on the latest biotechnology techniques ensured its swift approval. The R&D part of the new organization came to be known by its code name FERMENT. Its formation proved Brezhnev's determination to overtake the U.S. weapons program, both conventional and unconventional. The Politburo even went so far as to issue a decree stating that the purpose of the new program was to acquire modern biological weapons. Over the next few years, the Communist Party would amend and improve the decree to make its goals more ambitious.[11]

Harnessing and unleashing the destructive force of antibiotic resistance emerged as a major field of research. The State Research Center for Applied Microbiology conducted most of the work in weaponizing bacteria by making it impervious to any form of chemotherapeutic attack. Specifically, its subprogram Metol was a bacteria-only applied science wing that followed up on novel bacterial pathogens developed at the subprogram Bonfire.[12]

The center's focus, as dictated by the Ministry of Defense, revolved around weaponizing various bacterial pathogens. Its eight-floor building was arranged accordingly. Researchers on the second floor worked with *Yersinia pestis* (plague). The third floor was dedicated to *Francisella tularensis* (tularemia). The higher floors studied *Bacillus anthracis* (anthrax), *Burkholderia mallei* (glanders), and *Burkholderia pseudomallei* (melioidosis). For some time, Igor Domaradsky bore the responsibility of introducing antibiotic resistance genes into the various pathogens. The closest his team came to succeeding was with *F. tularensis*.[13]

Inserting resistance genes might have seemed easy on paper, and in practice, it was. The only problem—and it was a major one—was that every time the researchers succeeded in conferring resistance to a strain of bacteria, they found that its virulence plummeted, something called the pleiotropic effect. They found the antibiotic-resistant *F. tularensis* was no longer pathogenic. In other words, the transformed bacteria were useless for the Soviet military's purposes.[14]

Domaradsky described the experience: "Having become resistant to several antibiotics, the strain lost its virulence, which was unacceptable to the military. . . . The desired bioweapons strain had to be fully virulent and deliverable in aerosol form. One germ cell had to be enough to start a lethal infection in a monkey."[15]

The inability to solve the problem ended up costing Domaradsky his position and the freedom to choose his field of research. After his demotion, he was assigned work, something he considered a tremendous insult. A few years later, another researcher would achieve the goal that had eluded him and would give the Soviet military a man-made, multidrug-resistant, virulent strain of *F. tularensis*.[16]

Success simply whet the Ministry of Defense's appetite and proved that it could make demands of nature and be rewarded. The ministry ordered the center to develop genetically modified strains of *B. anthracis*, *B. mallei*, *B. pseudomallei*, and *Y. pestis*. It also demanded that each strain be resistant to no less than ten antibiotics. Soviet scientists never succeeded.[17]

Whether it was by design or an example of the grossest negligence possible, a number of BW research centers were located in the middle of or close to Russian cities. These centers were accidents waiting to happen. In 1979 an accident resulted in one of the most notorious examples of a man-made outbreak.

The eponymous Sverdlovsk Institute was centrally located in one of Russia's largest cities. It belonged to a larger collection of military compounds, most of which were not involved in BW research. The institute was housed in Compound 19 and was often referred to by that name. It stretched over an area of 495 acres and included living quarters as well as research buildings.[18]

During the 1970s, the Soviet BW program's administrators made the conscious decision to focus its resources on developing *B. anthracis* into its major biological weapon. According to researchers involved in the project, the shift took place after Soviet intelligence services purchased a copy of old "American plans" for researching and developing anthrax as a biological agent, though presumably for defensive purposes. According to a former worker, "Everything was connected with anthrax cultures. That is to say, all the scientific topics dealt with anthrax, and the equipment was designed to insert anthrax spores into munitions."[19]

One of the most important structures in Compound 19 was a building situated in the so-called special zone, where the most sensitive and secret work took place. That particular structure was responsible for the production of dry *B. anthracis*, which was manufactured specifically for offensive use. Each floor of the building played a specific role in the process. The basement served as a mixing station where the various chemicals, wet and dry, necessary for the fermentation process came together. The first floor contained the centrifuges that separated the spent biomass from the liquor containing the spores. Large stainless steel fermentation vats filled the next level, while the third floor contained smaller fermenters. The top floor of the building handled the ventilation equipment necessary to keep the lethal pathogens being grown in the building from being released into the densely populated city.[20]

On April 2, 1979, a massive plume rose over the dried anthrax production building. Something had gone wrong with the ventilation system, and spore-filled air that was supposed to be filtered shot out of one of the building's exhaust chimneys. The deadly dust filled the air around the building before a breeze gently swept the spores through the city. When the production night crew realized what had happened earlier in the day, the crewmen immediately informed their superiors, who then informed the appropriate officials in Moscow. In both instances, all received direct orders that forbade disclosing the accident to anyone else. Thus, nobody knew they were inhaling anthrax spores—not civilians walking the streets, not municipal officials responsible for their citizenry, not local public health officials, and not even members of the Communist Party who were unfortunate enough not to belong to the military.[21]

People who had been in the path of the moving cloud of anthrax began showing symptoms of infection two days later. The closer they had been to Compound 19 the quicker and the more severe their infections presented. Those with skin infections tended to fare better than those victims who had inhaled the spores. The weaponized strain of *B. anthracis*, known as strain 836, acted the way it had been designed—hyper infective and hyper virulent. Doctors threw everything they had at the infections. As a result of Communist Party obfuscation, the true number of casualties has yet to be established. According to one report, ninety-five people were infected; sixty-eight of them died. That's a 71.6 percent mortality rate. Just to provide some context, the 2014 *Zaire ebolavirus* outbreak in the Democratic Republic of the Congo featured a 74 percent fatality rate.[22]

The tragic incident in Sverdlovsk established, without question, the damage that could happen when genetically modified, weaponized pathogens escape into the environment. It proved that it was not a question of if but when.

THE SHINE CAME OFF antibiotic growth promoters pretty quickly for those who watched with honest eyes. Scientists and public health officials began to connect the dots between low-dose antibiotic use on farms and rising antibiotic resistance. Even in the face of mounting evidence that adding tetracycline or penicillin to animal feed had negative effects, "farmers" didn't stop using antibiotics to the fullest extent possible. Nor did this information discourage pharmaceutical companies from selling it. If they were going to forgo AGPs, the proof would have to be incontrovertible and convincing. Researchers hadn't hit that point yet.

E. S. "Andy" Anderson was one of the first members of the scientific community to dig in his heels and push back against the agricultural and pharmaceutical companies. Over the course of his career, he would shine a light on the dangers that subtherapeutic doses of antibiotics posed.

Since the early 1960s, the British public, government, and scientific community engaged in a healthy debate regarding the safety of AGPs. Groups as disparate as the Shropshire Federation of Women's Institutes to the Medical and Agricultural Research Councils expressed their views on the subject. The government convened a joint scientific inquiry headed by the president of the National Farmers' Union, James Turner, Lord Netherthorpe. Its aim was to bring the debate to a definitive resolution by having scientists establish the safety of feed additives.[23]

Rather unsurprising, the so-called Netherthorpe Committee declared the agricultural use of antibiotics to be safe and even recommended a loosening of restrictions on AGPs to fatten calves.

According to Robert Bud, "It was assumed that even if bacteria became resistant to the few drugs permitted for such uses, penicillin, oxy-tetracycline, and chlortetracycline, they would remain susceptible to other antibiotics." In not so many words, they argued that there was no proof linking antibiotic resistance in farm animals to human beings.[24]

While the findings of the Netherthorpe Committee failed to recognize the dangers of antibiotic resistance developing, it formalized the parameters of the debate and by doing so provided the structure that activist scientists would methodically undermine. Moving forward, researchers would employ the incremental nature of scientific discovery, gathering data one experiment at a time, until the case could be made one way or another.

In 1963 Andy Anderson, director of the Enteric Reference Laboratory at the Central Public Health Laboratory, began tracking antibiotic-resistant salmonella in the United Kingdom. Two years later, when he announced the results of his inquiry, Anderson documented how he had initially found salmonella that was resistant to streptomycin and various sulfonamides in calves; now he could add ampicillin and chloramphenicol to the list as well. The list of effective antibiotics was shrinking quickly. Making matters worse—as if that were possible—he added that the same strain of salmonella had been responsible for over five hundred bouts of illness that included six fatalities. Together with Bernard Dixon from the *New Scientist*, Anderson relied on the media to build awareness among the public and to pester and pressure the British government into taking action. As is so often the case, it took a tragedy to force the slightest movement from government and industry, which were historically tied at the hip.[25]

It started one day in November 1967 when two infants were admitted to the isolation ward of West Lane Hospital in Middlesbrough in northern England. They were suffering from a gastroenteritis caused by a resistant strain of *E. coli*. Eventually, babies in other hospitals fell sick with the same condition.[26] When health care professionals administered neomycin, the standard treatment, the babies' conditions did not improve; instead, they deteriorated. Other antibiotics proved just as powerless. In the end, ten children died.[27]

The public outcry and anxiety that accompanied the incident eventually led to the government's formation of the Swann Committee, whose final report was a milestone. Overall, it involved contributions from the scientific community, government researchers, pharmaceutical companies, and various industry groups. It linked twenty years of antibiotic-resistance research with more recent findings regarding plasmids and the use of growth promoters. In the process, the committee's report established the staggering amounts of antibiotics the agricultural industry used—over 185 tons of antibiotics per year. And that figure was for England alone; it did not count usage in Scotland, Wales, and Northern Ireland. Yet, despite the committee's findings, the smoking gun still had yet to be found.[28]

The debate among American researchers lagged that of their British counterparts, but a building unease festered in the minds of conscientious scientists. In 1972 the Food and Drug Administration attempted to get out in front of the AGP question by creating a task force of federal, university, and industry scientists to hold hearings regarding the issue. Farmers and agricultural groups were invited to testify in Washington. The task force issued a shorter version of the Swann Committee's report and proposed stringent controls on the use of AGPs. The verdict was far from unanimous, and half of its members penned a dissenting report that took issue with the official one. The usual suspects—congressmen together with pharmaceutical and agricultural companies—pressured the FDA. Even animal scientists from land-grant universities joined the beating. Cowed by the abuse they received, FDA officials offered a compromise: they would allow the pharmaceutical companies to sponsor and conduct their own research into the safety of using antibiotics in agriculture.[29]

In 1974 the Animal Health Institute, an agricultural lobby in Washington DC, hired Stuart D. Levy in the hopes his research would finally disprove the circumstantial link between antibiotic resistance in animals and humans. Levy knew antibiotics and possessed a deep understanding of tetracyclines. He had studies under his belt that identified genes responsible for antibiotic resistance and deciphered the mechanism that allowed bacteria to escape harm. He was also a relatively young researcher whom the Animal Health Institute may have felt it could nudge toward favorable conclusions, if not findings. After all, a little funding went a long way.[30]

Maryn McKenna summarized Levy's objectives in her book *Big Chicken*: "First, did the antibiotics in in feed cause resistant bacteria to emerge or multiply in the chickens receiving it? Second, did that resistance cross from those chickens to the rest of the flock? And third and most crucial, could it make the leap from chickens to humans?"[31]

To answer these questions, it was necessary to take the experiment outside the controlled environment of the academic lab and into the wild, so to speak. For decades, scientists had made assertions about the spread of antibiotic resistance from the farm to the consumer, while pharmaceutical firms and farmers wielded counter assertions that growth promoters were 100 percent safe. Without any conclusive data at hand, it was like a never-ending tennis match. The issue could only be settled in one place—on a farm.

Levy enlisted the help of the Downing family, which lived in a suburb outside of Boston, Massachusetts. The Downings had a cow and some pigs on their property but nothing elaborate. They also had a number of unused sheds and a big barn that would serve as perfect test sites to track the course of antibiotic resistance in an agricultural setting.[32]

Six wire pens were built. Four were placed inside the barn, fifty feet apart, and two were put outside. Pathogen-free eggs were purchased to ensure that the chickens weren't contaminated before the experiment even started. When the chicks hatched, they were placed in one of the pens on the farm and fed antibiotic-free feed until they were two months old. That was when the experiment began.[33]

Levy placed fifty chicks in each pen. Half of them were fed antibiotic-free feed, while the remainder were fed Pfizer's Terramycin-based animal feed. The feed mix consisted of 100 grams of antibiotic per ton, a dosage more in line with disease prophylaxis than growth promotion. In addition to the Downings' help in taking care of the chickens, neighbors living in the vicinity of the farm were asked to donate stool samples on a weekly basis.[34]

Before the chicks were fed the mixed feed, stool samples were taken from the birds, the animals, and the humans involved. They provided baseline readings that would be compared with the stool samples taken over the course of the experiment. At that point, the bacteria in their guts had very little resistance to tetracycline.[35]

Changes in the chickens' flora occurred in little over a day. By the time the experiment hit the two-week point, 90 percent of the chickens that had eaten the antibiotic-treated feed showed signs of harboring antibiotic resistance. The bacteria in those chickens that had been fed antibiotic-free feed did not show any changes. These findings affirmed what scientists had suspected in the past but lacked the proof to confirm: The low-dose administration had eliminated tetracycline-susceptible bacteria but were unable to destroy ones harboring genes coding for resistance. The surviving bacteria were able to replicate and form colonies with complete resistance to the antibiotic. No amount of tetracycline would be able to tilt the balance back to the baseline readings taken at the beginning of the experiment.[36]

A few weeks later, truly startling developments began to emerge. The chickens that had exhibited resistance to tetracycline continued to show it. However, when tested against other antibiotics such as sulfanilamides, neomycin, streptomycin, and chloramphenicol, the bacteria displayed resistance to them as well even though none of those drugs were included in the experiment. If that wasn't bad enough, the resistant bacteria had somehow colonized the guts of the chickens that were fed pure feed without antibiotics. They had navigated the fifty or more feet separating the pens. And just to prove that when things are bad, they can always get worse, the same multidrug-resistant bacteria began to show up in stool samples taken from the Downings. It was a twisted variation on the farm-to-table theme so popular in today's locavore parlance. When Levy brought the resistant bacteria back to his lab, he established one more discouraging finding: the genes for resistance were carried and transferred through plasmids, the extra-chromosomal snippets of DNA that bacteria passed on to each other, regardless of species. All in all, the facts painted a picture much worse than anything the Animal Health Institute could imagine.[37]

In September 1976 Stuart Levy published the results of the experiment at the Downing farm against his funders' wishes. A few months later, the FDA, led by Donald Kennedy, announced that the United

States planned on implementing a ban on agricultural antibiotic use similar to the ones in the United Kingdom. By this point, almost every food animal raised in the United States—close to 100 percent of the chickens and turkeys, 90 percent of veal calves and swine, 60 percent of cattle—was receiving antibiotics some time in its life. Once again, however, the pressure mounted by agricultural, pharmaceutical, and political groups proved too much, and the FDA was forced to walk back its decision. Antibiotics would continue being used in U.S. agriculture for decades to come. In an act of blatant negligence, a major factor in the rise of resistance—a fact proven by Levy's barnyard experiment—was allowed to continue and expand.[38]

DURING ANDY ANDERSON'S CAMPAIGN tracking incidents of salmonella infections across the United Kingdom, one of the nightmare scenarios he repeatedly mentioned was the potential emergence of chloramphenicol-resistant *Salmonella typhi*, the bacterium responsible for typhoid fever. (Chloramphenicol was considered the treatment of choice for *S. typhi* infections.) The combination of improved sanitation and modern antibiotics had relegated the disease to a rarity in developed countries. For developing countries with the wrong combination of shaky sanitation and unreliable access to antibiotics, typhoid fever continued to appear in the yearly cycles of disease. As early as 1950, chloramphenicol-resistant *S. typhi* had been reported. For the time being, it remained an isolated incident, but Anderson's warning became prophetic.[39]

In February 1972 an epidemic of chloramphenicol-resistant typhoid fever exploded in Mexico City and Pachuca. Over the next few months, the outbreak spread across central Mexico, ripping through cities such as Apizaco, Puebla, and Poza Rica at a dizzying pace. Newspapers soon picked up on the assault, particularly as other countries warned tourists against vacationing there. By the end of 1972, public health officials still struggled to get a grip on the outbreak. Clusters of new infections continued to surface well into the following year.[40]

During the first year of the epidemic, more than ten thousand confirmed cases of antibiotic-resistant typhoid fever were reported. Its most common victims were children between the ages of five and fourteen and young adults between fifteen and twenty-four years old. According to a contemporary study, "During the first 6 months of the outbreak, over 400 strains of *S. typhi* were recovered in seven different communities. Of these isolates, about 92% were multiply-resistant to chloramphenicol, tetracycline, streptomycin, and sulfonamides." They remained susceptible to ampicillin, colistin, and gentamicin among other antibiotics. The study cited the extensive use of chloramphenicol in the country as a major cause of the emergence of resistant strains of bacteria, suggesting that previous appearances of resistant *Shigella* and *E. coli* as sources of plasmid-mediated antibiotic resistance.[41]

Numerous outbreaks followed the Mexican epidemic in quick succession: India (1972), Vietnam (1972), and Korea (1977). During each of those outbreaks, the chloramphenicol-resistant strains also showed resistance to ampicillin. In 1975 a co-trimoxazole-resistant strain was reported in France. With strains impervious to all three first-line treatments in circulation, it was only a matter of time until a multidrug version appeared resistant to every first-line antibiotic. By the mid-1980s, the monster strain was in circulation. Multidrug-resistant strains of *S. typhi* first emerged in Southeast Asia; then it spread across the globe. Without the security of first-line defenses to fall back on, pediatricians were forced to use ciprofloxacin to treat typhoid fever, despite not even knowing whether it was safe for children. Luckily Cipro worked.[42]

During the late 1970s and 1980s, the pharmaceutical industry saw further consolidation of companies, and its overall drug R&D strategy underwent a dramatic change. The discovery of lovastatin (Mevacor), the first of the so-called statin cholesterol drugs, in 1976 caused drug companies to reconsider their business models. Rather than working to cure diseases, they transitioned to treating long-term chronic diseases that would provide a consistent payday for decades to come. This decision was the nail in the coffin for antibiotic research. Ironically, Mevacor production relied on the same deep tank fermentation methods pioneered during the development of penicillin.[43]

During the early 1980s, the industry took another stab at extending the shelf life of the old beta-lactam class of antibiotics by introducing third-generation cephalosporins. They were designed to be responses to the prevalence of beta-lactamases in organisms such as *E. coli* and *Klebsiella pneumoniae*. Once again, results were the same. They worked until they didn't. In fact, between 1960 and 2000, almost every antibiotic approved for clinical use was a synthetic derivative of an existing class. The four so-called scaffolds—such as 6-APA and 7-ACA—used were cephalosporins, penicillins, quinolones, and macrolides.[44]

The strategy of tweaking existing classes of antibiotics had a glaring weakness. Bacteria that were already resistant to a previous form tended to show resistance to the new version or to develop it at a dizzying pace. Beta-lactam antibiotics are the classic example. By 1983 researchers reported the discovery of plasmid-encoded beta-lactamases capable of disarming the recently introduced broad-spectrum cephalosporins. These newly resistant bacteria's enzyme was called extended-spectrum beta-lactamases.[45]

The resistance onslaught continued when a new crop of drug-resistant strains emerged, ravaging hospitals in the process. Many of the pathogens were commensal bacteria, found naturally in human flora, that were suddenly "weaponized" by the acquisition of antibiotic-resistant genes. They proved particularly deadly for patients recuperating in intensive care units.

As noted earlier, soon after methicillin was discovered, *S. aureus* developed a resistance to it, ushering what can be considered the next wave of the bacteria's assault on society and its medicine. Twenty years after the first appearance of methicillin-resistant *Staphylococcus aureus*, scientists discovered that the strains carry a specific gene, *mecA*, that encodes a protein that is bound to penicillin. Unlike the first wave of type 80/81 *S. aureus* that relied on an enzyme to survive but was narrow in scope, MRSA's strategy entails a physical change to the outer membrane and results in a much wider resistance.[46]

One of the earliest MRSA strains was isolated and studied in 1960. Known as COL, it was first discovered from a patient's culture at Colindale Laboratories in London and was a member of the "archaic" clones of MRSA. Since then, it has spread around the world and has the dubious distinction of belonging to one of the most successful MRSA lineages. During the 1970s, this strain circulated in hospitals throughout Europe. For the most part, the rest of the world escaped the effects of the COL strain, though isolated infections were reported in the United States. For reasons that remain uncertain, COL disappeared from European hospitals during the 1980s.[47]

The third wave of *Staphylococcus* occurred around the same time as the COL strain died away. These descendants of the archaic MRSA clone emerged in hospitals in the late 1970s and by the mid-1980s were endemic. These strains, which include the Iberian and Rome clones, spread through hospitals and long-term health care settings around the world and continue to this day. Their prevalence led to the use of vancomycin as an antibiotic of last resort. Unfortunately, vancomycin-resistant *S. aureus* neutralized the antibiotic's clinical use in the 2000s when it was isolated in a patient in Michigan.[48]

The fourth and latest phase, as defined by Henry Chambers and Frank DeLeo, involved MRSA's invasion of communities outside of health care settings. Strains of community-associated MRSA (CA-MRSA) were first isolated in the 1990s in Western Australia and were distinct from the strains of MRSA that were found in hospitals at the time. The first well-documented cases in the United States were reported in 1997 when otherwise healthy children fell sick. All died of overwhelming infection, suggesting that CA-MRSA was uniquely virulent. The American CA-MRSA outbreak, however, was ultimately traced to a Chicago outbreak in 1993–95.[49]

Multidrug-resistant and pan-drug-resistant gram-negative bacteria have also emerged that pose different but no less lethal threats than MRSA. *Acinetobacter baumannii, Escherichia coli, Klebsiella pneumoniae,* and *Pseudomonas aeruginosa* all belong to the group. They show resistance to just about every antibiotic available. Penicillins. Cephalosporins. Carbapenems. Monobactams. Quinolones. Aminoglycosides. Tetracyclines. Polymyxins. Unlike gram-positive bacteria such as *S. aureus,* these bacteria have an outer membrane that acts as a physical barrier to antibiotics. If the drugs are able to penetrate the bacteria's initial defense, a series of efflux pumps expel the potentially damaging medicine that made it through.[50]

Two bacteria played important roles as sources of resistance for other bacteria. *Klebsiella pneumoniae* was responsible for a number of diseases including pneumonia, urinary tract infections, and meningitis. Together with *E. coli*, it served as a major source of transferred extended-spectrum beta-lactamase resistance among bacteria. *Pseudomonas aeruginosa* formed impenetrable biofilm layers that sheltered bacteria from harm while at the same time providing a space for the exchange of antibiotic resistance genes. Scientists considered it one of two pangenomic gram-negative pathogenic species with an extraordinarily large scale of multidrug-resistant phenotypes.[51]

Meanwhile, *Acinetobacter baumannii* was widely believed to be susceptible to most antibiotics during the 1970s, but during the 1980s it emerged as a major antibiotic-resistant nosocomial pathogen in hospitals. Later, it gained a reputation as an infectious bacteria with a propensity for showing up during traumatic events such as wars, earthquakes, or terrorist attacks.[52]

Enterobacter spp. first came to the scientific community's attention when the bacteria exhibited resistance in 1969–70. Ampicillin, cephalothin, and carbenicillin no longer had any effect on it, but at that time, *Enterobacter* remained susceptible to gentamicin. During the mid-1970s, *Enterobacter* emerged as a significant nosocomial pathogen and, only a decade later, showed multidrug resistance to third-generation cephalosporins.[53]

Rounding out the emergent strains was *Enterococcus faecium*. Its arguably most significant resistant form emerged during the early 1980s with a resistance to vancomycin, which served as the antibiotic of last resort at the time. The bacteria's existence signaled to the scientific community that vancomycin's usefulness was on borrowed time.[54]

WHILE PUBLIC HEALTH OFFICIALS around the world wrestled with the implications of the explosion of antibiotic-resistant bacteria, a team of scientists at the Institute for Animal Disease Research at the Houghton Laboratory in England conducted the first research into phage therapy in decades. H. Williams Smith and Michael Huggins infected mice with *E. coli* O18:K1:H7; then they proceeded to treat them with mixtures containing different bacteriophages. Their thorough study established a few facts that dispelled some doubts surrounding phage therapy. First, they showed that the approach was at least as effective as antibiotics were in preventing mouse mortality when used correctly. This was important because Smith and Huggins also established that not all phages were successful against disease. In this case, they differentiated between the specific strains they used and grouped them according to effectiveness. The study also reinforced a notion that anecdotal evidence reported in the past; that is, survival rates declined significantly the later the treatment was initiated. According to a 2002 study that sought to replicate Smith and Huggins's experiment (successfully), "Perhaps most importantly, Smith and Huggins also provided information about the dynamics of phage treatment—the changes in bacterial and phage densities over the course of infection." Their controlled experiments and conclusions, offering robust information, helped bring attention to long-ignored phage therapy. The following year they followed up their research by conducting effectiveness studies in calves, piglets, and lambs with similarly promising results. Throughout the 1980s, they published more papers exploring therapeutic phage use in animal models.

Smith and Huggins laid the groundwork for further investigation in English-speaking science circles. As the antibiotic threat continued to grow and researchers searched for novel approaches of fighting bacterial infections, bacteriophage therapy started gaining traction again as a potential alternative. Access to the vast trove of knowledge contained in Eastern European and former Soviet institutions such as the Eliava Institute accelerated the "rediscovery" of phage therapy as pharmaceutical companies, in particular, sought to take advantage of decades' worth of research.[55]

Considering that Western scientific research returned to where it started over a half century before, it's difficult to see the interregnum between the papers published in the 1940s and those published in the 1990s (when experiments began in earnest) as anything but a missed opportunity.

IN THE MID-1980S, NEW York City experienced a sharp spike in antibiotic-resistant tuberculosis cases. For thirty years, the rates of infection had remained constant, but now something was causing the disease to spread throughout the city. The numbers were staggering and amounted to a 132 percent increase between 1980 and

1990. Making matters worse, nosocomial outbreaks of multidrug-resistant TB threatened hospitals and nursing homes. Rifampin and isoniazid, the first line of defense against the disease, had lost their potency. Gotham's creaky and underfunded health infrastructure showed signs of breaking.[56]

Entering the final decade of the twentieth century, New York City risked lurching backward to the chaos of the 1970s when the bankrupt city was left for dead by the Republican president Gerald Ford. In the 1980s public health services in the city struggled with shrinking budgets and a system taxed by the crack cocaine epidemic and an HIV/AIDS crisis that only seemed to be spinning further out of control. Crime and murders were reaching historic highs. It was a challenging time for a resilient metropolis.

Thomas Frieden, who would later go on to head the Centers for Disease Control, and his colleagues investigated the dramatic increase in antibiotic-resistant TB and published their findings in the *New England Journal of Medicine*. They found that besides patients with normal preconditions for the development of resistant TB (e.g., prior TB treatment, recent immigration, or cavitary lung disease), the strain was also isolated from a large number of individuals who did not meet established criteria. Frieden concluded that the spike resulted from people who were HIV-positive but were unaware of their infection. When they were treated for TB, their compromised immune systems not only hindered their treatment but also rendered them contagious for longer periods than normal. The combination went a long way toward explaining the spread of resistant TB and further proved that HIV/AIDS was allowing normally controlled conditions to become fatal.[57]

The arrival of HIV/AIDS in the United States is normally said to have come through Haiti. Current scientific consensus indicates that HIV first reached Haiti in the mid-1960s from Central Africa. A sizable portion of Haitians had fled there to escape the first wave of political repression during François Duvalier's presidency. At the same time, opportunities for French-speaking managers in business, health, and education fields opened in the newly independent nation of Zaire. (The Belgians had abandoned the country in a hurry and did not train any local citizens before leaving.) It was the perfect opportunity for Haitian professionals moving abroad. As more native Zaireans developed the necessary skills to take over administrative positions, Haitians returned home, where the political climate had eased considerably. Some of the managers returned with HIV in their bloodstreams.[58] Investigations of medical records and anecdotal evidence provided the first clues, as did the fact that while the Dominican Republic and Haiti share the same geographical island, their rates of HIV infection differ drastically. Later phylogenetic studies supported the theory that HIV was introduced to the United States by way of Haiti sometime around 1971. Five years later, the virus had made the leap across the country and became entrenched in gay communities in San Francisco. By the time Frieden had investigated the rise in antibiotic-resistant TB, HIV/AIDS had been circulating among New Yorkers for twenty years.[59]

While HIV/AIDS was ravaging the globe, the final act of the Cold War played out between two old American presidents and a younger Soviet premier. First, Ronald Reagan assumed a much more combative stance against the Soviet Union than his predecessor, Jimmy Carter, had. Rather than settling for peaceful coexistence, Reagan pushed the Soviet war production machine into the final throes of an arms race that stretched back decades. Mikhail Gorbachev inherited a country with a hobbled economy that could not hope to compete with that of the United States, much less match it missile for missile, plane for plane, and warhead for warhead. Long after Khrushchev's campaign to raise the standard of living in Russia, shortages still plagued the Soviet Union's markets. In the game of poker between the global superpowers, Reagan called the Soviet Union's bluff. To his credit, Gorbachev was a realist and understood something drastic needed to be done to save the union. The era of perestroika and glasnost opened the USSR to the West, unleashing forces very few people expected or knew how to control. It resulted in the dissolution of the Soviet Union and the Eastern bloc. By 1992 the Berlin Wall came down, and the Cold War drew to a close. The final spasm of the Cold War and antibiotic resistance played out in post-Communist Russia and the republics of the former USSR.

Prior to the end of Communism, the Soviet Union boasted an

extensive and effective tuberculosis treatment infrastructure. Screening for infections using roentgen flourography was implemented in the 1940s, and in 1943 streptomycin (purchased in the United States) was first used to treat the scientist Otto Schmidt. Streptomycin was being produced by 1947, thanks to the efforts of Zinaida Ermol'eva. In the 1960s, the Soviet TB program had over six thousand locations, sixteen thousand specialists, and over a quarter of a million hospital and sanatorium beds for patients. The bacille Calmette-Guérino vaccine was widely used as were mass screening techniques. Patients were granted up to ten months of disability support by the state and job protection that extended to a full year. According to one study, "The state provided patients with TB with extra living space, a remarkable benefit considering that most of the population lived in shared, congested apartments and barracks."[60]

And then the Soviet Union ceased to exist.

The breathtaking swiftness of Communism's demise caught most of the world flat-footed. The social and economic destabilization of the USSR led to its TB control program's being dangerously underfunded. As funding decreased, so did compensation for health care professionals involved in the field, resulting in an exodus of medical and research personnel. As the dominoes continued to fall, the lack of funds led to the cessation of screening, which is so important to controlling the spread of the disease. Most concerning, the broken infrastructure created shortages of antibiotics and irregular regimens. These results proved disastrous as TB incidence and mortality increased parabolically between 1991 and 2004. They also provided the perfect environment for resistance to arise, and it did.[61]

The penitentiary system suffered a serious epidemic of multidrug-resistant TB starting in the late 1990s. By 1999, 25 percent of Russia's total new infections were in prison populations. It took a decade's worth of concerted effort from the Russian government, nongovernmental organizations, and international health groups such as the World Health Organization to bring the epidemic under control. To this day, multidrug-resistant TB remains a serious problem in the Russian penitentiary system, though it is under control by prison officials and the Ministry of Public Health.[62]

THE COLD WAR IS a distant memory now. Most of the battle lines that divided East and West have either disappeared or been transformed and redefined. The economic and political skirmishes over antibiotics have given way to institutional apathy across the globe. And that's a problem that transcends orders and ideologies. As antibiotic resistance has grown in severity, the development of novel antimicrobials has dwindled. The so-called miracle drugs that the great powers jostled over have become an afterthought.

While the effectiveness of antibiotics has undoubtedly been weakened, they were also victims of their own success. By design, they are meant to cure and not prevent. The course of typical antibiotic treatment lasts for only a few days, whereas drugs such as Metformin (diabetes) and Humira (Crohn's disease) are meant to be taken for decades. The implications are drastic. If penicillin were developed today, it would be considered a money-losing proposition. As such, pharmaceutical companies would have steered clear of it. Indeed, that has proven to be the case. Antibiotic startups such as Achaogen and Aradigm have gone out of business in recent years. Even companies such as Melinta Therapeutics that successfully develop novel drugs have ultimately failed and filed for bankruptcy protection. In truth, the most debilitating blow to antibiotics may be one entirely outside of the scientific realm.

Ironically, after all of the ideological chest-thumping that occurred during the Cold War, the inability of pharmaceutical companies to figure out how to balance profit and necessity has exposed a weakness in the free market. Antibiotic resistance has raised an interesting question regarding current economic systems: when does the common good trump profits?

NOTES

Introduction

1. U.S. House of Representatives, "Combating Superbugs."

Chapter 1

1. Hastings, *Winston's War*.
2. Lax, *Mold in Dr. Florey's Coat*, chap. 6.
3. Lax, *Mold in Dr. Florey's Coat*, chap. 6.
4. Lax, *Mold in Dr. Florey's Coat*, chap. 6.
5. Lax, *Mold in Dr. Florey's Coat*, chap. 6.
6. Lax, *Mold in Dr. Florey's Coat*, chap. 7.
7. Hobby, *Penicillin*, 69–80.
8. Lax, *Mold in Dr. Florey's Coat*, chap. 8.
9. Lax, *Mold in Dr. Florey's Coat*, chap. 9.
10. Lax, *Mold in Dr. Florey's Coat*, chap. 9.
11. Lax, *Mold in Dr. Florey's Coat*, chap. 9.
12. Lax, *Mold in Dr. Florey's Coat*, chap. 9.
13. Khlevniuk, *Stalin*, chap. 5.
14. Roberts, *Stalin's Wars*, chap. 3.
15. Khlevniuk, *Stalin*, chap. 5.
16. O'Sullivan, *Harry Hopkins*, chap. 4.
17. O'Sullivan, *Harry Hopkins*, chap. 4.
18. O'Sullivan, *Harry Hopkins*, chap. 4.
19. O'Sullivan, *Harry Hopkins*, chap. 4.
20. Khlevniuk, *Stalin*, chap. 3.
21. O'Sullivan, *Harry Hopkins*, chap. 4.
22. Zachary, *Endless Frontier*.
23. Zachary, *Endless Frontier*, 89–118.
24. Zachary, *Endless Frontier*, 89–118.
25. Zachary, *Endless Frontier*, 89–118.
26. Lax, *Mold in Dr. Florey's Coat*, chap. 9.
27. Lax, *Mold in Dr. Florey's Coat*, chap. 9.
28. Lax, *Mold in Dr. Florey's Coat*, chap. 9.

29. Lax, *Mold in Dr. Florey's Coat*, chap. 9.

30. Lax, *Mold in Dr. Florey's Coat*, chap. 9.

31. Lax, *Mold in Dr. Florey's Coat*, chap. 9.

32. Lax, *Mold in Dr. Florey's Coat*, chap. 9.

33. Herrick to May, memo, October 9, 1941, Records of the Office of Science Research and Development, Record Group 227 (hereafter RG 227), National Archives and Records Administration (NARA), College Park MD.

34. Lax, *Mold in Dr. Florey's Coat*, chap. 9.

35. May to Northern Regional Research Laboratory, memo, October 9, 1941, RG 227, NARA, College Park MD.

36. Lax, *Mold in Dr. Florey's Coat*, chap. 9.

37. Brockman, *History of Penicillin Production*, 25–30.

38. Heatley to Knight, letter, September 29, 1941, RG 227, NARA, College Park MD.

39. Lax, *Mold in Dr. Florey's Coat*, chap. 9.

40. Lax, *Mold in Dr. Florey's Coat*, chap. 9.

41. Lax, *Mold in Dr. Florey's Coat*, chap. 9.

42. Lax, *Mold in Dr. Florey's Coat*, chap. 9.

43. Lax, *Mold in Dr. Florey's Coat*, chap. 9.

44. "Notes on penicillin," memo, June 13, 1945, RG 227, NARA, College Park MD.

45. Lax, *Mold in Dr. Florey's Coat*, chap. 9.

46. Pringle, *Murder of Nikolai Vavilov*.

47. Birstein, *Perversion of Knowledge*, part 4.

48. Birstein, *Perversion of Knowledge*, part 4.

49. Zachary, *Endless Frontier*, 89–118.

50. Bush, *Science, the Endless Frontier*, 135.

51. Stewart, *Organizing Scientific Research for War*, 105.

52. Stewart, *Organizing Scientific Research for War*, 35.

53. Stewart, *Organizing Scientific Research for War*, 35.

54. Stewart, *Organizing Scientific Research for War*, 59.

55. Stewart, *Organizing Scientific Research for War*, 123.

56. Herrick to May, memo, September 29, 1941, RG 227, NARA, College Park MD.

57. Herrick to May, memo, September 30, 1941, RG 227, NARA, College Park MD.

58. Conference on penicillin, minutes, Washington DC, October 8, 1941, RG 227, NARA, College Park MD.

59. Conference on penicillin, minutes, Washington DC, October 8, 1941, RG 227, NARA, College Park MD.

Chapter 2

1. Hayes, *Burdens of Disease*, chap. 4.

2. Conference on penicillin, minutes, Washington DC, October 8, 1941, RG 227, NARA, College Park MD.

3. Rosen, *Miracle Cure*, chap. 5.

4. Conference on penicillin, minutes, Washington DC, October 8, 1941, RG 227, NARA, College Park MD.

5. Conference on penicillin, minutes, Washington DC, October 8, 1941, RG 227, NARA, College Park MD.

6. Perlman, "Evolution," 25.

7. Hobby, *Penicillin*, 69–80.

8. Hobby, *Penicillin*, 75.

9. Conference on penicillin, minutes, Washington DC, October 8, 1941, RG 227, NARA, College Park MD.

10. Conference on penicillin, minutes, Washington DC, October 8, 1941, RG 227, NARA, College Park MD.

11. Conference on penicillin, minutes, Washington DC, October 8, 1941, RG 227, NARA, College Park MD.

12. A. N. Richards, telephone conversation with George Merck, November 14, 1941, RG 227, NARA, College Park MD.

13. A. N. Richards, telephone conversation with George Merck, November 14, 1941, RG 227, NARA, College Park MD.

14. Amyes, *Magic Bullets*, 1–21.

15. Amyes, *Magic Bullets*, 1–21.

16. Amyes, *Magic Bullets*, 1–21.

17. Amyes, *Magic Bullets*, 1–21.

18. Amyes, *Magic Bullets*, 1–21.

19. Amyes, *Magic Bullets*, 1–21.

20. A. N. Richards, telephone conversation with George Merck, November 14, 1941, RG 227, NARA, College Park MD.

21. A. N. Richards, telephone conversation with George Merck, November 14, 1941, RG 227, NARA, College Park MD.

22. Shama, "Zones of Inhibition?," 133–58.

23. Shama, "Zones of Inhibition?," 133–58.

24. Shama, "Zones of Inhibition?," 133–58.

25. Shama, "Zones of Inhibition?," 133–58.

26. Shama, "Zones of Inhibition?," 136.

27. Shama, "Zones of Inhibition?," 133–58.

28. Shama, "Pilzkrieg," 120–23.

29. Overy, *Russia's War*, chap. 4.

30. Overy, *Russia's War*, chap. 4.

31. Kutter et al., "Phage Therapy," 112-1–112-12.

32. Summers, "Strange History," 130–33.

33. Summers, "Strange History," 130–33.

34. Personal correspondence with Nina Chanishvili (Eliava Institute), February 2, 2018.

35. Personal correspondence with Nina Chanishvili (Eliava Institute), February 2, 2018.

36. Personal correspondence with Nina Chanishvili (Eliava Institute), February 2, 2018.

37. Personal correspondence with Nina Chanishvili (Eliava Institute), February 2, 2018.

38. Personal correspondence with Nina Chanishvili (Eliava Institute), February 2, 2018.

39. Borodin, *One Man*, 233–34.

40. Borodin, *One Man*, 233–34.

41. Borodin, *One Man*, 233–34.

42. Kaiser, *No End Save Victory*, chap. 3.

43. A. J. Moyer and N. G. Heatley, *Report of Cooperative Work on Penicillin Production*, RG 227, NARA, College Park MD.

44. Brockman, *History of Penicillin Production*, 18.

45. Abraham, "Beta-Lactams Antibiotics," 76–86.

46. Brockman, *History of Penicillin Production*, 33–36.

47. Brockman, *History of Penicillin Production*, 15–21.

Chapter 3

1. Williams, *Howard Florey*, 152–75.

2. Williams, *Howard Florey*, 152–75.

3. Williams, *Howard Florey*, 152–75.

4. Williams, *Howard Florey*, 152–75.

5. Williams, *Howard Florey*, 152–75.

6. Bickel, *Rise Up to Life*, 156–74.

7. Bickel, *Rise Up to Life*, 156–74.

8. Bickel, *Rise Up to Life*, 156–74.

9. Bickel, *Rise Up to Life*, 156–74.

10. Burns, Bennett, and van Dijck, "Code Name Bacinol," 25–32.

11. Burns, Bennett, and van Dijck, "Code Name Bacinol," 25–32.

12. Burns, Bennett, and van Dijck, "Code Name Bacinol," 25–32.

13. Roberts, *Stalin's Wars*, chap. 5.

14. Roberts, *Stalin's Wars*, chap. 5.

15. Werth, *Russia at War*, 441–507.

16. Kutter et al., "Phage Therapy," 112-1–112-12.

17. Carlton, "Phage Therapy," 267–74.

18. Carlton, "Phage Therapy," 267–74.

19. Carlton, "Phage Therapy," 267–74.

20. Carlton, "Phage Therapy," 267–74.

21. Carlton, "Phage Therapy," 267–74.

22. "Penicillin Research and Production in the USSR," top secret information report, October 14, 1948, CIA Records Search Tool (CREST), NARA, College Park MD.

23. Gall and Konashev, "Discovery of Gramicidin S," 137–50.

24. Gause and Brazhnikova, "Gramicidin S," 703.
25. Gause and Brazhnikova, "Gramicidin S," 703.
26. Gause and Brazhnikova, "Gramicidin S," 703.
27. Gall and Konashev, "Discovery of Gramicidin S," 137–50.
28. Dimbleby, *Destiny in the Desert*, chap. 23.
29. Dimbleby, *Destiny in the Desert*, chap. 23. Brackets in original.
30. Dimbleby, *Destiny in the Desert*, chap. 23.
31. Dimbleby, *Destiny in the Desert*, chap. 23.
32. Dimbleby, *Destiny in the Desert*, chap. 23.
33. Dimbleby, *Destiny in the Desert*, chap. 23.
34. Dimbleby, *Destiny in the Desert*, preface.
35. D'Este, *World War II*, chap. 1.
36. D'Este, *World War II*, 6.
37. D'Este, *World War II*, chap. 2.
38. D'Este, *World War II*, chap. 2.
39. Federal Trade Commission (FTC), *Economic Report*, 46–62.
40. Bickel, *Rise Up to Life*, 193–207.
41. Bickel, *Rise Up to Life*, 194.
42. Bickel, *Rise Up to Life*, 194.
43. Bickel, *Rise Up to Life*, 194.
44. Bickel, *Rise Up to Life*, 194.
45. "200 Die 100 Hurt as Flames Destroy Boston Night Club," *New York Herald Tribune*, November 29, 1942.
46. "Deaths Reach 433 in Boston Night Club Fire," *New York Herald Tribune*, November 30, 1942.
47. Homer Bigart, "Boston Recoils from Horror of Nightclub Fire," *New York Herald Tribune*, November 30, 1942.
48. Cope, "Treatment of the Surface Burns," 886.
49. Cope, "Treatment of the Surface Burns," 885–93.
50. "Jammed Door's Toll Is Stressed in Boston Fire," *New York Herald Tribune*, December 3, 1942.
51. Lombardino, "Brief History," 10–15.
52. Hobby, *Penicillin*, 182.
53. Brockman, *History of Penicillin Production*, 3–11.
54. Fraser, "Penicillin," 1723–25.
55. Williams, *Howard Florey*, 159.
56. Williams, *Howard Florey*, 174. Brackets in original.
57. Fraser, "Penicillin," 1723–25.
58. Fraser, "Penicillin," 1723–25.
59. Elder, *History of Penicillin Production*, 4.
60. Richards to Bush, "Penicillin," August 14, 1943, RG 227, NARA, College Park MD.

61. A. Baird Hastings and Michael B. Shimkin, "Report of American Representatives of Medical Research Mission to the Soviet Union," confidential report, April 17, 1944, RG 227, NARA, College Park MD.

62. Shimkin, "Roads to Oz," 572.

63. Shimkin, "Roads to Oz," 565–86.

64. Williams, *Howard Florey*, 196–218.

65. Williams, *Howard Florey*, 188.

66. Hastings and Shimkin, "Report of American Representatives," RG 227, NARA, College Park MD.

67. Myelnikov, "Alternative Cure," 402.

68. Myelnikov, "Alternative Cure."

69. Shimkin, "Roads to Oz," 565–86.

70. Williams, *Howard Florey*, 196–218.

71. Myelnikov, "Alternative Cure," 402.

72. Myelnikov, "Alternative Cure," 385–411.

73. Myelnikov, "Alternative Cure," 385–411.

74. Hastings and Shimkin, "Report of American Representatives," RG 227, NARA, College Park MD.

75. Brockman, *History of Penicillin Production*, 19.

76. Brockman, *History of Penicillin Production*, 19.

Chapter 4

1. Southard, *Nagasaki*, chap. 2.

2. Southard, *Nagasaki*, chap. 2.

3. Southard, *Nagasaki*, chap. 2.

4. Southard, *Nagasaki*, chap. 4.

5. Southard, *Nagasaki*, chap. 5.

6. Southard, *Nagasaki*, chap. 3.

7. Southard, *Nagasaki*, chap. 3.

8. Zinn, *The Bomb*, pt. 1.

9. Berinsky, "Assuming the Costs," 975–97.

10. Bocker and Knorre, "Antibiotica Research," 35–40.

11. American Embassy, Mexico, to Secretary of State, aerogram, February 29, 1944, RG 227, NARA, College Park MD.

12. Roy S. Koch to James Pilcher, letter, March 17, 1944, RG 227, NARA, College Park MD.

13. Thomas H. Locket to Cordell Hull, "Application to Mexican-American Commission for Economic Cooperation by E.R. Squibb & Sons de Mexico, S.A. for New Plant for Making Penicillin," memo, December 21, 1943, RG 227, NARA, College Park MD.

14. Locket to Hull, "Application," RG 227, NARA, College Park MD.

15. William Conkright to Cordell Hull, "Proposed Production of Penicillin in Mexico," memo, March 10, 1944, RG 227, NARA, College Park MD.

16. Conkright to Hull, "Proposed Production," RG 227, NARA, College Park MD.
17. Reinisch, *Perils of Peace*, 1–37.
18. Reinisch, *Perils of Peace*, chap. 1.
19. Reinisch, *Perils of Peace*, 31.
20. Reinisch, *Perils of Peace*, 41.
21. Reinisch, *Perils of Peace*, 159.
22. Reinisch, *Perils of Peace*, 152.
23. Sams, *Medic*, 103–4.
24. Green, Talbot, and Morton, "Control of Syphilis," 214–17.
25. Green, Talbot, and Morton, "Control of Syphilis," 214–17.
26. Rasnake et al., "History of U.S. Military," 61–65.
27. Rasnake et al., "History of U.S. Military," 61–65.
28. Sams, *Medic*, 103.
29. Roberts, "Price of Discretion," 1004.
30. Roberts, "Price of Discretion," 1002–30.
31. Roberts, "Price of Discretion," 1015.
32. Roberts, "Price of Discretion," 1002–30.
33. Roberts, "Price of Discretion," 1002–30.
34. Roberts, "Price of Discretion," 1002–30.
35. Morabia, "'East Side Story,'" 115.
36. Sams, *Medic*, 81–91.
37. Sams, *Medic*, 81–91.
38. Moberg, "René Dubos," 559–80.
39. Kingston, "Streptomycin," 441–62.
40. Pringle, *Experiment Eleven*, chap. 3.
41. Pringle, *Experiment Eleven*, chap. 4.
42. Pringle, *Experiment Eleven*, chap. 4.
43. Pringle, *Experiment Eleven*, chap. 4.
44. Pringle, *Experiment Eleven*, chap. 6.

Chapter 5

1. Sidney Shalett, "U.S. Was Prepared to Combat Axis in Poison-Germ Warfare," *New York Times*, January 3, 1946.
2. *U.S. Army Activities in the United States Biological Warfare Programs, 1942–1977*, vol. 1, iv, Records of the Central Intelligence Agency, Record Group 263 (hereafter RG 263), NARA, College Park MD.
3. *U.S. Army Activities*, RG 263, NARA, College Park MD.
4. *U.S. Army Activities*, RG 263, NARA, College Park MD.
5. George Merck, *Report to the Secretary of War by Mr. George Merck, Special Consultant for Biological Warfare*, 3, RG 263, NARA, College Park MD.
6. Merck, *Report to the Secretary of War*, RG 263, NARA, College Park MD.
7. Merck, *Report to the Secretary of War*, 5, RG 263, NARA, College Park MD.
8. Merck, *Report to the Secretary of War*, 5, RG 263, NARA, College Park MD.

9. Alibek, *Biohazard*.

10. Riddle, "Biological Warfare," 400–406.

11. Merck, *Report to the Secretary of War*, 5, RG 263, NARA, College Park MD.

12. Guillemin, *Hidden Atrocities*, chap. 1.

13. Harris, "Japanese Biological Warfare," 171–99.

14. Guillemin, *Hidden Atrocities*, chap. 1.

15. Guillemin, *Hidden Atrocities*, chap. 1.

16. Jeans, "Alarm in Washington," 411–39.

17. Gold, *Unit 731*, chap. 4.

18. Guillemin, *Hidden Atrocities*, chap. 1.

19. Guillemin, *Hidden Atrocities*, chap. 1.

20. Guillemin, *Hidden Atrocities*, chap. 1.

21. Harris, *Factories of Death*.

22. "Scientists See U.S. Very Vulnerable to Germ Warfare," *New York Times*, May 19, 1947; "Congressmen Reveal Germ Weapon Can Wipe out City at Single Blow," *New York Times*, May 25, 1946; Hanson W. Baldwin, "Destruction by Disease Looms as Rival to Atomic Bombs and Gases," *New York Times*, July 14, 1946; and "Bacteria Put above A-Bomb as Weapon," *New York Times*, October 16, 1947.

23. C. B. Allen, "Forrestal Scoffs at Idea of Germ 'Super-Weapon,'" *New York Herald Tribune*, March 13, 1949.

24. Newman, *Japan's Secret Weapon*.

25. Jeans, "Alarm in Washington," 411–39.

26. Jeans, "Alarm in Washington," 423.

27. Jeans, "Alarm in Washington," 423.

28. Sams, *Medic*, 92–101.

29. Sams, *Medic*, 92–101.

30. Albrecht, "Inherited Epidemic," 57–81.

31. Albrecht, "Inherited Epidemic," 57–81.

32. Sams, *Medic*, 92–101.

33. Sams, *Medic*, 92–101.

34. Albrecht, "Inherited Epidemic," 57–81.

35. Sams, *Medic*, 92–101.

36. FTC, *Economic Report*, chap. 3.

37. FTC, *Economic Report*, chap. 3.

38. FTC, *Economic Report*, chap. 3.

39. Raper, "Progress of Antibiotics," 49–57.

40. Brockman, *History of Penicillin Production*, 25–30.

41. Brockman, *History of Penicillin Production*, 25–30.

42. Robinson, "Chemistry of Penicillin," 274–76.

43. Steven Spencer, "The Great Penicillin Mystery," *Saturday Evening Post*, August 3, 1946, 11.

44. Spencer, "Great Penicillin Mystery," 11.

45. Spencer, "Great Penicillin Mystery," 11.
46. Abraham and Chain, "Enzyme from Bacteria."
47. Spencer, "Great Penicillin Mystery," 11.
48. Spencer, "Great Penicillin Mystery," 11.
49. Spencer, "Great Penicillin Mystery," 11.
50. Spencer, "Great Penicillin Mystery," 11.

Chapter 6

1. "Soviet Intelligence Targets in the United States," top secret information report, October 14, 1948, CREST, NARA, College Park MD.
2. Zelchenko, "Stealing America's Know-how."
3. Zelchenko, "Stealing America's Know-how."
4. Shama, "No New Thing," 1–4.
5. Borodin, *One Man*, 245–60.
6. "Penicillin Research and Production in the USSR," top secret information report, October 14, 1948, CREST, NARA, College Park MD.
7. Williams, *Howard Florey*, 176–95.
8. Williams, *Howard Florey*, 176–95.
9. Borodin, Philpot, and Florey, "Antibiotic from *Penicillium tardum*," 31–34.
10. "Penicillin Research and Production in the USSR," top secret information report, October 14, 1948, CREST, NARA, College Park MD.
11. "Soviet Intelligence Targets in the United States," top secret information report, October 14, 1948, CREST, NARA, College Park MD.
12. Gaddis, *George F. Kennan*, chap. 6.
13. George Kennan, "Long Telegram," February 22, 1946, Wilson Center Digital Archive, https://digitalarchive.wilsoncenter.org/document/116178.
14. Krementsov, *Stalinist Science*, 129–57.
15. Medvedev, *Rise and Fall*, 103–39.
16. Medvedev, *Rise and Fall*, 103–39.
17. Myelnikov, "Alternative Cure," 385–411.
18. "The Soviet BW Program," 51, secret report, RG 263, NARA, College Park MD.
19. "Conference with Byelorussian Ministry of Health," minutes, United Nations (UN), Archives and Records, New York.
20. Łotysz, "'Lasting Memorial,'" 70–91.
21. Eric Holland, *Penicillin Plant Project: Medical and Sanitation Supplies Division*, July 29, 1947, UN, Archives and Records, New York.
22. "Conference with Byelorussian Ministry of Health," March 26, 1947, 1, UN, Archives and Records, New York.
23. "Conference with Byelorussian Ministry of Health," March 26, 1947, 1, UN, Archives and Records, New York.
24. "Conference with Byelorussian Ministry of Health," UN, Archives and Records, New York.

25. Holland, *Penicillin Plant Project*, UN, Archives and Records, New York.
26. Łotysz, "'Lasting Memorial,'" 70–91.
27. Holland, *Penicillin Plant Project*, 4, UN, Archives and Records, New York.
28. Łotysz, "'Lasting Memorial,'" 70–91.
29. Łotysz, "'Lasting Memorial,'" 70–91.
30. "Drug Rushed to Save Boy," *New York Times*, November 24, 1946.
31. "Streptomycin Flown to Manila," *New York Times*, November 29, 1946.
32. "Pleas to Save Boy Fail," *New York Times*, April 10, 1946.
33. "Drug Rushed to Save Boy," *New York Times*, November 24, 1946.
34. Reinisch, *Perils of Peace*, chap. 5.
35. Reinisch, *Perils of Peace*, 214.
36. Reinisch, *Perils of Peace*, chap. 4.
37. "Penicillin—Issues to Displaced Persons and German Civil Population, for the Treatment of Disease Other than Gonorrhaea," August 13, 1946, 1, UN, Archives and Records, New York.
38. "Administrative Order No. 125-Penicillin," August 2, 1946, UN, Archives and Records, New York.
39. Plough, "Penicillin Resistance," 446–51.
40. Barber, "Staphylococcal Infection," 863.
41. Berg, "History of Genetics."
42. Weisfeld, "Importance of Discovery," 271–76.
43. Weisfeld, "Importance of Discovery," 271–76.
44. Weisfeld, "Importance of Discovery," 271–76.
45. Krementsov, *Soviet Science*, 97.
46. Weisfeld, "Importance of Discovery," 271–76.
47. Weisfeld, "Importance of Discovery," 271–76.
48. Medvedev, *Rise and Fall*, 115–21.
49. Medvedev, *Rise and Fall*, 115–21.
50. Krementsov, "'K.R.' Affair," 419–46.
51. Krementsov, "'K.R.' Affair," 419–46.
52. Krementsov, "'K.R.' Affair," 419–46.
53. Krementsov, "'K.R.' Affair," 432.
54. Krementsov, "'K.R.' Affair," 419–46.
55. Krementsov, "'K.R.' Affair," 419–46.
56. Medvedev, *Rise and Fall*, 117.
57. Berg, "History of Genetics."
58. Medvedev, *Rise and Fall*, 115–21.
59. Joravsky, *Lysenko Affair*, 97–143.
60. Capocci, "Chain Is Gonna Come," 61–80.
61. Capocci, "Chain Is Gonna Come," 61–80.
62. Borodin, *One Man*, 342.

Chapter 7

1. Kruger, *Logistics Matters*, 1–23.
2. Kruger, *Logistics Matters*, 1–23.
3. Kruger, *Logistics Matters*, 1–23.
4. Kruger, *Logistics Matters*, 1–23.
5. Kruger, *Logistics Matters*, 1–23.
6. Summers, "Strange History," 130–33.
7. Summers, "Strange History," 131.
8. Ho, "Bacteriophage Therapy," 1–16.
9. Ho, "Bacteriophage Therapy," 6.
10. Summers, "Strange History," 130–33.
11. Eaton and Bayne-Jones, "Bacteriophage Therapy," 1848.
12. Summers, "Strange History," 130–33.
13. Krueger and Scribner, "The Bacteriophage," 2269–77.
14. Krueger and Scribner, "The Bacteriophage," 2277.
15. Krueger and Scribner, "The Bacteriophage," 2277.
16. Krueger and Scribner, "The Bacteriophage," 2277.
17. Eli Lilly, *Elements of Biologics*, 143–48.
18. Eli Lilly, *Elements of Biologics*, 147.
19. Summers, "Strange History," 130–33.
20. Eli Lilly, *Elements of Biologics*, 143–48.
21. Kardos and Demain, "Ernst Chain," 6618.
22. Kardos and Demain, "Ernst Chain," 6613–22.
23. Kardos and Demain, "Ernst Chain," 6613–22.
24. Capocci, "Chain Is Gonna Come," 61–80.
25. Bundy, "There Was a Man."
26. Capocci, "Chain Is Gonna Come," 61–80.
27. Brockman, *History of Penicillin Production*, 45–50.
28. Brockman, *History of Penicillin Production*, 45–50.
29. Brockman, *History of Penicillin Production*, 45–50.
30. Łotysz, *Building a Lasting Monument*, 78.
31. Łotysz, *Building a Lasting Monument*, 80.
32. "Items under Unilateral U.S. Denial Policy to the Soviet Bloc," 2, RG 263, NARA, College Park MD.
33. Taroni, "Fabricca della Penicillina," 639–62.
34. Ernst Chain, "Banquet Speech," Stockholm, December 10, 1945, https://www.nobelprize.org/prizes/medicine/1945/chain/speech/.
35. Taroni, "Fabricca della Penicillina," 639–62.
36. Taroni, "Fabricca della Penicillina," 639–62.
37. Taroni, "Fabricca della Penicillina," 639–62.
38. Burns, Bennett, and van Dijck, "Code Name Bacinol," 31.
39. Burns, Bennett, and van Dijck, "Code Name Bacinol," 25–31.

40. Rane and Rane, "Aureomycin," 18–23.

41. Rane and Rane, "Aureomycin," 18–23.

42. Lombardino, "Brief History," 10–15.

43. Jones, "Effect of Antibiotic Substances."

44. Torres-Barceló and Hochberg, "Evolutionary Rationale," 249–56.

Chapter 8

1. "Proclamation of China's Communist Government (Transcript of Speech)," *New York Times*, October 3, 1949.

2. Cain, *Economic Statecraft*, 2.

3. Ernest M. Lippa, "I Was a Surgeon for the Chinese Reds," *Saturday Evening Post*, May 12, 1953.

4. Lippa, "I Was a Surgeon," 186.

5. Cain, *Economic Statecraft*, 14–26.

6. Cain, *Economic Statecraft*, 14–26.

7. Cain, *Economic Statecraft*, 5.

8. "Items under Unilateral U.S. Denial Policy to the Soviet Bloc," RG 263, NARA, College Park MD.

9. "Items under Unilateral U.S. Denial Policy to the Soviet Bloc," RG 263, NARA, College Park MD.

10. Cain, *Economic Statecraft*, 14–26.

11. Cain, *Economic Statecraft*, 7.

12. Cain, *Economic Statecraft*, 14–26.

13. Cain, *Economic Statecraft*, 14–26.

14. Cain, *Economic Statecraft*, 10.

15. Kruger, *Logistics Matters*, 2–24.

16. Kruger, *Logistics Matters*, 130–35.

17. Simpson, *Science of Coercion*, 219.

18. Simpson, *Science of Coercion*, 222.

19. Simpson, *Science of Coercion*, 3–75.

20. Kruger, *Logistics Matters*, 156.

21. Reinisch, *Perils of Peace*, 214.

22. "Soviet Production of Penicillin," secret report, RG 263, NARA, College Park MD.

23. Medvedev, *Rise and Fall*, 121. Parentheses in original.

24. Medvedev, *Rise and Fall*, 122.

25. Medvedev, *Rise and Fall*, 103–39.

26. Medvedev, *Rise and Fall*, 103–39.

27. Medvedev, *Rise and Fall*, 103–39.

28. "Soviet Widening Scientists' Purge," *New York Times*, September 23, 1948.

29. Łotysz, "'Lasting Memorial,'" 78.

30. Łotysz, "'Lasting Memorial,'" 70–91.

31. Łotysz, "'Lasting Memorial,'" 70–91.

32. Łotysz, "'Lasting Memorial,'" 70–91.
33. Łotysz, "'Lasting Memorial,'" 70–91.
34. "Russia Held Capable of Supplying Drugs," *New York Times*, March 8, 1949.
35. Łotysz, "'Lasting Memorial,'" 70–91.
36. Łotysz, "'Lasting Memorial,'" 70–91.
37. Harriman, *Mutual Defense*, 7.
38. Harriman, *Mutual Defense*.
39. Capocci, "Cold Drugs," 408.
40. Capocci, "Cold Drugs," 401–22.
41. Aminov, "History of Antimicrobial Drug," 4–19.
42. Aminov, "History of Antimicrobial Drug," 4–19.
43. Aminov, "History of Antimicrobial Drug," 4–19.
44. Aminov, "History of Antimicrobial Drug," 4–19.
45. Wang, "Cold War."
46. Wang, "Cold War."
47. Wang, "Cold War."
48. Wang, "Cold War."
49. Krementsov, "In the Shadow," 59.
50. Krementsov, "In the Shadow," 59.

Chapter 9

1. Haruki, *Korean War*, chap. 3.
2. Manring et al., "Treatment of War Wounds," 2168–91.
3. Murray, Hinkle, and Yun, "History of Infections," 221–31.
4. Murray, Hinkle, and Yun, "History of Infections," 221–31.
5. Murray, Hinkle, and Yun, "History of Infections," 221–31.
6. Sams, *Medic*, 209–30.
7. Sams, *Medic*, 217.
8. Cain, *Economic Statecraft*, 27–39.
9. Cain, *Economic Statecraft*, 13.
10. Cain, *Economic Statecraft*, 27–39.
11. Cain, *Economic Statecraft*, 14–26.
12. "The Antibiotic Industry in the Soviet Bloc," secret intelligence report, RG 263, NARA, College Park MD.
13. "The Antibiotic Industry in the Soviet Bloc," secret intelligence report, RG 263, NARA, College Park MD.
14. "The Antibiotic Industry in the Soviet Bloc," secret intelligence report, RG 263, NARA, College Park MD.
15. "The Antibiotic Industry in the Soviet Bloc," secret intelligence report, RG 263, NARA, College Park MD.
16. "The Antibiotic Industry in the Soviet Bloc," secret intelligence report, RG 263, NARA, College Park MD.

17. Kate Connolly, “Harry in the Shadows,” *Guardian*, July 9, 1999, https://www.theguardian.com/books/1999/jul/10/books.guardianreview10.

18. Connolly, “Harry in the Shadows.”

19. Santemases, “Long Postwar,” 615–38.

20. Kruger, *Logistics Matters*, 20.

21. Herbert Socks, “I Had to Be Heartless,” *Saturday Evening Post*, April 2, 1955, 30, 116.

22. Oskar Morgenstern, “Capitalist Oasis: On Rim of China's Red Desert, a Free Market Booms,” *Wall Street Journal*, November 30, 1954, 12.

23. Lai, “Historical Review.”

24. Philip Potter, “Suspense in Hong Kong: Booming Trade with Communist China,” *Manchester Guardian*, February 6, 1951.

25. Price Day, “The China Trade,” *Sun*, December 30, 1953, 12.

26. “The Antibiotic Industry in the Soviet Bloc,” 2, secret intelligence report, RG 263, NARA, College Park MD.

27. Morgenstern, “Capitalist Oasis,” 12.

Chapter 10

1. Tikhonov and Gregory, “Stalin's Last Plan,” 159–92.

2. “Antibiotics in the Soviet Bloc,” intelligence report, November 15, 1954, RG 263, NARA, College Park MD.

3. “Antibiotics in the Soviet Bloc,” intelligence report, November 15, 1954, RG 263, NARA, College Park MD.

4. A. I. Nesterov, “Analysis of Soviet Penicillin Sample,” information report, September 8, 1950, CREST, NARA, College Park MD.

5. Nesterov, “Analysis of Soviet Penicillin Sample,” information report, September 8, 1950, CREST, NARA, College Park MD.

6. “Production of Streptomycin at Jenapharm, Jena,” intelligence report, August 27, 1953, RG 263, NARA, College Park MD.

7. “Antibiotics in the Soviet Bloc,” intelligence report, November 15, 1954, RG 263, NARA, College Park MD.

8. “Antibiotics in the Soviet Bloc,” intelligence report, November 15, 1954, RG 263, NARA, College Park MD.

9. “Antibiotics in the Soviet Bloc,” intelligence report, November 15, 1954, RG 263, NARA, College Park MD.

10. “Effects of Western Embargo,” intelligence report, December 30, 1953, RG 263, NARA, College Park MD.

11. “Antibiotics in the Soviet Bloc,” intelligence report, November 15, 1954, 9, RG 263, NARA, College Park MD.

12. “Penicillin Production of the Jenapharm Plant,” intelligence report, March 26, 1951, RG 263, NARA, College Park MD.

13. “Personnel and Production, Zeus's, Jena,” intelligence report, October 16, 1950, RG 263, NARA, College Park MD.

14. Horst Willim, "Political—Sabotage," intelligence report, December 10, 1953, RG 263, NARA, College Park MD.

15. Myelnikov, "Alternative Cure," 408.

16. Mudd, "Staphylococcus Problem," 41–45.

17. Mudd, "Staphylococcus Problem," 41–45.

18. Bud, *Penicillin*, 61.

19. FTC, *Economic Report*, 199–223.

20. FTC, *Economic Report*, 199–223.

21. FTC, *Economic Report*, 199–223. In 2009 alone, anti-infective substances derived from this bacteria accounted for $79 billion and a total of roughly 166 antibiotics. Among all bioactive compounds, 45 percent are produced by actinomycetes and 38 percent by fungi, and 17 percent by unicellular eubacteria.

22. Philpot, "Penicillin-like Substance," 725.

23. Cook and Lacey, "Kojic Acid," 790.

24. Chen et al., "Antibiotic Substance," 234.

25. Falagas and Kasaikou, "Colistin," 1333–41.

26. Umemura, *Japanese Pharmaceutical Industry*, chap. 3.

27. Umemura, *Japanese Pharmaceutical Industry*, chap. 3.

28. Umemura, *Japanese Pharmaceutical Industry*, chap. 3.

29. Leitenberg, "New Russian Evidence," 185–99.

30. Leitenberg, "New Russian Evidence," 185–99.

31. Leitenberg, "New Russian Evidence," 185–99.

32. Leitenberg, "New Russian Evidence," 185–99.

33. Leitenberg, "New Russian Evidence," 185–99.

34. Leitenberg, "New Russian Evidence," 185–99.

35. Leitenberg, "New Russian Evidence," 185–99.

36. Leitenberg, "New Russian Evidence," 185–99.

Chapter 11

1. Harry B. Price and Roy E. Foulke, interview with Gen. George C. Marshall, Truman Library, February 18, 1953.

2. Harry B. Price and Roy E. Foulke, interview with Gen. George C. Marshall, Truman Library, February 18, 1953.

3. George C. Marshall, "European Initiative Essential to Economic Recovery: Remarks by the Secretary of State," Harvard University, June 5, 1947, in *Record of the Week*, June 15, 1947, 1160, Truman Library, https://www.trumanlibrary.gov/library/research-files/speech-george-c-marshall-european-initiative-essential-economic-recovery.

4. George C. Marshall, "European Initiative Essential to Economic Recovery."

5. Applebaum, *Iron Curtain*, chap. 9.

6. Applebaum, *Iron Curtain*, chap. 9.

7. Applebaum, *Iron Curtain*, chap. 9.

8. Applebaum, *Iron Curtain*, chap. 9.

9. Applebaum, *Iron Curtain*, chap. 9.

10. "Project Number 5: Streptomycin Plant for Société des Usines Chimiques Rhône-Poulenc," RG 263, NARA, College Park MD.

11. Macekura, "Point Four Program," 126–60.

12. Macekura, "Point Four Program," 141.

13. Macekura, "Point Four Program," 143.

14. Macekura, "Point Four Program," 147.

15. Macekura, "Point Four Program," 148.

16. Macekura, "Point Four Program," 148.

17. McKenna, *Big Chicken*, chap. 2.

18. McKenna, *Big Chicken*, chap. 2.

19. Macekura, "Point Four Program," 126–60.

20. Macekura, "Point Four Program," 126–60.

21. FTC, *Economic Report*, 65–107.

22. Chas. Pfizer, "Annual Report," 1950, 8–9.

23. Chas. Pfizer, "Annual Report," 1950, 8–9.

24. Boyd, "Making Meat," 631–64.

25. Boyd, "Making Meat," 631–64.

26. Boyd, "Making Meat," 631–64.

27. Boyd, "Making Meat," 631–64.

28. Boyd, "Making Meat," 652.

29. Boyd, "Making Meat," 631–64.

30. Boyd, "Making Meat," 657.

31. FTC, *Economic Report*, 148–98.

32. FTC, *Economic Report*, 148–98.

33. FTC, *Economic Report*, 46–62.

34. FTC, *Economic Report*, 92.

35. FTC, *Economic Report*, 148–98.

36. Macekura, "Point Four Program," 143.

37. "Information of Antibiotics," memo, Records of Foreign Assistance Agencies, Record Group 469 (hereafter RG 469), NARA, College Park MD.

38. R. W. Lipton (Lederle) to Clayton Whipple (Point Four), letter, May 29, 1953, RG 469, NARA, College Park MD.

39. Ray Johnson to E. N. Holmgreen, letter, March 10, 1953, RG 469, NARA, College Park MD.

40. Philippines: Annual Livestock Report, January 1953, RG 469, NARA, College Park MD.

41. Philippines: Annual Livestock Report, January 1953, RG 469, NARA, College Park MD.

42. Philippines: Annual Livestock Report, January 1953, RG 469, NARA, College Park MD.

43. E. N. Holmgreen to Ray Johnson, letter, January 26, 1953, RG 469, NARA, College Park MD.

44. E. N. Holmgreen to Ray Johnson, letter, January 26, 1953, RG 469, NARA, College Park MD.

45. Ray Johnson to E. N. Holmgreen, letter, March 10, 1953, RG 469, NARA, College Park MD.

46. Ray Johnson to E. N. Holmgreen, letter, March 10, 1953, RG 469, NARA, College Park MD.

47. "Poultry Feed Imports," report, May 26, 1953, RG 469, NARA, College Park MD.

48. R. W. Linton to Merrill Abbey, letter, June 3, 1953, RG 469, NARA, College Park MD.

Chapter 12

1. Jayaraman, "Joshua Lederberg's Legacy," 716–29.

2. Jayaraman, "Joshua Lederberg's Legacy," 716–29.

3. Lederberg and Lederberg, "Replica Plating," 399–406.

4. Lederberg and Lederberg, "Replica Plating," 309.

5. Lederberg and Lederberg, "Replica Plating," 399–406.

6. Lederberg and Lederberg, "Replica Plating," 399–406.

7. Jayaraman, "Joshua Lederberg's Legacy," 716–29.

8. Jayaraman, "Joshua Lederberg's Legacy," 716–29.

9. Rubenstein, *Last Days of Stalin*, chap. 7.

10. Shama, "No New Thing," 1–4.

11. Myelnikov, "Alternative Cure," 385–411.

12. "USSR Scientist Reports on 1955 Warsaw International Conference on Antibiotics," intelligence report, n.d., RG 263, NARA, College Park MD.

13. "USSR Scientist Reports," intelligence report, RG 263, NARA, College Park MD.

14. "USSR Scientist Reports," intelligence report, RG 263, NARA, College Park MD.

15. "USSR Scientist Reports," intelligence report, RG 263, NARA, College Park MD.

16. "Recent USSR Work in the Field of Antibiotics," intelligence report, February 10, 1953, RG 263, NARA, College Park MD.

17. "USSR Progress in the Field of Antibiotics during 1951–1953," 2, intelligence report, RG 263, NARA, College Park MD.

18. Korzbski, Kowszyk-Gindifer, and Kurlowicz, *Antibiotics*.

19. McKenna, "Last Resort," 394.

20. Umezawa, "Kanamycin," 20–26.

21. Aminov, *History of Antimicrobial Drug*, 4–19.

22. Tyabji, "Gaining Technical Know-how," 331.

23. Tyabji, "Gaining Technical Know-how," 331–49.

24. Tyabji, "Gaining Technical Know-how," 334.

25. Tyabji, "Gaining Technical Know-how," 331–49.

26. Tyabji, "Gaining Technical Know-how," 331–49.

27. Tyabji, "Gaining Technical Know-how," 331–49.

28. Tyabji, "Gaining Technical Know-how," 331–49.

29. Tyabji, "Gaining Technical Know-how," 331–49.

30. Tyabji, "Gaining Technical Know-how," 331–49.
31. Tyabji, "Gaining Technical Know-how," 339.
32. Tyabji, "Gaining Technical Know-how," 340.
33. Tyabji, "Gaining Technical Know-how," 331–49.
34. Tyabji, "Gaining Technical Know-how," 331–49.
35. Tyabji, "Gaining Technical Know-how," 331–49.
36. Mudd, "Staphylococcus Problem," 41–45.
37. Rountree and Freeman, "Infections Caused," 157–61.
38. Wentworth, Miller, and Wentworth, "Staphylococcal Infections," 287–98.
39. Wentworth, Miller, and Wentworth, "Staphylococcal Infections," 287–98.
40. Barber, "Hospital Infection," 2–10.
41. Mudd, "Staphylococcus Problem," 41–45.
42. Mudd, "Staphylococcus Problem," 41–45.
43. Mudd, "Staphylococcus Problem," 41–45.
44. Podolsky, *Antibiotic Era*, 146.
45. Mudd, "Staphylococcus Problem," 41–45.
46. Kutter et al., "Phage Therapy," 945–56.
47. Kutter et al., "Phage Therapy," 112-8.
48. Lawrence Osborne, "A Stalinist Antibiotic Alternative," *New York Times*, February 6, 2000.
49. Joravsky, *Lysenko Affair*, 171–73.
50. Joravsky, *Lysenko Affair*, 171–73.
51. Joravsky, *Lysenko Affair*, 171–73.
52. Joravsky, *Lysenko Affair*, 171–73.
53. Joravsky, *Lysenko Affair*, 171–73.
54. Schneider, "Michurinist Biology," 529.
55. Schneider, "Michurinist Biology," 525–56.
56. Schneider, "Michurinist Biology," 525–56.
57. Schneider, "Michurinist Biology," 525–56.
58. Schneider, "Michurinist Biology," 525–56.
59. Schneider, "Michurinist Biology," 525–56.
60. Schneider, "Michurinist Biology," 525–56.
61. Schneider, "Michurinist Biology," 544.
62. Schneider, "Michurinist Biology," 525–56.
63. Schneider, "Michurinist Biology," 525–56.

Chapter 13

1. Pfizer advertisement, *New York Herald Tribune*, March 31, 1957, 116.
2. Podolsky and Greene, "Combination Drugs," 488–91.
3. "One+One=Three: New Weapons to Attack Stubborn Disease Germs," *Los Angeles Times*, April 14, 1957.
4. "Pfizer Says Sigmamycin Drug Fights More Types of Germs than Others," *Wall Street Journal*, September 13, 1956, 24.

5. Podolsky, *Antibiotic Era*, 69.

6. Podolsky, *Antibiotic Era*, 69.

7. Podolsky, *Antibiotic Era*, 71.

8. Podolsky, *Antibiotic Era*, 71.

9. Podolsky, *Antibiotic Era*, 71.

10. Bud, "Antibiotics, Big Business," 329.

11. Brown, "M.D.s Who Didn't Exist," 42.

12. See the Federal Trade Commission's website, FTC.com.

13. "FTC Clears Pfizer; Drops Charge of Misleading Advertising of Antibiotic," *New York Times*, June 6, 1960.

14. Tobbell, *Pills, Power, and Policy*, chap. 4.

15. "S.S. Hope Beached to Prevent Sinking after Tug Ramming," *New York Times*, February 11, 1975.

16. Tobbell, *Pills, Power, and Policy*, chap. 4.

17. Tobbell, *Pills, Power, and Policy*, chap. 4.

18. Tobbell, *Pills, Power, and Policy*, chap. 4.

19. Tobbell, *Pills, Power, and Policy*, chap. 4.

20. Tobbell, *Pills, Power, and Policy*, chap. 4.

21. Tobbell, *Pills, Power, and Policy*, chap. 4.

22. Tobbell, *Pills, Power, and Policy*, chap. 4.

23. Tobbell, *Pills, Power, and Policy*, chap. 4.

24. Tobbell, *Pills, Power, and Policy*, chap. 4.

25. Abraham, "Beta-Lactam Antibiotics," 76–87.

26. Abraham, "Beta-Lactam Antibiotics," 76–87.

27. Abraham, "Beta-Lactam Antibiotics," 76–87.

28. Abraham, "Beta-Lactam Antibiotics," 76–87.

29. Abraham, "Beta-Lactam Antibiotics," 76–87.

30. Aminov, *History of Antimicrobial Drug*, 4–19.

31. Bo, "Giuseppe Brotzu," 6–8.

32. Abraham, "Beta-Lactam Antibiotics," 76–87.

33. Aminov, *History of Antimicrobial Drug*, 4–19.

34. Aminov, *History of Antimicrobial Drug*, 4–19.

35. Shaffir, "Flashback."

36. Applebaum, *Iron Curtain*, chap. 8.

37. Berg, "History of Genetics," 46.

38. Hale-Dorrell, *Corn Crusade*, 13.

39. Berg, "History of Genetics."

40. Medvedev, *Rise and Fall*, 181.

41. Joravsky, *Lysenko Affair*, 293–305.

42. Joravsky, *Lysenko Affair*, 282–93.

43. Taubman, *Khrushchev*.

44. Kirchhelle, "Pharming Animals," 4.

45. Kirchhelle, "Pharming Animals," 1–13.

46. Chas. Pfizer, "Annual Report," 1960.
47. Chas. Pfizer, "Annual Report," 1960.
48. Kirchhelle, "Pharming Animals," 1–13.
49. Kirchhelle, "Pharming Animals," 1–13.
50. Kirchhelle, "Pharming Animals," 1–13.
51. Kirchhelle, "Pharming Animals," 1–13.
52. McKenna, *Big Chicken*, chap. 4.
53. Kirchhelle, "Pharming Animals," 1–13.
54. Barber, "Hospital Infection," 2–10.
55. Summers, "Strange History," 130–33.
56. Rose, "New Penicillins," 66–71.
57. Rose, "New Penicillins," 66–71.
58. Chambers and DeLeo, "Waves of Resistance," 629–41.

Chapter 14

1. Joseph, *For Whom the Dogs Spy*, chap. 5.
2. Greene, *The Comedians*.
3. Abbott, *Haiti*, chap. 5.
4. Abbott, *Haiti*, chap. 5.
5. Abbott, *Haiti*, chap. 5.
6. Abbott, *Haiti*, chap. 5.
7. Samame, "Treponematosis Eradication," 897–910.
8. Hopkins, "Yaws in the Americas," 548–54.
9. Abbott, *Haiti*, chap. 4.
10. Abbott, *Haiti*, chap. 4.
11. Joseph, *For Whom the Dogs Spy*, chap. 5.
12. Lentz, *Heads of States*, 354.
13. Watanabe, "Infective Heredity," 87–115.
14. Watanabe, "Infective Heredity," 87–115.
15. Watanabe, "Infective Heredity," 87–115.
16. Watanabe, "Infectious Drug Resistance," 19–27.
17. Watanabe, "Infectious Drug Resistance," 19–27.
18. Mudd, *Staphylococcus Problem*, 41–45.
19. Aminov, *History of Antimicrobial Drug*, 4–19.
20. Abraham, Newton, and Loder, "Cephalosporin C Nucleus," 408–16.
21. Andriole, "Quinolones," s113–s119.
22. Felsenfeld, "Some Observations," 289–96.
23. Wallace et al., "1961 Cholera Epidemic," 795–810.
24. Felsenfeld, "Some Observations," 289–96.
25. Mandal, Mandal, and Pal, "Cholera," 573–80.
26. Mukerjee, "Cholera El Tor," 546–48.

27. As of this writing, the seventh pandemic is still raging and has circled the globe.

28. Sayamov, "Treatment and Prophylaxis," 361–67.

29. Summers, "Cholera and Plague," 275–301.

30. Sayamov, "Treatment and Prophylaxis," 361–67.

31. Monsur et al., "Effect of Massive Doses," 723–32.

32. Marčuk et al., "Clinical Studies," 82.

33. It is worth noting that during this time, the Eliava Institute had conducted what is considered "one of the most, if not the most extensive studies evaluating the utility of therapeutic phages for prophylaxis of infectious diseases" in Tbilisi. See Sulakvelidze, Alavidze, and Morris, "Bacteriophage Therapy," 649–59.

34. Kennedy, "Anglo-French Rivalry," 199–215.

35. Ringer, "Convicts and Conservation," 221.

36. "Tiger Cages of Viet Nam," *Life*, July 17, 1970.

37. Kim, "Penile Necrosis," 541–61.

38. Baby, "White Cong."

39. Acar and Röstel, "Antimicrobial Resistance," 797–810.

40. Cokie Roberts and Steven V. Roberts, "The Venereal Disease Pandemic," *New York Times*, November 7, 1971, SM62.

41. Davis, "Multidrug-Resistant Acinetobacter," 1218.

42. Blythe et al., "Lessons of War," 228–35.

43. Blythe et al., "Lessons of War," 228–35.

44. Hell, "Characteristics of the Ideal," 164–69.

45. Taubman, *Khrushchev*, chap. 19.

46. Joravsky, *The Lysenko Affair*, 163.

Chapter 15

1. Medvedev, *Rise and Fall*, 142.

2. Leitenberg and Zilinskas, *Soviet Biological Weapons Program*, chap. 2.

3. Leitenberg and Zilinskas, *Soviet Biological Weapons Program*, chap. 2.

4. Leitenberg and Zilinskas, *Soviet Biological Weapons Program*, chap. 2.

5. Leitenberg and Zilinskas, *Soviet Biological Weapons Program*, chap. 2.

6. Leitenberg and Zilinskas, *Soviet Biological Weapons Program*, chap. 2.

7. Leitenberg and Zilinskas, *Soviet Biological Weapons Program*, chap. 2.

8. Leitenberg and Zilinskas, *Soviet Biological Weapons Program*, chap. 2.

9. Leitenberg and Zilinskas, *Soviet Biological Weapons Program*, chap. 2.

10. Leitenberg and Zilinskas, *Soviet Biological Weapons Program*, chap. 2.

11. Leitenberg and Zilinskas, *Soviet Biological Weapons Program*, chap. 2.

12. Leitenberg and Zilinskas, *Soviet Biological Weapons Program*, chap. 2.

13. Leitenberg and Zilinskas, *Soviet Biological Weapons Program*, chap. 2.

14. Leitenberg and Zilinskas, *Soviet Biological Weapons Program*, chap. 2.

15. Leitenberg and Zilinskas, *Soviet Biological Weapons Program*, chap. 2.

16. Leitenberg and Zilinskas, *Soviet Biological Weapons Program*, chap. 2.
17. Leitenberg and Zilinskas, *Soviet Biological Weapons Program*, chap. 2.
18. Leitenberg and Zilinskas, *Soviet Biological Weapons Program*, chap. 2.
19. Meselson et al., "Sverdlovsk Anthrax Outbreak," 1202–8.
20. Meselson et al., "Sverdlovsk Anthrax Outbreak," 1202–8.
21. Meselson et al., "Sverdlovsk Anthrax Outbreak," 1202–8.
22. Meselson et al., "Sverdlovsk Anthrax Outbreak," 1202–8.
23. Kirchhelle, "Swan Song," 317–50.
24. Bud, *Penicillin*, 175.
25. Bud, *Penicillin*, 163–91.
26. Bud, *Penicillin*, 163–91.
27. Bud, *Penicillin*, 163–91.
28. Bud, *Penicillin*, 163–91.
29. McKenna, *Big Chicken*, chap. 5.
30. McKenna, *Big Chicken*, chap. 5.
31. McKenna, *Big Chicken*, chap. 5.
32. McKenna, *Big Chicken*, chap. 5.
33. McKenna, *Big Chicken*, chap. 5.
34. McKenna, *Big Chicken*, chap. 5.
35. McKenna, *Big Chicken*, chap. 5.
36. McKenna, *Big Chicken*, chap. 5.
37. McKenna, *Big Chicken*, chap. 5.
38. McKenna, *Big Chicken*, chap. 5.
39. Zakinthos and Karande, "Multidrug-Resistant Typhoid Fever," 324–37.
40. Olarte and Galindo, "*Salmonella typhi* Resistant," 597–601.
41. Olarte and Galindo, "*Salmonella typhi* Resistant," 597–601.
42. Olarte and Galindo, "*Salmonella typhi* Resistant," 597–601.
43. Andrew Jack, "The Fall of the World's Best-Selling Drug," *Financial Times*, November 28, 2009.
44. Aminov, *History of Antimicrobial Drug*, 4–19.
45. Saga and Yamaguchi, "History of Antimicrobial Agents," 103–8.
46. Chambers and DeLeo, "Waves of Resistance," 629–41.
47. Chambers and DeLeo, "Waves of Resistance," 629–41.
48. Chambers and DeLeo, "Waves of Resistance," 629–41.
49. Chambers and DeLeo, "Waves of Resistance," 629–41.
50. Boucher et al., "Bad Bugs," 1–12.
51. Boucher et al., "Bad Bugs," 1–12.
52. Boucher et al., "Bad Bugs," 1–12.
53. Boucher et al., "Bad Bugs," 1–12.
54. Boucher et al., "Bad Bugs," 1–12.
55. Bull et al., "Dynamics of Success," 35.
56. Frieden et al., "Emergence of Drug-Resistant Tuberculosis," 521–26.

57. Frieden et al., "Emergence of Drug-Resistant Tuberculosis," 521–26.

58. Molez "Historical Question," 273–76.

59. Gilbert et al., "Emergence of HIV/AIDS," 18566–70.

60. Yablonskii et al., "Tuberculosis in Russia," 373.

61. Yablonskii et al., "Tuberculosis in Russia," 372–76.

62. Yablonskii et al., "Tuberculosis in Russia," 372–76.

BIBLIOGRAPHY

Archives

National Archives and Records Administration, College Park MD.
Records of Allied Operational and Occupation Headquarters, World War II, Record Group 331.
Records of Foreign Assistance Agencies, Record Group 469.
Records of the Central Intelligence Agency, Record Group 263.
Records of the Office of Science Research and Development, Record Group 227.
United Nations, Archives and Records, New York.
United States National Library of Medicine, Bethesda MD.
Joshua Lederberg Papers.

Published Sources

Abbott, Elizabeth. *Haiti: A Shattered Nation*. New York: Harry Abrams, 2011. Ebook.

Abraham, E. P. "The Beta-Lactam Antibiotics." *Scientific American* 244, no. 6 (June 1981): 76–87.

Abraham, E. P., and E. Chain. "An Enzyme from Bacteria Able to Destroy Penicillin." *Nature* 146 (1940): 837.

Abraham, E. P., E. Chain, C. M. Fletcher, A. D. Gardner, N. G. Heatley, M. A. Jennings, and H. W. Florey. "Further Observations on Penicillin." *Lancet* 238, no. 6155 (1941): 177–89.

Abraham, E. P., G. G. F. Newton, and Bronwen Loder. "The Cephalosporin C Nucleus (7-Aminocephalosporanic Acid) and Some of Its Derivatives." *Biochemical Journal* 79, no. 2 (1961): 408–16.

Acar, J., and B. Röstel. "Antimicrobial Resistance: An Overview." *Revue Scientifique et Technique (International Office of Epizootics)* 20, no. 3 (2001): 797–810.

Albrecht, Bailey Kirsten. "The Inherited Epidemic: A History of Tuberculosis in Occupied Japan." PhD diss., University of Illinois, 2014.

Alexander, T. W., L. J. Yanke, E. Topp, M. E. Olson, R. R. Read, D. W. Morck, and T. A. McAllister. "Effect of Subtherapeutic Administration of Antibiotics on the Prevalence of Antibiotic-Resistant Escherichia coli Bacteria in Feedlot Cattle." *Applied and Environmental Microbiology* 74, no. 14 (2008): 4405–16.

Alibek, Ken. *Biohazard: The Chilling True Story of the Largest Covert Biological Weapons Program in the World, Told from the Inside by the Man Who Ran It.* New York: Delta, 1999.

Altemeier, William A., Robert P. Hummel, and Edward O. Hill. "Staphylococcal Enterocolitis Following Antibiotic Therapy." *Annals of Surgery* 157, no. 6 (1963): 847.

Ambrose, Stephen. *The Supreme Commander: The War Years of General Dwight D. Eisenhower*. New York: Anchor Books, 2012.

Aminov, Rustam. "History of Antimicrobial Drug Discovery: Major Classes and Health Impact." *Biochemical Pharmacology* 133 (2017): 4–19.

Amyes, Sebastian. *Magic Bullets, Lost Horizons: The Rise and Fall of Antibiotics.* London and New York: Taylor & Francis, 2001.

Andriole, Vincent T. "The Quinolones: Past, Present, and Future." *Clinical Infectious Diseases* 41, Supplement 2 (2005): s113–s119.

Applebaum, Anne. *Gulag: A History*. New York: Anchor Books, 2010.

———. *Iron Curtain: The Crushing of Eastern Europe, 1944–1956*. New York: Doubleday, 2012. Ebook.

Baby, John S. "White Cong and Black Clap: The Ambient Truth of Vietnam War Legendary." In *The Viet Nam Generation Big Book*, edited by Dan Duffy and Kali Tal. Woodbridge CT: Viet Nam Generation Press, 1994.

Bain, R. J. *The Arsenal of Democracy*. Boston: Houghton Mifflin Harcourt, 2014.

Baquero, F., J. Martínez Beltrén, and E. Loza. "A Review of Antibiotic Resistance Patterns of Streptococcus pneumoniae in Europe." *Journal of Antimicrobial Chemotherapy* 28, Supplement C (1991): 31–38.

Barber, Mary. "Hospital Infection Yesterday and Today." *Journal of Clinical Pathology* 14, no. 2 (1961): 2–10.

———. "Staphylococcal Infection due to Penicillin-Resistant Strains." *British Medical Journal*, November 29, 1947, 863–65.

Barber, Mary, and Pamela M. Waterworth. "Antibacterial Activity of the Penicillins." *British Medical Journal* 1, no. 5286 (1962): 1159.

Berg, Raissa L. "On the History of Genetics in the Soviet Union: Science and Politics; the Insight of a Witness." Final Report to National Council for Soviet and East European Research. St. Louis MO: Washington University, August 1, 1983.

Berinsky, Adam. "Assuming the Costs of War: Events, Elites, and American Public Support for Military Conflict." *Journal of Politics* 69, no. 4 (November 2007): 975–97.

Bickel, Leonard. *Rise Up to Life: A Biography of Howard Walter Florey Who Gave Penicillin to the World.* London: Angus and Robertson, 1972.

Birstein, Vadim. *The Perversion of Knowledge: The True Story of Soviet Science.* New York: Basic Books, 2004.

Blythe, Dana, H. C. Yun, D. R. Tribble, and C. K. Murray. "Lessons of War: Combat-Related Injury Infections during the Vietnam War and Operation Iraqi and

Enduring Freedom." *Journal of Trauma and Acute Care Surgery* 79, Supplement 2 (October 2015): 228–35.

Bo, G. "Giuseppe Brotzu and the Discovery of Cephalosporins." *Clinical Microbiology and Infectious Diseases* 6, Supplement 3 (2000): 6–8.

Bocker, Harald, and Wolfgang A. Knorre. "Antibiotica Research in Jena from Penicillin and Nourseothricin to Interferon." In *History of Modern Biotechnology II*, edited by Armin Fiechter, 35–40. New York: Springer, 2000.

Borodin, Nikolai. *One Man in His Time*. New York: Macmillan, 1955.

Borodin, N., F. J. Philpot, and H. W. Florey. "An Antibiotic from *Penicillium tardum*." *British Journal of Experimental Pathology* 28, no. 1 (February 1947): 31–34.

Boucher, H., G. H. Talbot, J. S. Bradley, J. E. Edwards, D. Gilbert, L. B. Rice, M. Scheld, B. Spellberg, and J. Barlett. "Bad Bugs, No Drugs: No ESKAPE! An Update from the Infectious Diseases Society of America." *Clinical Infectious Diseases* 48, no. 1 (January 2009): 1–12.

Boyd, William. "Making Meat: Science, Technology and American Poultry Production." *Technology and Culture* 42, no. 4 (October 2001): 631–64.

Brecht, Bertolt. *War Primer*. Translated by John Willett. London: Verso, 2017.

Brockman, Maxwell. *The History of Penicillin Production*. New York: American Institute of Chemical Engineers, 1970.

Brown, Herb, ed. "The M.D.s Who Didn't Exist." *Changing Times: The Kiplinger Magazine*, September 1959.

Buchanan, Tom. "The Courage of Galileo: Joseph Needham and the 'Germ Warfare' Allegations in the Korean War." *History* 86, no. 284 (2001): 503–22.

Bud, Robert. "Antibiotics, Big Business, and Consumers: The Context of Government Investigations into the Postwar American Drug Industry." *Technology Culture* 46, no.2 (April 2005): 329.

———. *Penicillin: Triumph and Tragedy*. New York: Oxford University Press, 2007.

Bulgakov, Mikhail. *A Country Doctor's Notebook*. Translated by Michael Glenny. Brooklyn: Melville House, 2013.

Bull, J. J., Bruce R. Levin, Terry DeRouin, Nina Walker, and Craig A. Bloch. "Dynamics of Success and Failure in Phage and Antibiotic Therapy in Experimental Infections." BMC *Microbiology* 2 (2002): 35.

Bundy, Amanda Melaine. "There Was a Man of UNRRA: Internationalism, Humanitarianism, and the Early Cold War in Europe, 1943–1947." PhD diss., Ohio State University, 2017.

Burns, Marlene, J. W. Bennett, and Piet W. M. van Dijck. "Code Name Bacinol." ASM *News* 69, no. 1 (2003): 25–31.

Buruma, Ian. *The Wages of Guilt: Memories of War in Germany and Japan*. New York: New York Review of Books, 2015.

———. *Year Zero*. New York: Penguin Press, 2013.

Bush, Vannevar. *Science, the Endless Frontier: A Report to the President on the Program for Postwar Scientific Research*. Washington DC: National Science Foundation, 1945.

Butler, Susan. *Roosevelt and Stalin: Portrait of a Partnership*. New York: Alfred Knopf, 2015.

Cain, Frank. *Economic Statecraft during the Cold War: European Responses to the US Trade Embargo*. New York: Routledge, 2007.

Cantoni, Roberto. "Breach of Faith? Italian-Soviet Cold War Trading and ENI's International 'Oil Scandal.'" *Quaestio Rossica* 4 (2015): 180–98.

Capocci, M. "A Chain Is Gonna Come: Building a Penicillin Plant in Post-War Italy." In *Circulation of Antibiotics: Journeys of Drug Standards*, edited by Ana Romero, Christoph Gradmann, and Maria Santesmases, 61–80. Madrid: European Science Foundation, 2010.

———. "Cold Drugs, Circulation, Production and Intelligence of Antibiotics in Post-WWII Years." *Medicina Nei Secoli: Arte e Scienza* 26, no. 2 (2014): 401–22.

Carlton, Richard. "Phage Therapy: Past History and Future Prospects." *Archivum Immunologiae et Therapiae Experimentalis* 47 (1999): 267–74.

Chain, Ernst, Howard W. Florey, Arthur D. Gardner, Norman G. Heatley, Margaret A. Jennings, Jean Orr-Ewing, and A. Gordon Sanders. "Penicillin as a Chemotherapeutic Agent." *Lancet* 236, no. 6104 (1940): 226–28.

Chambers, Henry, and Frank DeLeo. "Waves of Resistance: Staphylococcus aureus in the Antibiotic Era." *Nature Reviews Microbiology* 7, no. 9 (2009): 629–41.

Chang, Iris. *Rape of Nanking: The Forgotten Holocaust of World War II*. New York: Basic Books, 2011.

Chang, Jung. *Mao: The Unknown Story*. New York: Anchor Books, 2006.

Chas. Pfizer & Co., Inc. "Annual Report." Brooklyn: Chas. Pfizer & Co., 1950.

———. "Annual Report." Brooklyn: Chas. Pfizer & Co., 1960.

Chen, S. L., B. L. Cheng, W. K. Cheng, and P. S. Tang. "An Antibiotic Substance in the Chinese Water-chestnut, *Eleocharis tuberosa*." *Nature* 156, no. 3956 (1945): 234.

Choy, Bong-youn. *Korea: A History*. Rutland VT: Charles E. Tuttle, 1971.

Clark, Ronald W. *The Life of Ernst Chain: Penicillin and Beyond*. London: Weidenfeld & Nicholson, 1995.

Colley, Rupert. *The Siege of Leningrad*. London: HarperPress, 2012.

Cook, A. H., and M. S. Lacey. "Kojic Acid and the Antibiotic Action of Species of *Aspergillus*." *Nature* 155, no. 3948 (1945): 790.

Cope, Oliver. "The Treatment of the Surface Burns." *Annals of Surgery* 117, no. 6 (June 1943): 885–93.

Cozzoli, Daniele. "Penicillin and the Reconstruction of Japan." *Medicina nei secoli: Arte e Scienza* 26, no. 2 (2014): 469–84.

Cronkite, Walter. *Cronkite's War: His World War II Letters Home*. Washington DC: National Geographic Society, 2013.

Davis, K. A. "Multidrug-Resistant Acinetobacter Extremity Infections in Soldiers." *Emerging Infectious Diseases* 11, no. 8 (August 2005): 1218.

Davis, Margaret A., Katherine N. Baker, Lisa H. Orfe, Devendra H. Shah, Thomas E. Besser, and Douglas R. Call. "Discovery of a Gene Conferring Multiple-

Aminoglycoside Resistance in *Escherichia coli*." *Antimicrobial Agents and Chemotherapy* 54, no. 6 (2010): 2666–69.

Demain, Arnold L., and Sergio Sanchez. "Microbial Drug Discovery: 80 Years of Progress." *Journal of Antibiotics* 62, no. 1 (2009): 5.

Department of the Army. *U.S. Army Activity in the U.S. Biological Warfare Programs, 1942–1977*. Vol. 1. Washington DC: Department of the Army, 1977.

D'Este, Carlo. *World War II in the Mediterranean, 1942–1945*. Chapel Hill: Algonquin Books, 1990. Ebook.

Dimbleby, Jonathan. *Destiny in the Desert: The Road to El Alamein—the Battle That Turned the Tide of World War II*. New York: Pegasus Books, 2012. Ebook.

Djelic, Marie-Laure, and Rolv Petter Amdam. "Americanization in Comparative Perspective: The Managerial Revolution in France and Norway, 1940–1990." *Business History* 49, no. 4 (2007): 483–505.

Dower, John. *Embracing Defeat: Japan in the Wake of World War II*. New York: W. W. Norton, 1999.

Dudley-Cash, B. "AGPs in Ag: History, Mode Discussed." *Feedstuffs*, 2005, 10.

Eaton, Monroe, and Stanhope Bayne-Jones. "Bacteriophage Therapy: Review of the Principles and Results of the Use of Bacteriophage in the Treatment of Infections." *Journal of the American Medical Association* 103 (1934): 1847–53.

Elder, Albert. "The Role of the Government in the Penicillin Program." In Brockman, *History of Penicillin Production*, 3–11.

Eli Lilly and Company. *The Elements of Biologics*. Indianapolis: Eli Lilly, 1917.

Endo, Mieko. "Douglas MacArthur's Occupation of Japan: Building the Foundation of U.S.-Japan Relationship." Thesis, University of Montana, 2006.

Fair, Richard J., and Yitzhak Tor. "Antibiotics and Bacterial Resistance in the 21st Century." *Perspectives in Medicinal Chemistry* 6 (2014): PMC-S14459.

Falagas, Matthew E., and Sofia K. Kasaikou. "Colistin: The Revival of Polymyxins for the Management of Multidrug-Resistant Gram-Negative Bacterial Infections." *Clinical Infectious Diseases* 40 (2005): 1333–41.

Federal Trade Commission (FTC). *Economic Report on Antibiotics Manufacture*. Washington DC: U.S. Government Printing Office, 1958.

Fehrenbach, T. R. *This Kind of War*. New York: Open Road Integrated Media, 2014.

Feldblum, Paul, and Michael Rosenberg. "A Historical Perspective on Condoms." In *Condoms in the Prevention of Sexually Transmitted Diseases: Proceedings of a Conference Held in February 1987 in Atlanta, Georgia*, 1–3. Research Triangle Park NC: American Social Health Association, U.S. Centers for Disease Control, and Family Health International, 1989.

Felsenfeld, Oscar. "Some Observations on the Cholera (El Tor) Epidemic in 1961–62." *Bulletin of the World Health Organization* 28 (1963): 289–96.

Florey, Howard W. "Penicillin: A Survey." *British Medical Journal* 2, no. 4361 (1944): 169.

Fraser, Ian. "Penicillin: Early Trials in War Casualties." *British Medical Journal* 289 (December 22–29, 1984): 1723–25.

Frieden, Thomas R., T. Sterling, A. Pablos-Mendez, J. O. Kilburn, G. M. Cauthen, and S. W. Dooley. "The Emergence of Drug-Resistant Tuberculosis in New York City." *New England Journal of Medicine* 328, no. 8 (February 25, 1993): 521–26.

Gaddis, John Lewis. *George F. Kennan: An American Life*. New York: Penguin Press, 2011. Ebook.

Gailey, Harold. *War in the Pacific*. Novato CA: Presidio, 1995.

Gall, Tasha M., and Mikhail Konashev. "The Discovery of Gramicidin S: The Intellectual Transformation of G. F. Gause from Biologist to Researcher of Antibiotics and on Its Meaning for the Fate of Russian Genetics." *History and Philosophy of the Life Sciences* 23 (2001): 137–50.

Gause, G. F., and M. G. Brazhnikova. "Gramicidin S and Its Use in the Treatment of Infected Wounds." *Nature* 154 (December 1944): 703.

Gelpi, Adriane, and Joseph Tucker. *A Cure at Last? Penicillin's Unintended Consequences on Syphilis Control, 1944–1964. Sexually Transmitted Infections* 91, no. 1 (February 2015): 70.

Gilbert, M. Thomas P., Andrew Rambaut, Gabriela Wlasiuk, Thomas J. Spira, Arthur E. Pitchenik, and Michael Worobey. "The Emergence of HIV/AIDS in the Americas and Beyond." *Proceedings of the National Academy of Sciences* 104, no. 47 (November 20, 2007): 18566–70.

Gold, Hal. *Unit 731: Testimony*. North Clarendon VT: Tuttle, 1997. Ebook.

Goldsworthy, Peter, and Alexander McFarlane. "Howard Florey, Alexander Fleming and the Fairy Tale of Penicillin." *Medical Journal of Australia* 176, no. 4 (February 2002): 176–78.

Graham, Loren. *Science in Russia and the Soviet Union: A Short History*. New York: Cambridge University Press, 1993.

Green, T., M. Talbot, and R. S. Morton. "The Control of Syphilis: A Contemporary Problem, a Historical Perspective." *Sexually Transmitted Infections* 77 (2001): 214–17.

Greene, Graham. *The Comedians*. New York: Viking Press, 1966. Ebook.

Grossman, Vassily. *A Writer at War*. New York: Vintage Books, 2013.

Guillemin, Jeanne. *Hidden Atrocities: Japanese Germ Warfare and American Obstruction of Justice at the Tokyo Trial*. New York: Columbia University Press, 2017. Ebook.

Hale-Dorrell, Aaron T. *Corn Crusade: Khrushchev's Farming Revolution in the Post-Stalin Soviet Union*. New York: Oxford University Press, 2019.

Hamilton, Nigel. *The Mantle of Command: FDR at War, 1941–1945*. Boston: Houghton Mifflin Harcourt, 2014.

Harriman, Averell. *Mutual Defense Assistance Control Act, Public Law 213—82d Congress: First Report to Congress*. Washington DC: U.S. Mutual Security Agency, 1952.

Harris, Sheldon. *Factories of Death: Japanese Biological Warfare, 1932–1945, and the American Cover-Up*. New York: Routledge, 2002.

———. "Japanese Biological Warfare Experiments and Other Atrocities in Manchuria, 1932–1945, and the Subsequent United States Cover Up: A Preliminary Assessment." *Crime, Law and Social Change* 15 (1991): 171–99.

Haruki, Wada. *The Korean War: An International History*. Translated by Frank Baldwin. Latham MD: Rowman & Littlefield, 2013. Ebook.

Hassan, Jonathan. *Near and Distant Neighbors: A New History of Soviet Intelligence*. New York: Farrar, Straus and Giroux, 2015.

Hastings, Max. *Winston's War: Churchill, 1940–1945*. New York: Penguin, 2010. Ebook.

Hayes, J. N. *The Burdens of Disease: Epidemics and Human Response in Western History*. New Brunswick NJ: Rutgers University Press. Ebook.

Hell, Konrad. "Characteristics of the Ideal Antibiotic for Prevention of Wound Sepsis among Military Forces in the Field." *Reviews of Infectious Diseases* 13, Supplement 2 (1991): 164–69.

Higgins, Marguerite. *War in Korea: The Report of a Woman Combat Correspondent*. New York: Doubleday, 1951.

Ho, Karen. "Bacteriophage Therapy for Bacterial Infections: Rekindling a Memory from the Pre-Antibiotics Era." *Perspectives in Biology and Medicine* 44 (2001): 1–16.

Hobby, Gladys. *Penicillin: Meeting the Challenge*. New Haven CT: Yale University Press, 1985.

Hopkins, Donald R. "Yaws in the Americas, 1950–1975." *Journal of Infectious Diseases* 156, no. 4 (October 1977): 548–54.

Hotta, Eri. *Japan 1941: Countdown to Infamy*. New York: Alfred Knopf, 2013.

Jayaraman, R. "Joshua Lederberg's Legacy to Bacterial Genetics." *Resonance* 13, no. 8 (August 2008): 716–29.

Jeans, Roger B., Jr. "Alarm in Washington: A Wartime 'Exposé' of Japan's Biological Warfare Program." *Journal of Military History* 71, no. 2 (April 2007): 411–39.

Jones, Doris. "The Effect of Antibiotic Substances upon Bacteriophage." *Journal of Bacteriology* 50, no. 3 (September 1945): 341–48.

Joravsky, David. *The Lysenko Affair*. Chicago: University of Chicago Press, 1970.

Joseph, Raymond. *For Whom the Dogs Spy: Haiti—from the Duvalier Dictatorships to the Earthquake, Four Presidents, and Beyond*. New York: Arcade Publishing, 2014. Ebook.

Kaiser, David. *No End Save Victory: How FDR Led the Nation into War*. New York: Basic Books, 2014. Ebook.

Kardos, Nelson, and Arnold L. Demain. "Ernst Chain: A Great Man of Science." *Applied Microbiology and Biotechnology* 97, no. 15 (August 2013): 6613–22.

Keefer, Chester S., Francis G. Blake, E. Kennerly Marshall Jr., John S. Lockwood, and W. Barry Wood Jr. "Penicillin in the Treatment of Infections: A Report of 500 Cases." *Journal of the American Medical Association* 122, no. 18 (1943): 1217–24.

Kennedy, B. E. "Anglo-French Rivalry in Southeast Asia 1763–93: Some Repercussions." *Journal of Southeast Asian Studies* 4, no. 2 (1973): 199–215.

Khlevniuk, Oleg. *Stalin: New Biography of a Dictator*. New Haven CT: Yale University Press, 2015. Ebook.

Kim, Jane S. H. "Penile Necrosis, Military Medicine, and South Korean Participation in the Vietnam War, 1964–1973." *East Asian Science, Technology and Society* 11, no. 4 (December 2017): 541–61.

Kingston, William. "Streptomycin, Schatz v. Waksman, and the Balance of Credit for Discovery." *Journal of History of Medicine and Allied Sciences* 59, no. 3 (July 2004): 441–62.

Kirchhelle, Claas. "Pharming Animals: A Global History of Antibiotics in Food Production (1935–2017)." *Palgrave Communications* 4, no. 96 (August 2018). DOI: 10.1057/s41599-018-0152-2.

———. "Swan Song: Antibiotic Regulation in British Livestock Production (1953–2006)." *Bulletin of the History of Medicine* 92, no. 2 (Summer 2018): 317–50.

Kolchinsky, Eduard I. "Nikolai Vavilov in the Years of Stalin's 'Revolution from Above' (1929–1932)." *Centaurus* 56, no. 4 (2014): 330–58.

Korzybski, Tadeusz, Zuzanna Kowszyk-Gindifer, and Wlodzimierz Kurylowicz. *Antibiotics*. Vol. 2, *Origin, Nature, and Properties*. Oxford: Pergamon Press, 1967.

Krementsov, Nikolai. "Big Revolution, Little Revolution: Science and Politics in Bolshevik Russia." *Social Research* 73, no. 4 (Winter 2006): 1173–1204.

———. "In the Shadow of the Bomb: U.S.-Soviet Biomedical Relations in the Early Cold War, 1944–1948." *Journal of Cold War Studies* 9, no. 4 (Fall 2007): 41–67.

———. "The 'K.R.' Affair: Soviet Science on the Threshold of the Cold War." *History and Philosophy of the Life Sciences* 17 (1995): 419–46.

———. *Stalinist Science*. Princeton NJ: Princeton University Press, 1996.

Krueger, Albert Paul, and E. Jane Scribner. "The Bacteriophage: Its Nature and Its Therapeutic Use." *Journal of the American Medical Association* 116 (1941): 2269–77.

Kruger, Lee. *Logistics Matters and the U.S. Army in Occupied Germany, 1945–1949*. New York: Palgrave Macmillan, 2017.

Kurtz-Phelan, Daniel. *The China Mission: George Marshall's Unfinished War, 1945–1947*. New York: W. W. Norton, 2018.

Kutter, Elizabeth, Sarah Kuhl, Zemphira Alavidze, and Bob Blasdel. "Phage Therapy: Bacteriophages as Natural, Self-Limiting Antibiotics." In *Textbook of Natural Medicine*, 4th ed., edited by Joseph Pizzorno and Michael T. Murray. New York: Elsevier Churchill Livingstone, 2012.

Lai, Ding-Kee. "A Historical Review of Smuggling in Hong Kong." PhD diss., University of Hong Kong, 1995.

Landas, Marc. *The Fallen: A True Story of American POWs and Japanese Wartime Atrocities*. Hoboken NJ: Wiley, 2004.

Lax, Eric. *The Mold in Dr. Florey's Coat: The Story of the Penicillin Miracle*. New York: Henry Holt, 2016. Ebook.

Lederberg, Joshua, and Ethel Lederberg. "Replica Plating and Indirect Selection of Bacterial Mutants." *Bacteriology* 63, no. 3 (1952): 399–406.

Leitenberg, Milton. "New Russian Evidence on the Korean War Biological Warfare Allegations: Its Background and Analysis." *Cold War International History Project Bulletin* 11 (Winter 1998): 185–99.

Leitenberg, Milton, and Raymond A. Zilinskas. *The Soviet Biological Weapons Program: A History*. Cambridge MA: Harvard University Press, 2012. Ebook.

Lelyveld, Joseph. *His Final Battle: The Last Months of Franklin Roosevelt*. New York: Alfred Knopf, 2015.

Lentz, Harris M., III. *Heads of States and Governments since 1945*. London: Routledge, 1996.

Lombardino, Joseph. "A Brief History of Pfizer Central Research." *Bulletin for the History of Chemistry* 25, no. 1 (2000): 10–15.

Łotysz, Slawomir. "A 'Lasting Memorial' to the UNRRA? Implementation of the Penicillin Plant Programmer in Poland, 1946–1949." *ICON: Journal of the International Committee for the History of Technology* 12, no. 2 (2014): 70–91.

Lysenko, Trofim. *Agrobiology*. Moscow: Foreign Languages Publishing House, 1954.

MacDonogh, Giles. *After the Reich: The Brutal History of the Allied Occupation*. New York: Basic Books, 2009.

Macekura, Stephen. "The Point Four Program and U.S. International Development Policy." *Political Science Quarterly* 128, no. 1 (2013): 127–60.

Manchester, William. *American Caesar: Douglas MacArthur, 1880–1964*. Boston: Little Brown, 1978.

Mandal, Shyamapada, Manisha Deb Mandal, and Nishith Kumasi Pal. "Cholera: A Great Global Concern." *Asia Pacific Journal of Tropical Medicine* (2011): 573–80.

Manring, M. M., Alan Hawk, Jason H. Calhoun, and Romney C. Andersen. "Treatment of War Wounds: A Historical Review." *Clinical Orthopaedics and Related Research* 467, no. 8 (2009): 2168–91.

Marčuk, L. M., V. N. Nikiforov, Ja. F. Ščerbak, T. A. Levitov, R. I. Kotljarova, M. S. Naumšina, S. U. Davydov, et al. "Clinical Studies of the Use of Bacteriophage in the Treatment of Cholera." *Bulletin of the World Health Organization* 48 (1971): 77–83.

Mayers, David. "Destruction Repaired and Destruction Anticipated: United Nations Relief and Rehabilitation Administration (UNRRA), the Atomic Bomb, and US Policy 1944–46." *International History Review* 38, no. 5 (2016): 961–83.

McKenna, Maryn. *Big Chicken: The Incredible Story of How Antibiotics Created Modern Agriculture and Changed the Way the World Eats*. Washington DC: National Geographic, 2017. Ebook.

———. "The Last Resort." *Nature* 499, no. 7459 (2013): 394.

Medvedev, Zhores. *The Rise and Fall of T.D. Lysenko*. Translated by Michael Lerner. Garden City NY: Anchor Books, 1971.

Meselson, Matthew, J. Guillemin, M. Hugh-Jones, A. Langmuir, I. Popova, A. Shelokov, and O. Yampolskaya. "The Sverdlovsk Anthrax Outbreak of 1979." *Science* 226, no. 5188 (1994): 1202–8.

Moberg, Carol L. "René Dubos, a Harbinger of Microbial Resistance to Antibiotics." *Perspectives in Biology and Medicine* 42, no.4 (Summer 1999): 559–80.

Molez, Jean-François. "The Historical Question of Acquired Immunodeficiency Syndrome in the 1960s in the Congo River Basin Area in Relation to Cryptococcal Meningitis." *American Journal of Tropical Medicine and Hygiene* 58, no. 3 (1998): 273–76.

Monsur, K. A., M. A. Rahman, F. Huq, M. N. Islam, R. S. Northrup, and N. Hirschhorn. "Effect of Massive Doses of Bacteriophage on Excretion of Vibrios, Duration of Diarrhoea, and Output of Stools in Acute Cases of Cholera." *Bulletin of the World Health Organization* 42 (1970): 723–32.

Moorhouse, Roger. *The Devil's Alliance: Hitler's Pact with Stalin, 1939–1941*. London: Bodley Head, 2014.

Morabia, Alfredo. "'East Side Story': On Being an Epidemiologist in the Former USSR, an Interview with Marcus Klingberg." *Epidemiology* 17, no.1 (January 2006): 115–19.

Mudd, Stuart. "The Staphylococcus Problem." *Scientific American* 200, no. 1 (January 1959): 41–45.

Mukerjee, S. "Cholera El Tor in Calcutta." *British Medical Journal* 2 (1964): 546–48.

Murray, Clinton, Mary Hinkle, and Heather Yun. "History of Infections Associated with Combat-Related Injuries." *Journal of Trauma, Injury, Infection, and Critical Care* 64, (2008): 221–31.

Murray, Clinton K., H. C. Yun, M. E. Griffith, D. R. Hospenthal, and M. J. Tong. "Acinetobacter Infection: What Was the True Impact during the Vietnam Conflict?" *Clinical Infectious Diseases* 43 (August 1, 2006): 383–84.

Myelnikov, D. "An Alternative Cure: The Adoption and Survival of Bacteriophage Therapy in the USSR, 1922–1955." *Journal of the History of Medicine and Allied Sciences* 73, no. 4 (October 2018): 385–411.

Newman, Barclay Moon. *Japan's Secret Weapon*. Edited by Peter Greenleaf. New York: Current Publishing Company, 1944.

Olarte, Jorge, and Emma Galindo. "*Salmonella typhi* Resistant to Chloramphenicol, Ampicillin, and Other Antimicrobial Agents: Strains Isolated during an Extensive Typhoid Fever Epidemic in Mexico." *Antimicrobial Agents and Chemotherapy* 4, no. 6 (1973): 597–601.

O'Sullivan, Christopher D. *Harry Hopkins: FDR's Envoy to Churchill and Stalin*. Lanham MD: Rowman & Littlefield, 2015. Ebook.

Overy, Richard. *Russia's War: Blood upon the Snow*. New York: Penguin Books, 1997. Ebook.

Palmer, Adam C., and Roy Kishony. "Understanding, Predicting and Manipulating the Genotypic Evolution of Antibiotic Resistance." *Nature Reviews Genetics* 14, no. 4 (2013): 243.

Parker, Barry. *The Physics of War: From Arrows to Atoms*. Amherst NY: Prometheus Books, 2014.

Peraino, Kevin. *A Force So Swift: Mao, Truman, and the Birth of Modern China*. New York: Crown Publishing, 2017.

Perlman, D. "The Evolution of Penicillin Manufacturing Processes." In Brockman, *History of Penicillin Production*, 23–30.

Philippon, Alain, Roger Labia, and George Jacoby. "Extended-Spectrum Beta-Lactamases." *Antimicrobial Agents and Chemotherapy* 33, no. 8 (1989): 1131.

Philpot, Flora J. "A Penicillin-like Substance from Aspergillus giganteus Wehm." *Nature* 152, no. 3868 (1943): 725.

Plough, Harold H. "Penicillin Resistance of Staphylococcus aureus and Its Clinical Implications." *American Journal of Clinical Pathology* 15 (1945): 446–51.

Podolsky, Scott. *The Antibiotic Era: Reform, Resistance, and the Pursuit of a Rational Therapeutics*. Baltimore: Johns Hopkins University Press, 2015.

Podolsky, Scott, and Jeremy Greene. "Combination Drugs—Hype, Harm, and Hope." *New England Journal of Medicine* 365, no. 6 (August 11, 2011): 488–91.

Pringle, Peter. *Experiment Eleven: Dark Secrets behind the Discovery of a Wonder Drug*. New York: Walker, 2012. Ebook.

———. *The Murder of Nikolai Vavilov: The Story of Stalin's Persecution of One of the Great Scientists of the Twentieth Century*. New York: Simon & Schuster, 2016.

Rammelkamp, Charles H., and Chester S. Keefer. "The Absorption, Excretion, and Distribution of Penicillin." *Journal of Clinical Investigation* 22, no. 3 (1943): 425–37.

Rane, Leo, and Dora S. Rane. "Aureomycin." *Scientific American* 180, no. 4 (April 1949): 18–23.

Raper, Kenneth B. "The Progress of Antibiotics." *Scientific American* 186, no. 4 (1952): 49–57.

Rasnake, Mark, N. G. Conger, K. McAllister, K. K. Holmes, and E. C. Tramont. "History of U.S. Military Contributions to the Study of Sexually Transmitted Diseases." *Military Medicine* 170, no. 4 (April 2005): 61–65.

Rayfield, Donald. *Stalin and His Hangmen: The Tyrant and Those Who Killed for Him*. New York: Random House, 2005.

Reinisch, Jessica. "'Auntie UNRRA' at the Crossroads." *Past & Present* 218, Supplement 8 (2013): 70–97.

———. *Perils of Peace: The Public Health Crisis in Occupied Germany, 1943–1945*. Oxford: Oxford University Press, 2013.

Reynolds, Herbert E. "Back to the Beginning for the Eighth Evacuation Hospital in Morocco during World War II: 70 Years Ago." *Transactions of the American Clinical and Climatological Association* 125 (2014): 154–69.

Riddle, Stefan. "Biological Warfare and Bioterrorism: A Historical Review." *Baylor University Medical Center Proceedings* 17, no. 4 (2004): 400–406.

Ringer, Greg. "Convicts and Conservation: Con Dao National Park, Vietnam." In *Sustainable Tourism: A Global Perspective*, edited by Rob Harris, Peter Williams, and Tony Griffin. New York: Routledge, 2002.

Roberts, Geoffrey. *Stalin's Wars: From World War to Cold War, 1939–1953*. New Haven CT: Yale University Press, 2006. Ebook.

Roberts, Mary Louise. "The Price of Discretion: Prostitution, Venereal Disease, and the American Military in France, 1944–1946." *American Historical Review* 115, no. 4 (October 2010): 1002–30.

Robinson, F. A. "The Chemistry of Penicillin." *Analyst* 72 (1947): 274–76.

Rose, Anthony. "New Penicillins." *Scientific American* 204, no. 3 (1961): 66–71.

Rosen, William. *Miracle Cure: The Creation of Antibiotics and the Birth of Modern Medicine*. New York: Penguin Books, 2017. Ebook.

Rountree, Phyllis, and Barbara Freeman. "Infections Caused by a Particular Phage Type of Staphylococcus aureus." *Medical Journal of Australia* 42, no. 5 (July 30, 1955): 157–61.

Rubenstein, Joshua. *The Last Days of Stalin*. New Haven: Yale University Press: 2016. Ebook.

Saga, Tomoo, and Keizo Yamaguchi. "History of Antimicrobial Agents and Resistant Bacteria." *Japan Medical Association Journal* 52, no. 2 (2009): 103–8.

Samame, G. E. "Treponematosis Eradication, with Special Reference to Yaws Eradication in Haiti." *Bulletin of the World Health Organization* 15 (1956): 897–910.

Sams, Crawford. *Medic: The Mission of an American Military Doctor in Occupied Japan and Wartorn Korea*. Armonk NY: M. E. Sharpe, 1998.

Santesmases, Maria Jesus. "The Long Postwar and the Politics of Penicillin: Early Circulation and Smuggling in Spain, 1944–1954." *Medicina Nei Secoli: Arte e Scienza* 26, no. 2 (2014): 615–38.

Sayamov, R. M. "Treatment and Prophylaxis of Cholera with Bacteriophage." *Bulletin of the World Health Organization* 28 (1963): 361–67.

Schneider, Laurence. "Michurinist Biology in the People's Republic of China, 1948–1956." *Journal of the History of Biology* 45, no. 3 (Fall 2012): 525–56.

Sebald, W. G. *On the Natural History of Destruction*. Translated by Anthea Ball. New York: Random House, 2003.

Seymour, Morris, Jr. *Supreme Commander: MacArthur's Triumph in Japan*. New York: Harper, 2014.

Shaffir, Kimberlee. "Flashback: *Face the Nation* Goes to Moscow." CBS News, June 1, 2017. https://www.cbsnews.com/news/flashback-face-the-nation-goes-to-moscow-russia-ussr-nikita-khrushchev/.

Shaikh, Sibhghatulla, Jamale Fatima, Shazi Shakil, Syed Mohd Danish Rizvi, and Mohammad Amjad Kamal. "Antibiotic Resistance and Extended Spectrum Beta-Lactamases: Types, Epidemiology and Treatment." *Saudi Journal of Biological Sciences* 22, no. 1 (2015): 90–101.

Shalamov, Varlam. *Kolyma Tales*. Translated by John Glad. London: Penguin 1994.

Shama, Gilbert. "No New Thing under the Sun (?): On Claims to the Discovery of Penicillin prior to 1928." *Journal of Pharmaceutical Microbiology* 3, no. 1 (2017): 1–4.

———. "Pilzkrieg: The German Wartime Quest for Penicillin." *Microbiology Today*, no. 30 (August): 120–23.

———. "Zones of Inhibition? The Transfer of Information Relating to Penicillin in Europe during World War II." In *Advances in Applied Microbiology*, vol. 69, edited by Allen I. Larkin, 133–58. Amsterdam: Elsevier, 2009.

Shimkin, Michael B. "Roads to Oz. I. A Personal Account of Some U.S.-U.S.S.R. Medical Exchanges and Contacts, 1942–1962." *Perspectives in Biology and Medicine* 22, no. 4 (Summer 1979): 565–86.

Short, Philip. *Mao: The Man Who Made China*. London: I. B. Tauris, 2017.

Showalter, Dennis. *Armor and Blood: The Battle of Kursk, the Turning Point of World War II*. New York: Random House: 2013.

Silver, L. L., and K. A. Bostian. "Discovery and Development of New Antibiotics: The Problem of Antibiotic Resistance." *Antimicrobial Agents and Chemotherapy* 37, no. 3 (1993): 377.

Simpson, Christophe. *Science of Coercion: Communication Research and Psychological Warfare, 1945–1960*. New York: Oxford University Press, 1994.

Smith, Jean Edward. *Eisenhower: In War and Peace*. New York: Random House, 2012.

———. *FDR*. New York: Random House, 2007.

Sneader, Walter. *Drug Discovery: A History*. Hoboken NJ: John Wiley & Sons, 2005.

Snyder, Timothy. *Blood Lands: Europe between Hitler and Stalin*. New York: Basic Books, 2010.

Sonneborn, T. M. "The Cytoplasm in Heredity." *Heredity* 4 (1950): 11–36.

Southard, Susan. *Nagasaki: Life after Nuclear War*. New York: Penguin Books, 2016. Ebook.

Spalding, Elizabeth. *The First Cold Warrior: Harry Truman, Containment, and the Remaking of Liberal Internationalism*. Lexington: University of Kentucky Press, 2006.

Spence, Jonathan. *Mao Zedong*. New York: Viking, 1999.

Starr, Paul. *The Social Transformation of American Medicine*. New York: Basic Books, 1982.

Stewart, Irvin. *Organizing Scientific Research for War: The Administrative History of the Office of Scientific Research and Development*. Boston: Little, Brown, 1948.

Sulakvelidze, A., Z. Alavidze, and J. G. Morris Jr. "Bacteriophage Therapy." *Antimicrobial Agents and Chemotherapy* 45, no. 3 (March 2001): 649–59.

Summers, William. "Cholera and Plague in India: The Bacteriophage Inquiry of 1927–1936." *Journal of the History of Medicine and Allied Sciences* 48 (1993): 275–301.

———. "The Strange History of Phage Therapy." *Bacteriophage* 2, no. 2 (2012): 130–33.

Svoboda, Terese. "U.S. Courts-Martial in Occupation Japan: Rape, Race, and Censorship." *Asia-Pacific Journal* 7, no. 21 (May 2009): 1–9.

Sze, Szeming. "Today's Global Frontiers in Public Health: II. Regional Health Organization in the Far East." *American Journal of Public Health and the Nation's Health* 35, no. 2 (1945): 96–99.

Szinicz, Ladislaus. "History of Chemical and Biological Warfare Agents." *Toxicology* 214, no. 3 (2005): 167–81.

Talbot, David. *The Devil's Chessboard: Allen Dulles, the CIA, and the Rise of America's Secret Government*. New York: Harper, 2015.

Taroni, Francesco. "The Fabricca della Penicillina in Postwar Italy: An Institutionalist Approach." *Medicina nei Secoli: Arte e Scienza* 26, no. 2 (2014): 639–62.

Taubman, William. *Khrushchev: The Man and His Era*. New York: W. W. Norton, 1990.

Tikhonov, Aleksei, and Paul R. Gregory. "Stalin's Last Plan." In *Behind the Façade of Stalin's Command Economy: Evidence from the Soviet State and Party Archives*, edited by Paul Gregory. Stanford CA: Hoover Institute Press, 2001.

Tillman, Barrett. *D-Day Encyclopedia: The Normandy Invasion A–Z*. Washington DC: Brassey's, 2004.

Tobbell, Dominique. *Pills, Power, and Policy: The Struggle for Drug Reform in Cold War America and Its Consequences*. Berkeley: University of California Press, 2011. Ebook.

Torres-Barceló, Clara, and Michael E. Hochberg. "Evolutionary Rationale for Phages as Complements of Antibiotics." *Trends in Microbiology* 24, no. 4 (January 2016): 249–56.

Tyabji, Nasir. "Gaining Technical Know-how in an Unequal World: Penicillin Manufacture in Nehru's India." *Technology and Culture* 45, no. 2 (April 2004): 331.

Umemura, Maki. *The Japanese Pharmaceutical Industry: Its Evolution and Current Challenges*. London: Routledge, 2011. Ebook.

Umezawa, Hamao. "Kanamycin: Its Discovery." *Annals of the New York Academy of Sciences* 76, no. 2 (1958): 20–26.

U.S. House of Representatives. "Combating Superbugs: U.S. Public Health Responses to Antibiotic Resistance, Hearing Before the Subcommittee on Oversight and Investigations of the Committee on Energy and Commerce." 114th Cong., June 14, 2016. Washington DC: U.S. Government Printing Office, 2017. https://www.govinfo.gov/content/pkg/CHRG-114hhrg21484/html/CHRG-114hhrg21484.htm.

Ventola, C. Lee. "The Antibiotic Resistance Crisis: Part 1: Causes and Threats." *Pharmacy and Therapeutics* 40, no. 4 (2015): 277.

Wainwright, Milton, and Harold T. Swan. "CG Paine and the Earliest Surviving Clinical Records of Penicillin Therapy." *Medical History* 30, no. 1 (1986): 42–56.

Wallace, Craig, Anastasia Fabie, Ophelia Mangubat, Emma Velasco, Corazon Juninho, and Robert Phillips. "The 1961 Cholera Epidemic in Manila, Republic of the Philippines." *Bulletin of the World Health Organization* 30 (1964): 795–810.

Wang, Zuoyue. "The Cold War and the Reshaping of Transnational Science in China." In *Science and Technology in the Global Cold War*, edited by Naomi Oreskes and John Krige. Cambridge MA: MIT Press, 2014. Ebook.

Watanabe, Tsutomu. "Infectious Drug Resistance." *Scientific American* 217, no. 6 (December 1967): 19–27.

———. "Infective Heredity of Multiple Drug Resistance in Bacteria." *Bacteriological Reviews* 27, no. 1 (March 1963): 87–115.

Weathersby, Kathryn. "Deceiving the Deceivers: Moscow, Beijing, Pyongyang, and the Allegations of Bacteriological Weapons Use in Korea." *Cold War International History Project Bulletin* 11 (Winter 1998): 176–85.

Weisfeld, Larissa I. "Importance of Discovery of I.A. Rapoport of Chemical Mutagenesis in the Study of Mechanism of Cytogenic Effect of Mutagens." In *Ecological Consequences of Increasing Crop Productivity: Plant Breeding and Biotic Diversity*, edited by Anatoly Iv. Opalko, Larissa I. Weisfeld, Sarra A. Bekuzarova, Nina A. Bome, and Gennady E. Zaikov, 271–76. Toronto: Apple Academic Press, 2015.

Wentworth, Frederick H., Adah L. Miller, and Berttina B. Wentworth. "Staphylococcal Infections in the Hospital and Community: Observations Relative to the Nature and Control of Epidemic Staphylococcal Disease." *American Journal of Public Health and the Nation's Health* 48, no. 3 (1958): 287–98.

Werth, Alexander. *Russia at War, 1941–1945*. New York: Skyhorse Publishing, 1964.

Wheelis, Mark, and Malcolm Dando. "On the Brink: Biodefence, Biotechnology and the Future of Weapons Control." *CBW Conventions Bulletin* 58 (2002): 3–7.

Wiener, Tim. *Legacy of Ashes: The History of the CIA*. New York: Anchor Books, 2008.

Williams, Trevor. *Howard Florey: Penicillin and After*. Oxford: Oxford University Press, 1984.

Yablonskii, Peter K., Alexandr A. Vizel, Vladimir B. Galkin, and Marina V. Shulgina. "Tuberculosis in Russia: Its History and Its Status Today." *American Journal of Respiratory and Critical Care Medicine* 191, no. 4 (February 15, 2015): 372–76.

Zachary, G. Pascal. *Endless Frontier: Vannevar Bush, Engineer of the American Century*. New York: Free Press, 1997.

Zakinthos, Syed Ahmed, and Sunil Karande. "Multidrug-Resistant Typhoid Fever: A Review." *Journal of Infection in Developing Countries* 5, no. 5 (2011): 324–37.

Zelchenko, Henry L. "Stealing America's Know-how: The Story of AMTORG." *American Mercury* 74, no. 338 (February 1952): 75–84.

Zinn, Howard. *The Bomb*. San Francisco: City Lights Books, 2010.

INDEX